A BODY OF WORK

Also Available from Bloomsbury

The Bloomsbury Companion to Contemporary Philosophy of Medicine
Edited by James Marcum

Hurt and Pain: Literature and the Suffering Body
By Susannah B. Mintz

A BODY OF WORK

AN ANTHOLOGY OF POETRY AND MEDICINE

Edited by Corinna Wagner and Andy Brown

Bloomsbury Academic
An imprint of Bloomsbury Publishing Plc

BLOOMSBURY
LONDON · OXFORD · NEW YORK · NEW DELHI · SYDNEY

Bloomsbury Academic

An imprint of Bloomsbury Publishing Plc

50 Bedford Square	1385 Broadway
London	New York
WC1B 3DP	NY 10018
UK	USA

www.bloomsbury.com

BLOOMSBURY and the Diana logo are trademarks of Bloomsbury Publishing Plc

First published 2016

British Library Cataloguing-in-Publication Data
A catalogue record for this book is available from the British Library.

ISBN: HB: 978-1-4725-1181-2
PB: 978-1-4725-1329-8

Library of Congress Cataloging-in-Publication Data
A catalog record for this book is available from the Library of Congress.

Typeset by Deanta Global Publishing Services, Chennai, India

CONTENTS

EXTENDED CONTENTS

Medical Writing:

Chapter 2   Nerves, Mind and Brain

Medical Writing:

Chapter 3   Consuming

Medical Writing:

Chapter 4   Illness, Disease and Disability

Medical Writing:

Chapter 5   Treatment

Medical Writing:

Chapter 6 Hospitals, Practitioners and Professionals

Medical Writing:

Chapter 7   Sex, Evolution, Genetics and Reproduction

Chapter 8 Aging and Dying

Medical Writing:

ILLUSTRATIONS

FOREWORD AND
ACKNOWLEDGEMENTS

We would like first to say a few words about why we have produced this anthology. Quite simply, one impetus was sheer necessity: like other lecturers and writers who teach and research in the growing field of the medical humanities, we found ourselves spending precious time searching for and gathering poetry and medical writing from a wide variety of sources. Another motivation for this project was the considerable public interest in this subject area. This anthology demonstrates that, historically, there has been a perennial curiosity about the anatomy and functioning of the body, ailments and diseases, doctors and patients, and medical discoveries and new technologies. The chronological range of poems and medical writing reveals sometimes surprising historical continuities, not least the way medicine is bound up with the human compulsion, if not need, to create narratives and to tell stories about the physical and psychological experience of living in a body.

And yet, there is also something about this particular historical moment. In universities and medical schools, the medical humanities (or health humanities) have become a growing, lively field. In literature and film, there has been an unprecedented interest in writing about, reading about, or visually representing the sick body, the enhanced body, the modified body, the disabled body, etc. New genres have developed, such as pathography (illness narrative), and graphic autobiography (comics about disease or psychological distress). Films with titles like *Contagion* or *Virus* are part of the thriving genre of outbreak movies. In the visual arts – whether found in galleries and museums, or on billboards and screens – we are surrounded by an extraordinarily wide array of bodies and bodily conditions. In the last few decades there has been an explosion of body art, of which only two out of countless examples are Marc Quinn's 'portrait' of *Sir John Edward Sulstan* (2001), a sample of the sitter's DNA in agar jelly mounted in a stainless steel frame, and Katharine Dowson's 3-D glass laser etchings of her brain, entitled *My Soul* (2005). In the world of museums, the Wellcome Collection galleries in London have been hugely successful, and the Hunterian Museum has undergone a significant and impressive transformation. Across America and Europe, there is considerable public interest in the pathological objects on display and the interpretive programs on offer at the Mütter Museum in Philadelphia or the Museum Vrolik in Amsterdam. In popular culture, Gunther von Hagens' Body Worlds exhibitions of human anatomy have drawn huge crowds, whilst in Brooklyn, New York, visitors are treated to a full calendar of events at the recently opened Morbid Anatomy Museum. It is as if there is something in the water.

Why now? Is this fascination with the body a fashion? Or a matter of urgency? Should we view the art-humanities-medicine nexus as a new phenomenon or part of a longer history of engagement between these fields? These are only a few of the larger questions that motivate this project. We focus here on how poetry in particular has been in dialogue with medicine and continues to participate in debates about the body and well-being. It is a literary form, we believe, that has and is now making important interventions in how we understand and experience disease, illness and disability. Poetic language, which is typically distilled and more spare than prose, focuses closely on the meanings that inhere in single words – words like 'terminal', 'abnormal', 'pain' or 'ankylosing spondylitis' – and in phrases like 'quality of life' or 'declining condition'. We hope this anthology shows that poetry, in all its many forms, is a manner of narrativizing or storytelling that is particularly adaptable to making sense of our experiences with living and dying in a body.

We are very grateful for the many colleagues and collaborators, from whom we have learned enormously. Respondents at conferences, symposiums and receptions, in Britain, America, Europe, India and China have given us valuable insights into the relationship between the arts and sciences more generally.

Special thanks are due to Professor Mark Jackson at the University of Exeter's Centre for Medical History and to the University's 'Medical Humanities' strand of the Humanities and Social Sciences (HASS) research strategy, for the support to initiate exploration in this area. In addition, the editors have benefitted from funding from the University of Exeter's International Office to travel to universities in Northern India, and Peking University and Fudan University, China. The global exchange of ideas has enhanced our understanding of current projects on epidemics, sanitation, literature and the architectural reform of cities.

We owe a debt of gratitude to our Research Assistant, Dr Ben Smith, who has worked tirelessly on this volume. In particular, he has had the unenviable task of seeking permissions. We need to say something here, too, about the generosity of poets, friends and colleagues who, having seen the value of this project, have given permission to reprint their poems gratis. We also thank publishers and agents who negotiated with us – it would otherwise have been impossible to include the wonderful range of modern poetry we have here. It is often difficult to reconcile one's artistic and intellectual vision with economic reality. In addition, and as usual, we thank the Wellcome Trust: their policy of open access and their championing of the medical humanities is an absolute boon to academics, artists and interested members of the public.

Lastly, we would like to thank our commissioning editor at Bloomsbury, David Avital, for immediately recognizing the value of this project, to Mark Richardson, for his fortitude and professional eye, to Joanne Murphy for a smooth production, and Divya Bardhan for efficient copyediting.

NOTE ON TEXT

We have been guided by two general editorial principles. First, we have made minimal textual alteration, particularly with the poetry. Obvious printers' errors have been silently corrected and, in keeping with modern tastes and our desire to appeal to a wide audience, the more conspicuous archaisms have been modernized. This is particularly the case where those archaisms do not contribute to the tone or meaning of a passage. Spelling is largely normalized to American standards for selections originally published there, and to British standards elsewhere. There are exceptions; for instance, we have made no changes to Mary Carey's 'Upon the Sight of my Abortive Birth the 31st December 1657', which was an unpublished poem, written in her personal correspondence. We hope readers will glean the emotion and meaning that comes through the irregular style, as well as get a sense of early modern language and conventions. Eighteenth- and nineteenth-century referencing was often inconsistent and idiosyncratic, so unless they serve a particularly significant purpose, authorial notes and in-text references are omitted in the medical writing. Many of the bibliographic references in texts on early obstetrics or diet, for example, are unlikely to be of great interest to general readers.

Our second editorial principle concerns choice of editions, chronology and dating. For both the poetry and medical writing, we have typically chosen the first edition and ordered them by that initial date of publication. By doing so, we hope to lend readers a sense of how the poems relate to one another and how they respond to developments in the history of medicine. Arranging them chronologically, by theme, reveals important continuities and changes in approaches toward health, disease, ethics, and bodily and psychological well-being.

Having said that, there are notable exceptions. In the case of some selections of eighteenth-century poetry and medical writing, we have not always opted for first editions, when later editions are widely expanded or substantially revised. For instance, there were many versions of 'Dialogue between a Blind-man and Death' and the wildly popular *Aristotle's Masterpiece,* the latter of which was published from the late seventeenth century through to the twentieth, and had various pirated sections and more than one contributing author. In cases like this, we have chosen a later edition to give a sense of its evolution and its long-standing appeal. In a very few other cases, we have ordered a poem according to its date of composition, rather than publication, when the latter occurs posthumously or after a significant passage of time (for example, John Wilmott, the Earl of Rochester's 'A Song of a Young Lady to her Ancient Lover'). The poems included here from Whitman's *Leaves of Grass* come from various editions, depending on scholarly consensus about preferred versions. For instance, 'I Sing the Body Electric' is taken from the 1865 edition, when the term 'electric' first came into use. Generally, our rule has been to choose an edition that best expresses the medical priorities and problems of its moment.

Introduction

'People Bleed Stories': Illness, Medicine and Poetry

CORINNA WAGNER[1]

> Verse is for healthy
> arty-farties. The dying
> and surgeons use prose.
>
> (Peter Reading, from C, 1984)

In this poem, a haiku, Peter Reading raises the age-old division between art and science. 'Verse' stands here for imagination, creativity, art and poetry, while 'prose' stands for fact, rationality, empiricism and medicine. There are at least two opposing ways to read these three simple lines. One way is to take it at face value: when health scares and serious illness stop daily life in its tracks, verse becomes a luxury that is quickly superseded by the certainty of forthright and factual prose. When confronted with disease and debility, we often seek assurance from the language of analysis, machines, medications and operations. Scientific prose seems to penetrate the body's surface, uncovering the unseen sources of disorders and promising cures. Poetry can do nothing of the kind.

Yet we can understand Reading's poem another way: we may assume that his tongue is set firmly in his cheek. Verse *is* the language of the sick and dying; *in extremis*, we reach for a literary form that is particularly able to express the silences and eruptions of emotion attendant upon trauma, anger and fear. The spare language and restrained form of the haiku offer a different kind of assurance in the face of uncertainty. When a body goes wrong, the mind can gather strength from reflection. We may consider the successes and failures of our lives, the states of our relationships or the beauty of the natural world – subjects particularly suited to poetic expression. Faced with his impending death from ocular cancer, the neurologist and writer Oliver Sacks describes how he suddenly found himself caring very little about the daily political affairs that had always interested him. Instead his thoughts had shifted to focus on the 'enormous privilege and adventure' of having 'been a sentient being, a thinking animal, on this beautiful planet' (2015: A25). Our experience as reflective, expressive beings, living in an endlessly intriguing and evolving world – this is the very stuff of poetry.

---

[1] With Andy Brown.

Perhaps Peter Reading's poem makes yet another claim: that there is much more coherence between medical prose and poetic language than we may commonly assume. The sociologist Arthur Frank identifies a similar type of overlap. He points out that we tend to think of *disease* as biochemistry, and thus expressed in medical prose; at the same time, we think of *illness* as personal, and thus expressed through autobiographical genres (2014: 14). In reality however, the relationships between disease and illness, prose and poetry, and the professional objectivity of the physician and the personal experiences of the patient, are much more muddled. For pathographies (or illness autobiographies) are informed by hard science, and the human experience of illness unquestionably feeds back into medical knowledge and treatment. Even if we examine the experience of disease and illness from the perspective of the patient alone, we notice that 'by the time disease is imagined, it has already become illness' (Frank 2014: 14). The mind and body exist symbiotically, and so disease and illness are always 'conjoined', as Frank notes; in fact, they could only be separated if the mind could miraculously locate 'itself outside the body' (2014: 15). How patients manage their recoveries, their bodies and their lives in the face of hard medical facts is informed by a range of emotions – among them anxiety, anger, denial, resignation, hope and sometimes hopelessness.

I THE TWO CULTURES REVISITED (AGAIN)

The dichotomies – or false dichotomies, as the case may be – that we have identified here between medical prose and 'arty-farty' poetry is underpinned by a more foundational opposition, between medicine and the humanities. Taken at face value, Peter Reading's verse encapsulates (and perhaps targets) a general attitude, famously voiced by the scientist and novelist C. P. Snow, in his 1959 Rede lecture at Cambridge. Snow's theme, on the irreconcilable differences between the humanities and the sciences, has spawned numerous newspaper articles and books on this topic.[2] An in-depth engagement with this still provoking argument is beyond the remit of this introduction, and others have taken up its challenge admirably.[3] We only want to re-raise Snow's spectre here in the hopes of contributing in some small way to healing the remaining rift. This anthology, and further sections of this introduction, should show clearly that poetry and medicine have not always been so historically divided, and that even in the wake of Snow's challenge there has been considerable collaboration between the two cultures.

In the supposed contest between the humanities and science, Snow came down firmly on the side of science. The Western world had entered a new political and

---

[2]*The Times Literary Supplement* included the subsequent publication of Snow's lecture, *The Two Cultures and the Scientific Revolution*, among the 100 post-Second World War books that have most influenced Western public discourse.

[3]See Stefan Collini's essay on this contest (2013) and his two introductions to recent editions of Snow (2012) and Leavis (2013). Also, see individual essays in *From Two Cultures to No Culture: C P Snow's 'Two Cultures' Lecture Fifty Years On* (Whelan 2009).

scientific era and he worried that 'the rate of change' had 'increased so much that our imagination can't keep up' ([1959] 2012: 42–3). Science and the humanities responded to the demands of a speedily shifting world in markedly different ways. The scientists had 'the future in their bones,' he claimed, but 'traditional culture', by which he meant the humanities and the arts, wished 'the future did not exist' ([1959] 2012: 10–11). According to Snow, nostalgic arty-farties only hid their heads in the sand, while scientists, medics and researchers got on with the progressive stuff that would pull Britain ahead in the global race for intellectual, technological and political might.

Literary don F. R. Leavis was utterly incensed. In 1962, he responded to Snow and his claims with an almost equally famous, and rather scathing counter-attack. Leavis accused Snow of being a hack – 'as a novelist he doesn't exist; he doesn't begin to exist. He can't be said to know what a novel is' – as well as a fairly poor scientist who put on 'a show of knowledgeableness' ([1962] 2013: 57, 59). Fighting words these may be, but in many ways they ring true. On the count that Snow was a failed novelist, most literary critics would agree, for his novels are widely acknowledged to be pedestrian, with stilted dialogue, formulaic plots and flat characters. On the second count, that Snow was a second-rate scientist, Leavis may have been ungentlemanly, but again there is support for his opinion. Snow spoke as science's great defender, but his own contributions could be described as less than stellar. At any rate, the strident tone and personal nature of Leavis's attack should not overshadow his most important point, that the culture of capital had created a society where image trumped substance, and indiscriminate self-promotion was the name of the game. Privileging neither the sciences nor the arts, Leavis called for a thinking public, properly educated in a system where profit did not determine policy and economics did not drive education ([1962] 2013: 84–5; 108–18).[4]

Since Leavis's call for a balanced approach to the disciplines, others have pointed out the historical inaccuracy of Snow's description of the humanities as traditional, nostalgic, anti-rational and both 'unscientific' and 'anti-scientific' (2012: 11). Even a perfunctory understanding of history teaches us quite the opposite lesson, for as Roger Kimball puts it, 'there's not much anti-scientific aroma emanating' from a Western intellectual tradition in the humanities that includes the work of Aristotle, Galileo, Descartes, Newton, Locke and Kant (2009: 37). In addition, Snow's claim that scientists had 'the future in their bones', while artists, writers and philosophers were 'natural Luddites', ignores or misses an extraordinarily long and varied tradition of dissent ([1959] 2012: 10–11; 22–30). Throughout history, and across the globe, artists and poets have challenged authority, dogma, injustice, superstition, and false, unethical beliefs. Those same poet-philosophers and artist-anatomists, among history's most forward-looking and inventive individuals, would not recognize our concept of the two cultures. Arguably, until the beginnings of

---

[4] It is worth remembering that the Snow-Leavis conflict is a product of specific mid-century political, social and educational crises – among them, the first phase of the Cold War, economic austerity and the creation of the post-war welfare state.

a divide began to show in the nineteenth century, generations of thinkers worked within a *one*-culture model of knowledge.[5]

II CONSILIENT CULTURES

At the beginning of the nineteenth century, the scientist, inventor, poet, painter and one-time president of the Royal Society, Sir Humphry Davy saw commonality between art and science, and identified continuities between history and the present. In an 1805 essay on the 'Parallels between Art and Science', he wrote:

> The perception of truth is almost as simple a feeling as the perception of beauty; and the genius of Newton, of Shakespeare, of Michael Angelo, and of Handel, are not very remote in character from each other. Imagination, as well as reason, is necessary to perfection in the philosophical mind. A rapidity of combination, a power of perceiving analogies, and of comparing them by facts, is the creative source of discovery ([1805] 1840: 308).

Davy celebrates artists like Michelangelo and scientists like Newton who were receptive, imaginative and dared to follow the counter-intuitive path. They shared an ability to innovate by recognizing significant correspondences between things, where at first none was obvious. In other words, they were consilient thinkers.

Consilience is a belief in the unity of knowledge: the methods of chemistry and medicine, history and literature, should produce analogous and equally valuable results.[6] A consilient thinker himself, Davy collaborated not just with fellow scientists, such as the surgeon (and poet) Thomas Beddoes, the naturalist Sir Joseph Banks, and the chemist Michael Faraday, but also with the inventor and engineer James Watt and the Romantic poets Samuel Taylor Coleridge and Robert Southey. The consilient, investigative mind is not confined to a specific discipline: Coleridge, who commented that Davy could have been a great poet, attended Davy's scientific lectures in order to pick up new metaphors, while Beddoes studied 'historical criticism', at the same time that he experimented with gases and developed novel bovine treatments for tuberculosis. (Although it must be said that Beddoes was rather less successful in these experiments than Edward Jenner was with his cowpox vaccination against smallpox.)

A particularly salutary example of a career characterized by consilient thinking is that of the Victorian doctor and early anaesthetist John Snow, celebrated today for his identification of the source of cholera. During the 1854 cholera epidemic, Snow set out to identify the local origin of the disease in the hard-hit neighbourhood of Soho, London. The dominant medical paradigm of the day, miasma theory, conceived of

---

[5]In another Rede Lecture, in 1882, the critic Matthew Arnold considered whether a classical education was still relevant in an age of great scientific and technological advance. In his lecture on 'Literature and Science', Arnold responded to an earlier lecture by the writer and scientist T. H. Huxley, who argued that science offered as rigorous an intellectual training as the (then privileged) study of the classics (Arnold [1882] 1974).

[6]For more on consilience see Slingerland and Collard (2012) and Wilson (1998).

disease as originating in filth, damp and decay, and then spreading via contaminated air. But Snow rejected this airborne paradigm, based upon evidence, which he had gathered from listening to people, observing their habits and understanding their relationships. In addition, Snow collaborated with the local cleric of St Luke's Church in Soho, Henry Whitehead, to construct a demographic picture of the cholera-hit neighbourhood, and to trace the outbreak to contaminated drinking water. His findings were then plotted on his famous map (see Figure 2, p. 231), which gives a bird's-eye view of where cholera occurred. The unmistakable black bars, their thicknesses indicating numbers of deaths, clearly ring the Broad Street Pump, and taper off as the eye moves away from this locus. The map confronts viewers with truths made visible, which they otherwise could not, or would not see. It shows us the *where* and *who* of disease, and thus also indicates something of the all-important *how*. So, despite the technological limitations in microscopy at the time, which meant that he could not see and therefore prove the existence of the bacterium *Vibrio cholerae*, Snow deduced correctly, through sociological methods, that cholera was waterborne.

We raise this particular historical anecdote in order to underscore the importance of consilient thinking. Snow was a working physician, a medical researcher and one of the founders of epidemiology, but he was also a sociologist, an anthropologist and a geographer. This anthology shows that contrary to popular misconception, in the past 300 years, poets and doctors did not speak diametrically opposed languages. Throughout history, knowledge about the functioning of the body, new methods of diagnoses, innovative treatments and changing ideas about the prevention of disease migrated between medicine and literature. In fact, scientific writing and poetry very often shared a common language. In the eighteenth century, there existed a medico-poetic discourse quite simply because many doctors were poets. In the age of

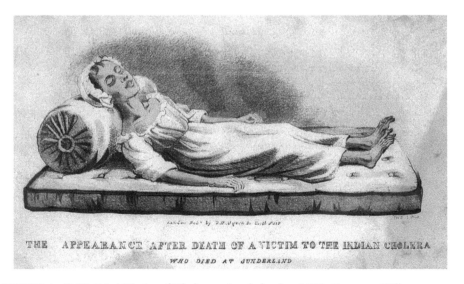

FIGURE 1: 'I. W. G.', *A Victim of Cholera at Sunderland*, c. 1832. Courtesy Wellcome Library, London.

Enlightenment, a well-respected medical man was very often a man of letters. This was the case with, for example, Erasmus Darwin (1731–1802); Oliver Goldsmith (1728–74); Edward Jenner (1749–1823) and Friedrich von Schiller (1759–1805). In addition, some eighteenth-century doctors, such as John Armstrong (1709–79), composed full medical treatises in verse. Almost invariably, of course, this is an all-male realm, but there are some quite wonderful exceptions, such as Jane Barker's 1688 poetic musings on anatomy or Lady Mary Wortley Montagu's prose writing on smallpox inoculation (see them in this anthology).

At the turn of the nineteenth century, the priorities of the professionalizing medical establishment sometimes meshed less seamlessly with literary ones. This is the case, for instance, with the Romantic poet-physician John Keats (1795–1821), who turned away from the triumphs of progressive medicine to resurrect in poetry the classical and medieval worlds he associated with humanistic virtues – virtues he feared were under threat in modern society. Yet, Keats had a continuing interest in medicine and a unified understanding of the natural world and human culture, as he expresses in one May 1818 letter. 'Every department of knowledge we see excellent and calculated towards a great whole,' he wrote, 'I am so convinced of this, that I am glad at not having given away my medical Books, which I shall again look over to keep alive the little I know' (1958: 277). Other writers used poetry as a means of entering more directly into medical debates on issues surrounding madness, hospitals, evolution and genetics. The American federal judge and writer Francis Hopkinson, for instance, promotes anatomical dissection in a poem written about a dispute between a professor of anatomy and a lecturer in Philadelphia in 1789. And, the Victorian philosopher of science Constance Woodhill Naden combined Darwinian theories of evolution and natural selection with the private intimacies of everyday life in her poetry.[7]

At the dawn of the twentieth century, poet-physicians such as Sir Oliver Wendell Holmes (1809–94), Sir Ronald Ross (1857–1932), Havelock Ellis (1859–1939) and Gottfried Benn (1886–1956) lauded the importance of humanistic values, sometimes as a counter to the demands of rationality, empiricism and professional objectivity. The Canadian bibliophile, writer and 'Father of Modern Medicine', William Osler used the past to bring about what has been termed a 'rehumanisation of medicine'.[8] A founder of Johns Hopkins Hospital, Osler contributed to reinstate the model of the gentleman-physician, for whom a liberal arts education was as vital as practical medicine. Today, we continue to grapple with the problems that Osler identified and responded to, including overspecialization, commercialization and apathy.

In spite of the predominance of the two-culture model in the twentieth century, many poet-physicians seemed as comfortable in the 'white coat' as the 'purple coat', to use Dannie Abse's distinctions.[9] Besides Abse (1923–2014), were William Carlos

---

[7]Selections by Hopkinson and Naden are included in this anthology, see pp. 307–11 and 400–02.
[8]As early as 1889, professor of medical history at Vienna, Theodor Puschmann agitated for a rehumanization of the physician in an age of science, and Osler would pick up this torch. See Warner, 'Humanizing', 322–32.
[9]Abse titled his 1989 poetry collection 'White Coat, Purple Coat'.

Williams (1883–1963), Miroslav Holub (1923–98), Gael Turnbull (1928–2004), John Stone (1936–2008), Raymond Tallis (b.1946) and Rafael Campo (b. 1964). Twentieth- and twenty-first-century medical poetry often contends with competing demands, and expresses a wide-ranging approach to the body and its care. Abse captures this by imagining how a doctor and a poet would respond to the fall of the mythical Icarus. The doctor would attempt to help; the poet would write a poem; but a poet-doctor 'must do both'.[10] This collection celebrates those who recognize the importance of both fixing and creating, healing and crafting, and it honours those who refuse to sacrifice a comprehensive view of the medical arts in the face of specialization. We should 'be impatient' with the 'two cultures', the biographer Richard Holmes urges, and like Beddoes and his curious, speculating friends, we should embrace a 'wider, more generous, more imaginative perspective' (2010: 469). We hope this book will encourage just that.

III THE EMERGENCE AND EVOLUTION OF MEDICAL HUMANITIES

The growing field of medical humanities – made up of contributing disciplines and sub-disciplines including sociology, cultural studies, history, art history, human geography, fine art, music and drama – has been notoriously difficult to define. We have no intention of attempting definitions here, both because we appreciate the indeterminacy of a field that continues to shape itself as it responds to issues in medicine, health and well-being, and also because this is a task others have ably taken on.[11] Here, we wish only to give the briefest overview of the history of this field. The term 'medical humanities', coined by George Sarton in 1947, referred at that time mainly to efforts in the United States and the United Kingdom to use art as medical therapy and to 'humanize' medical curricula. Former director of the Institute for the Medical Humanities at the University of Texas, Ronald A. Carson, identifies the consumerist – but also reactively anti-authoritarian and anti-capitalist – decade of the 1960s as a time when medical professionals turned to the humanities for input into medical training and patient care (2007: 322). Director of a similar program at Colorado's Center for Bioethics and Humanities, Therese Jones points to the 1970s as a decade when organ transplantation and in vitro fertilization raised new ethical issues that required contributions from philosophers, historians and social scientists (2014: 29). In subsequent decades, literature, history, philosophy, as well as the social sciences, have all contributed to developing innovative methods of care.

More recently, there has been a move to use the descriptor 'health humanities' rather than medical humanities, so as to better capture the wide, inclusive and

---

[10]Qtd. in 'Dannie Abse - Obituary,' *The Telegraph*, 24 August 2015.
[11]Scholars have wrangled over whether to call medical or health humanities a 'multidiscipline', 'interdiscipline', 'transdiscipline', 'circumdiscipline' or 'field'. Those interested in this discussion should see, for instance, Bates, Bleakley and Goodman (2014); Evans and Mcnaughton (2000) and Jones, Wear and Friedman (2014).

interdisciplinary nature of this field. Daniel Goldberg, for instance, suggests that efforts 'should be directed to health and human flourishing rather than to the delivery of medical care' even though both aims are clearly 'of great worth' (2012). Whichever term we choose to use, we agree with Victoria Bates and Sam Goodman's recent plea that the medical humanities be inclusive, broad and reciprocal (2014: 5). This inclusivity and reciprocity is captured in the Wellcome Trust's definition of medical humanities as 'a variety of disciplines that explore the social, historical and cultural dimensions of scientific knowledge, clinical practice and healthcare policy' (web).[12] Inclusivity demands that we recognize the consilient value and utility of disciplinary backgrounds that are not our own and that we consider the significant ways that history and culture have shaped, and continue to shape, medicine.

Over the years, researchers and teachers in humanities disciplines have been challenged to defend what they do. More specifically, those in medical humanities have been asked: What can historians, artists, and literary critics add to public understanding of medical issues, to care of the ailing, or to the training, ethical decision-making and daily practices of doctors, nurses, surgeons, medical researchers and therapists?[13] Clearly, this is another huge, multi-sided debate, and one which we cannot possibly do justice to here. We only wish to situate this anthology as part of the exciting, still emerging and perennially evolving field, by outlining its main areas of activity.

1 Narrative Medicine

One argument, posed early on by Joanne Trautmann Banks, the first literary scholar hired by a medical school (in 1972) and Rita Charon, the founder and executive director of the program in Narrative Medicine at Columbia University, is that there is clinical utility in the study of novels, plays and poetry.[14] Such literary training teaches healthcare professionals how to interpret ambiguities in language and to understand the social contexts behind the personal narratives of their patients. Importantly, narrative competence is not inherent; we are not born with it. Just as would-be engineers and architects must train to obtain a set of specific skills, so too must one learn how to gain narrative competence, which 'requires a combination of textual skills (identifying a story's structure, adopting its multiple perspectives, recognizing metaphors and allusions), creative skills (imagining many interpretations, building curiosity, inventing multiple endings), and affective skills (tolerating uncertainty as a story unfolds, entering the story's mood)' (Charon 2004: 862). These literary competencies are not frills, added on to 'real' medical training; the skills Charon outlines are fundamental to the business of diagnosis.

In *How Doctors Think*, Jerome Groopman makes the point that medicine is an uncertain business, and the majority of diagnostic errors are the result of settling on a particular diagnosis and/or treatment too soon (2007). Accurate narrative interpretation is what medical professionals are required to do, whether that is

---

[12]See the Wellcome Trust website http://www.wellcome.ac.uk/Funding/Humanities-and-social-science/index.htm
[13]See for instance, Jones, Wear and Friedman (2014).
[14]See Charon (2006), Charon and Montello (2002) and Charon (2003).

diagnosing symptoms, unravelling patient case histories or deciphering X-rays, scans and MRIs. Learning how to read a character's psychology, motivation and desire are skills that transfer directly to understanding those patient histories and symptoms. The writer and paediatrician Mark Vonnegut may seem to overstate things when he claims that 'the arts are about as extra' to medicine 'as breathing', but in light of the fact that 'Huck Finn, Lady Chatterley, Willy Loman, and Ophelia ... will all come to see you disguised as patients,' literary study would seem to fit the bill (2014: ix). Undoubtedly, it is one way of making an uncertain business less so.

As in literary and historical studies more generally, the best kind of narrative medical approach also considers larger, overarching issues – public health and social justice, for example – at the same time that it pays heed to individual, interpersonal experiences. Narration of personal experience of illness, treatments and clinics 'reaches beyond the individual', as Arthur Frank puts it, and enters 'into the consciousness of the community' (1997: 63–4). Likewise important research in the humanities not only pays close attention to the nuances of texts (whether they are poems, eyewitness accounts or court documents), but also raises big questions from them and draws larger conclusions about the structure and function of society, politics, science and culture.

2 The Ethical Approach: Compassion, Humanitarianism and Medical Training

The focus on narrative competence is allied to the view that literary study fulfils a distinctly humanistic or ethical role in the training of medical professionals. For advocates of this approach, training in the humanities is a positive counterbalance to clinical training in objectivity and professional distance. According to Rita Charon, acquiring skills in narrative interpretation and evaluation also trains our emotions, increases our capacity for compassion, and encourages us to be 'moved by the stories of illness' (2008: vii).[15] Others working in this area have suggested that an arts-based curriculum encourages medical students to feel empathy and to recognize their own prejudices.[16]

This is deeply contested terrain, and a variety of criticisms and cautions have been levied against casting the humanities as a humanizing force. In a 1998 *Lancet* article, 'More Than a Green Placebo', Dannie Abse contended that

> in an attempt to justify one's trade as a poet, it is no longer possible to resort to arguing the moral nature of poetry. Those 19th century claims that 'Poetry strengthens the faculty which is the organ of the moral nature of man in the same manner as exercise strengthens a limb' ('A Defence of Poetry', P. B. Shelley) seem hollow now post Auschwitz and Hiroshima. Even T. S. Eliot's 'poetry refines the dialect of the tribe' seems in all its ambiguities to be a grandiose assertion, if not a dubious one (362).

---

[15]See also Charon (2001) and DasGupta and Charon (2004).
[16]See for instance Stokes (1980); Downie, Hendry and Macnaughton (1997); Rees (2010) and Perry, Maffulli and Willson (2011).

Abse looks back on Romantic and modernist defences of poetry through a sceptical lens, in the twilight of the twentieth century. World wars and many other political, ideological and religious conflicts have made moderns less sanguine than their ancestors about the civilizing effects of the arts. Even art's greatest advocates hesitate to make claims about how paintings and poetry can contribute to the creation and maintenance of a just, equitable and liberal society.

Literary critics have also expressed doubts about the idea that engaging with literature can lead to empathic feeling and compassionate action. In a playfully insightful article, renowned critic Geoffrey Hartman expresses strong doubts about the ability of literature, or more specifically, storytelling and illness narratives, to mobilize real human emotion. In light of the prevailing faith in neuroscience and the penchant for prescribing drugs to cure what ails, he poses an apposite and timely set of questions. Apart from 'a chemical intervention', he asks, how can people be made 'to feel for other people'? 'Short of pharmaceutical treatment ... can there be empathy management, as we now have pain management?' (2004: 339).[17] Speaking more widely of the disciplines, the literary theorist Jonathan Culler rejects the 'traditional strategy of justification', which links humanities with '*humanistic* thinking and even *humane* behaviour' (2005: 38). This view accords with that of Anne Hudson Jones who, some decades ago, argued that there was no 'guarantee' that literature or art would necessarily inspire empathy, fairness or understanding, nor should this be the 'burden' or sole purview of the humanities (1984: 32). The point is that many thoughtful, caring surgeons and lab technologists did not get that way through the study of literature. Moreover, there have been some rather hard-hearted poets and artists who, in spite of their proximity to great literature and fine art, have held reprehensible political views. Of course, the hope is that a humanities education *will* inspire empathy and fairness; it is only that a love of classical music, the poems of Emily Dickinson or the paintings of Vincent Van Gogh will not guarantee it.

This emphasis on humanizing often leads to instrumental justifications for the inclusion of humanities subjects in both medical education and in considerations of patient care. The danger is that in the effort to make 'physicians more understanding people' and thus 'more effective physicians', the medical humanities becomes increasingly 'product oriented' (Gillis 2008: 7). With this orientation comes a pressure to produce measureable outcomes, thereby forcing the humanities to conform to a market model. In addition, there have been concerns that this model relegates the humanities to a nonthreatening, supplementary position, a tool of medicine, rather than an equally weighted and independent voice (Macneill 2011; Greaves and Evans 2000; Bishop 2008). Johanna Shapiro calls what is described here 'a model of acquiescence', and she uses the terms 'instrumental' and 'ornamental' to encapsulate the view of the medical humanities as a softening and humanizing force that equips medical students and physicians to better perform their stressful, demanding jobs (Shapiro 2012: 3; also Greaves 2001). Again, some of these aims and outcomes are tremendously positive, yet the arts and humanities

---

[17]Also on the question of literary studies specifically, see Suzanne Keen (2007).

should not simply be made functional or reduced to an instrument of market forces.

3 Therapy and/or Aesthetics?

Yet another approach, related to the two described above, shifts focus from the education of medical professionals to the care of the patient. Charon's work in narrative competence also emphasizes this therapeutic component, which is clearly illustrated by one of her case studies, worth reproducing here:

> A 36-year-old Dominican man with a chief symptom of back pain comes to see me for the first time. As his new internist, I tell him, I have to learn as much as I can about his health. Could he tell me whatever he thinks I should know about his situation? And then I do my best not to say a word, not to write in his chart, but to absorb all that he emits about his life and his health. I listen not only for the content of his narrative, but for its form – its temporal course, its images, its associated subplots, its silences, where he chooses to begin in telling of himself, how he sequences symptoms with other life events. I pay attention to the narrative's performance – the patient's gestures, expressions, body positions, tones of voice. After a few minutes, he stops talking and begins to weep. I ask him why he cries. He says, 'No one has ever let me do this before' (2004: 862).

Charon's anecdote captures how important it is for the practitioner to listen for information about symptoms that would not otherwise be forthcoming. Charon is trained to process subtle signposting about lived experiences that may have triggered illness, yet these same skills and techniques can also lead to therapeutic benefits for the patient. Diagnosis is 'encoded in the narratives patients tell of symptoms'; at the same time, listening attentively and critically provides 'deep and therapeutically consequential understandings of the persons who bear symptoms' (2004: 862). Moreover, these benefits also go beyond the clinical encounter, when mobilized in practical forms of healing, including drama, music and writing therapies.

Creative arts therapies for patients with, for instance, dementia, aphasia or a terminal prognosis, would seem to be anything but objectionable; yet there are issues too, about the instrumentalization of the arts. Angela Wood rightly cautions against viewing art therapies 'as an expert-therapeutic-pedagogic "service" provided to the client-patient-student with the goal of enhancing individual wellbeing' (2014: 1). Surveying current writing in this area, she observes that 'too often, treatises on the merits of the medical humanities' that emphasize practical therapies can 'appear either oddly evangelical or cagey, anxious and defensive in tone' (2014: 1). In some respects, this is due to the fact that, as Jane Macnaughton et al. point out, the arts in health movement began life as 'small, local and poorly resourced' (2005: 337). Yet even as this movement has become more supported, diverse and well-connected, it has produced rather less successful research and writing in which, as Woods observes, 'rigorous reflexivity is bracketed in favour of reflections on the humanisation of healthcare' (2015: 1). It seems to us that this is often the case when defences of art, music and writing therapy are not underpinned by, or at the very least informed by historical research or theoretical models. It is worth mentioning again that the use of arts in healing and well-being is a very good thing, but insisting that the arts perform to an agenda, or casting the arts as solely an instrument of therapy limits what writing, painting, music and performance can do. One group that has addressed these problems in commendable ways is the Centre for Research into Reading, Literature and Society (CRILS) at the University of Liverpool. Led by literary scholar Philip Davis, the Centre has developed literature-based programs for older people living with dementia, and other vulnerable groups. For them, shared reading has intrinsic value, in that it stimulates the patient's mental involvement and cognitive processes as well as fostering feelings of community. Importantly, they suggest that shared reading might be 'therapeutic for not being therapy' and 'useful precisely by not being instrumental' (39).[18] The point is that the arts and humanities should fully participate, in a variety of ways, in debates about wellness, public health and the intersection of social issues and medicine. (We will examine this issue more closely in a later section.)

Even accomplished or 'professional' medical poetry has not always ranked highly aesthetically. When the editor of a 1945 anthology of medical poetry, Mary Lou McDonagh surveyed her own collection, she admitted that medical poetry was often seen as 'poetry in quotation marks and much of it . . . feeble stuff', but she defended her collection on the grounds that it reflected 'the spirit of helpfulness which gives to the medical profession its value to humanity.'[19] More recently, the poet-physician Jack Coulehan echoed McDonagh's verdict about the low aesthetic standards of medical poetry. On the NYU School of Medicine's *Literature, Arts, and Medicine Database* he describes McDonagh's anthology as a collection of poems that mostly 'have no enduring literary value'. In light of the fact that Coulehan refers to work by professional, published poet-physicians (some of whom are also included in his anthology), what shall we say about the poetry of the untrained and uninitiated? It can be difficult to reconcile the whole enterprise of critical judgement with the heartfelt, good-intentioned, even necessitous poetry of illness, which may also be, if we are honest, simply not very good.

Difficult, but not impossible. The writer and literary critic Anatole Broyard, who wrote about his experiences with prostate cancer, sought to square the tension between aesthetics and healing. It is not enough for illness to be a story, he argues, it must be a *good* story, and constructing a good story requires the knowledge and skills that come from reading, writing and practice in evaluation and analysis, as are taught in humanities subjects (1992: 45). Picking up from Broyard's argument, Arthur Frank underscores the importance of these skills for the wounded storyteller: 'The humanities have extraordinary resources', he argues, 'that can help ill people first

---

[18]Quoted in 'Cultural Value: Assessing the intrinsic value of The Reader Organisation's Shared Reading Scheme,' A Report from the Centre for Research into Reading, Literature and Society (CRILS), University of Liverpool.

[19]McDonagh gives no reference for this quote, but it is from Dr William Osler's *Medical Incunabula*, quoted in Harvey Cushing's 1940 *The Life of Sir William Osler*, vol. 2 (Hamburg: Severus Verlag) rpt. 2013, p. 1081.

to tell good stories and then in the telling to *become* good stories'; moreover, these extraordinary resources become 'necessary resources' for sick people who 'try to live illness as more than bare disease' (Frank 2014: 14). Reading and writing can open new imaginative worlds for a patient, thereby expanding 'what illness has contracted' (2014: 17).[20] For Broyard, writing fills the silence that otherwise surrounds diagnosis and treatment. Illness causes the patient 'to bleed stories' but those 'stories are antibodies against illness and pain' (1992: 21, 20).

Part of this sense of expansion and imaginative engagement can come through process, rather than product; in other words, the actual process of learning how to be a properly good writer, to pursue excellence, can be incredibly therapeutic. Communicating new imaginative worlds in effective and engaging ways requires that writers learn the differences between hackneyed, clichéd poetry and innovative, insistent poems. For illness to be a good story it should challenge readers in some way; it should demand something from them, whether that be emotion, introspection, action, a change of opinion, greater understanding or something else. Very good writing about the body is often difficult and full of discord; like the poems of Emily Dickinson, they can be fragmented; like the poems of Robert Graves, there can be semantic confusion. But the disquiet we get from these poems – their refusal to assure us – can be another form of therapy. It is worth mentioning, too, that one learns how to be a good writer through the practice of reading. The selections in this anthology, perhaps some more aesthetically sophisticated than others, provide access to a wide variety of human encounters with illness and communicate diverse experiences of living in a body. We hope that readers, whether professionals or patients, scholars or practitioners, healthy or otherwise, will find these poems pleasurable, reassuring and/or challenging.

4 History and Debate

Another school of thought insists that humanities subjects are not simply supplementary to the real business of medicine, but actively contribute to debates about the body and its treatment. A previous editor of the *British Medical Journal*, Richard Smith terms the former the 'additive view', which sees the humanities as softening the hard edges of medicine, and the latter as the 'integrated view' which more ambitiously shapes the 'nature, goals and knowledge base' of medicine (1999: 319, 0a).[21] Historians in particular have taken up the integrated view, although other humanities disciplines have as well; in fact, medical historians David S. Jones, Jeremy A. Greene, Jacalyn Duffin and John Harley Warner recently produced a manifesto of sorts, in which they argue that among other things, history in medical education offers 'essential insights about the causes of disease' and demonstrates 'the contingency of medical knowledge and practice amid the social, economic, and

---

[20]Frank expands here on a William James's 1906 lecture, in which he argued that humans failed to live up to their potential, that they lived 'contracted' lives. This is especially the case, Frank proposes, when living with a demoralizing illness.
[21]See also, in the same issue, Evans and Greaves (1999), Evans and Mcnaughton (2000).

political contexts of medicine' (17). History should be considered, they suggest, as legitimate a part of medical school curricula as anatomy or pathophysiology. This group of historians are keen to carve out a distinct role for their discipline and to make a particular case for it as 'an essential component of medical knowledge, reasoning, and practice' (2014: 1). As such, they resist identifying themselves under the medical humanities umbrella, choosing not to affiliate with humanities scholars who aim to foster medical professionalism (2014: 1).

These medical historians makes a strong case for their discipline; however almost the same strong case could be made for literary studies – after all, poems, paintings, novels and films are historical artefacts. They reveal as much about how we have approached the body in the past as the more obvious historical documents like medical treatises and court documents. More to the point, as art historian Ludmilla Jordanova succinctly puts it, 'medicine may productively be considered as a form of culture' (2014: 43). This has been demonstrated and recognized time and again: 'The truth is', Oliver Wendell Holmes stated unequivocally in 1860, 'that medicine, professedly founded on observation, is as sensitive to outside influences, political, religious, philosophical, imaginative, as is the barometer to the changes of atmospheric density'.[22] This refrain has since received widespread agreement – and literature is an important part of the cultural milieu that informs and is informed by medicine. Literature not only reveals how culturally specific anxieties and priorities influenced medical practices that often claim objective, value-free status; it also engages in debates with medicine about its priorities and values.

Jordanova has made a convincing case, along these lines, for visual culture specifically. She outlines 'a hefty agenda for the medical humanities', which includes exploration of such topics as:

> the medicalization of selfhood, the visualization of medicine, the somatization of sexuality, the rebellion against conventions surrounding the body, the sensational display of bodily phenomena and the commercialization of suffering (2014: 61).

This ambitious, expansive agenda is not confined to visual art, for what she describes – the medicalization of selfhood, the rebellion against conventions – is also the stuff of literature. These themes are equally present in 'misery memoirs' or disability literature. The visualization of medicine or the sensational display of bodily phenomena occurs in genres that combine text and visual representation, such as graphic pathographies (autobiographical comics about illness), neuroscientific/theatrical collaborations, or the huge realm of performance art that uses the body as a text.

5 History, Debate and Literature

This anthology is informed by an inclusive approach to the medical humanities, which is why medical writing – historical documents proper – is included alongside poems. The poems should be approached as legitimate historical texts, as well as

---

[22]See page 367 of this anthology.

aesthetic objects and as forms of engagement and protest (but more about that later). The poems and medical texts in this anthology, which span from the Enlightenment to the present day, reveal significant moments of historical and aesthetic change, as well as surprising continuities. Religious beliefs, political events and prevailing cultural attitudes affect the aetiology, classification, diagnosis and treatment of disease (and what even counts as disease). Certain cultural influences on medical science reach down through generations, sometimes even in spite of radical alterations to definitions and treatments of disease. At the same time, new medical knowledge can bring about profound transformations in culture – instigating changes in religious belief or social attitudes toward addictions, sex, reproduction or contagion, for instance.

A chronological survey of any of the chapters reveals how the medical themes of the poems change over time – as do the diseases and conditions that plague human communities. In the eighteenth century, poems and medical treatises recount the horrors of syphilis and quack treatments; in the same century, poems about smallpox recount not only the deadly effects of a virus that claimed lives and left others blinded or permanently debilitated, but also the aftermath of living permanently with facial scars. The cholera that arrived in England in the autumn of 1831, as part of the second great pandemic, and then in 1848–49, 1853–54 and 1866, generated a body of poetry replete with images of dampness, fog, mildew and poisoned air. That cholera had bubbled up from the mangrove swamps of the Sunderbans on the Bay of Bengal, then wound itself along trade routes, across oceans, and down the Thames to infect the heart of the capital, produced a whole realm of anxieties. As the sample of Victorian poetry on cholera included here reveals, those anxieties gave rise to a considerable number of poetic tropes about foreign invasion and the dark side of imperialism.

Cholera was the most frequently mapped disease of the nineteenth century – the same century in which medical mapping emerged as an important tool for understanding both the global and local relations between disease, people and place. So, for instance, American poets and physicians wrote about yellow fever, or in the vernacular of the South, 'Yellow Jack', at roughly the same time that British writers were fixating on 'King Cholera'. Lady Mary Wortley Montagu's writing on smallpox inoculation is a case in point about the global circulation of medical ideas. In 1717, she spent two years in the Ottoman Empire with her husband, the British ambassador to Istanbul. There she observed the Turkish women practice 'engrafting', that is, introducing pus from a smallpox lesion into an incision on the arm of a healthy person. It was believed that this inoculation against smallpox – also called 'variolation' – would then render that person immune to the disease. Montagu had her son inoculated in Turkey, and on her return to London, promoted the practice to friends, as well as to an unyielding medical establishment who would not support a foreign, Eastern practice. Montagu's poetry and prose, like that on the topic of cholera, give us a sense of medico-geographical differences, and the medical changes that are brought about through inter-cultural contact. We are reminded of the long-standing relationship between health and space, and the unevenness of the medical terrain, geographically and chronologically. Clearly, this anthology contains mostly

British and American writing, reflecting the lively transatlantic exchange of ideas and styles. We do not have the room or the expertise to include many selections from around the world, but we would urge interested readers to seek specialist collections for poetry from farther afield.

The frameworks for understanding illness are also constantly evolving. In the nineteenth century, for instance, the contamination model of disease posited that morbid matter was transmitted between individuals. Doctor-poets such as John Armstrong wrote of how, particularly in cities, contaminated lungs breathed out 'contagious matter' that was inhaled by other sets of lungs. This model of disease posited an 'invisible threat' and placed responsibility for the health of the wider community with individuals, which led to disciplinary measures against those who were seen as unhygienic or polluted by poverty, alcohol or immoral sexual habits (Wagner 2013: 143). The poems and medical writing on cholera are also informed by the prevailing belief in miasma theory in the long nineteenth century, which conceived of disease as originating in bad air or vapours filled with particles of decomposed matter (miasmata). The miasma framework was replaced by the germ theory of disease in the second half of the nineteenth century, following the epidemiological studies of John Snow, Louis Pasteur, Robert Koch and others. This change in medical understanding elicited new literary paradigms: microscopic vision, metaphors of infection and updated plague narratives with active, dangerously intelligent microbes as the new enemy.

The idea of evolving and shifting paradigms structures the work of French theorist Michel Foucault, who has shown us that facts, knowledge and even physical realities like disease are deeply embedded in culture, and vice versa. Through his genealogical method, he investigated cultural assumptions surrounding sexuality, madness and disease, and in the process demonstrated that phenomena which appear natural or 'without history' actually have very complicated cultural histories (139–40). Foucault has influenced the work of many literary and cultural historians who have addressed 'the role of the literary imagination in the cultural framing of disease', to use David Shuttleton's phrase (2012: 3). This is not to deny the material reality of illness or to suggest that culture invented disease: one need only read Fanny Burney's account of experiencing a mastectomy before the days of anaesthetic, X-ray and germ theory to realize how misguided that would be (see pp. 292–99). Nevertheless cultural assumptions, discourses and beliefs affect the way illnesses are imagined, treated, written about, visually represented and known – by medical professionals and the general public. As Shuttleton points out, it was once thought that smallpox could be contracted by fear, and since women were thought to be naturally nervous, it was believed they were more susceptible to infection. In *The Adventures of David Simple* (1753), the eighteenth-century novelist Sarah Fielding satirized this belief through her portrayal of the manipulative, socially aspirational character, Mrs. Ratcliffe, who fakes a fear of becoming infected through the upsetting words of a letter. As Shuttleton points out, 'this satirical depiction relied for its reach upon the reader's own morally freighted associations between the imagination, femininity and the risk of contagion by conceit' (2012: 39). This example reminds us that medical knowledge is historically contingent, and shaped by prevailing beliefs about race, ethnicity, class, gender and sexuality.

There are many similar examples of evolving beliefs and attitudes in *Body of Work*, but as things change, so they stay the same. The gender biases of previous centuries that are so obvious in the bawdy poems of the popular eighteenth-century sex handbook *Aristotle's Masterpiece,* or John Marten's anti-masturbation treatise *Onania* (1723) are very different from the gendered perceptions expressed in Fleur Adcock's 1971 pro-masturbation poem 'Against Coupling' or Haki R. Madhubuti's 1997 poem 'Abortion'. At the same time, however, some of the gender biases that seem so apparent in *Aristotle's* bawdy poems are also more subtly expressed in the professional, supposedly objective medical findings of Havelock Ellis's 1905 *Sexual Selection in Man*. In fact, readers will also notice how aims, attitudes and anxieties about the body often remain surprisingly consistent. The ambiguity and anguish that inform Anne Finch's 1701 poem 'The Spleen' also informs Edward Thomas's 1915 poem 'Melancholy', two hundred years later. Despondency also crosses gender and racial divides, appearing in Anne Sexton's 1960 'Noon Walk on the Asylum Lawn' and Michael S. Harper's 1973 'Maalox Bland Diet Prescribed'. For all the differences between these poems, there are connections to be made between modern struggles to represent depression as a legitimate illness and the defensiveness of the eighteenth-century narrator of Anne Finch's poem, who is unfairly accused of 'pretended Fits.' The perennial sense of uncertainty surrounding a condition that has been known variously as 'spleen', 'depressed spirits', 'melancholy' or 'depression', also crosses disciplinary borders. Many of the feelings, fears and ideas expressed in poetry can be detected in medical and psychological treatises such as Robert Whyte's 1765 work on hysteria and nervous disorders, George Miller Beard's *American Nervousness: Its Causes and Consequences* (1881) and Sigmund Freud's *Mourning and Melancholia* (1917).

We could do this same exercise – mapping changes and continuities – with terms such as 'contagion', 'cancer' or 'pain'. We could also trace how tenacious certain conditions and discourses are, as well as how unstable are others. What changes and what remains the same, for example, between British poet John Greenleaf Whittier's 'The Fat Man' of 1832 and the Ghana-born, Jamaica-raised Kwame Dawes's 'Fat Man' of 2003? How have our attitudes toward body size or 'excess' evolved? Or, what are the differences between poetic and medical representation of addiction? What is at stake when 'monstrosity' becomes replaced with the word 'curiosity', later jettisoned in favour of 'handicap', and then for very good reasons, replaced with 'disability'?

In addition, this collection reveals how aesthetic traditions have both endured through centuries but have also developed in new directions. In the opening to his long peripatetic essay of 1821, 'Confessions of an English Opium-Eater', Thomas De Quincey writes that there is nothing 'more revolting to English feelings, than the spectacle of a human being obtruding on our notice his moral ulcers or scars'. Part of the golden age of English essay writing, De Quincey recognized that although the eighteenth-century novel of sensibility had introduced readers to character interiority, they was a reticence about committing to paper one's nightmarish experiences 'chasing the dragon.' There were successors to De Quincey's *Confession*: in his own *Confessions* (1782), Jean Jacques Rousseau told of his homoerotic encounters with monks, his desire to be spanked, and his urge to flash unsuspecting women. But unlike De Quincey's text, Rousseau's confessions rationalize his transgressions and excuse his sometimes repugnant behaviour. Samuel Taylor Coleridge's opium dream of Xanadu, 'Kubla Khan', was written under the drug's effect, but not about his personal experiences of it, and while Coleridge's 'The Pains of Sleep' represents withdrawal, addiction and nightmares that bleed into waking hours, it is nothing like De Quincey's frank, gritty urban prose. De Quincey was the new modern flaneur, who meshed personal confessions about addiction with rational, incisive observations about nineteenth-century society.

Almost a century and a half later, D. J. Enright's poem 'Confessions of an English Opium Smoker' (1962), is haunted by the spectres of Coleridge and De Quincy.

> I offer to recall those images:
> Damsel, dome and dulcimer,
> Portentous pageants, alien altars,
> Foul unimaginable imagined monster,
> Façades of fanfares, Lord's Prayer
> Tattooed backwards on a Manchu fingernail,
> Enigma, or a dread too well aware,
> Swirling curtains, almond eyes or smell?

De Quincey's 'unutterable monsters' become Enright's 'Foul unimaginable imagined monster', here in a twentieth-century version of Romantic English-Orientalist visions of Chinese, Indian, Turkish apparitions. De Quincey's experiences of being solitary and invisible in the midst of the nineteenth-century urban multitude are resurrected in Enright's description of being 'rocked by the modern traffic of the town'. But, the abrupt juxtaposition of English and Orientalist scenes reflects a contracted world – Enright lived and worked in Egypt, Japan, Thailand and Singapore – in which the foreign and the local were in closer proximity. His images of common English people, common English objects and common English streets portray a degenerating society; demoralized people living in grubby shacks signal the long slow decline of Empire and Britain's downgraded status on the world stage. This is a poem informed by the past, but its poetic form and its take on contemporary events indicate a cultural, geographical, medical and historical specificity.

6 Activism and Protest

Crucially, literary texts are more than artefacts that provide evidence of the preoccupations and prevailing ideologies of a people. A poem is an aesthetic object that can also shape and, more to the point, *challenge* those ideologies. Walt Whitman's 'Wound-Dresser' (1865; 1881–82), one of his civil war poems, is an articulation of his experience conveying and attending the wounded, from the battlefields to Washington hospitals. Yet more than a personal account, 'Wound-Dresser' is a declaration against the bloody waste of war and a condemnation of politicians who weigh up the cost of goods and land but not individual life. Whitman's poem is as much a form of protest as a strongly worded polemic, but does so through poetic language and by creating striking images of crushed heads and death-glazed eyes.

On a completely different subject, if we again think of the poems and medical writing about sex that were addressed in the previous section, we see how poets can write against the weight of history. Fleur Adcock's poem 'Against Coupling' (1971) could be read as something of a declaration against contemporary sexual hang-ups that have their foundation in the beliefs of earlier centuries (as expressed, for instance, in John Marten's 1723 treatise *Onania*). Adcock's poem challenges the powerful legacy of the medical designations *normal, deviant* or *perverse*; it also protests the way religion has influenced medical knowledge in problematic ways.

Some decades ago, the early historian of medicine Henry Sigerist claimed that the study of history would equip doctors to combine health care with social action. 'If we want to act consciously and intelligently', he argued, we must be able to trace the historical origins of contemporary 'developments and trends' (1939: 659). Since then, medical historians making similar claims have produced work that examines social injustice, uncovers the mechanisms and processes of oppression, and integrates protest with institutional politics. Yet, this is not the purview of medical historians only. Seventy-five years on, Therese Jones echoes Sigerist's sentiments, but rather than singling out any particular discipline, she highlights the radical potential and democratizing energies of the humanities as a *whole*. As a body of thinkers, we are renowned, she writes, for our 'fearless questioning of representations', our willingness to confront 'abuses of authority' and our 'steadfast refusal' to acknowledge the division that medicine has traditionally set 'between biology and culture' (2014a: 28–9). Ultimately, these are precisely the qualities that link the various disciplines in the arts and humanities. These are also the qualities that make literary critics, historians, philosophers and artists so important as key players – and protesters – in debates about the relationship between biology and culture.

Investigations of the ways discourses determine how we deal with material reality have been particularly fruitful. In *Illness as Metaphor* (1978) and *AIDS as Metaphor* (1989), Susan Sontag interrogates the mythologies that attach to illness. The frightening physical reality of cholera in the nineteenth century – which very quickly turned people into shrunken, dehydrated, blue skinned figures – has left its trace in today's language. In French, the phrase for overpowering fear is *une peur bleue* ([1989] 2002: 121). Sontag explores how historically, the most feared diseases, such as leprosy, syphilis and cholera, have been those that 'transform the body into something alienating' ([1989] 2002: 131). These diseases, she argues, have been understood in the cultural imagination as forms of biblical plagues, as retributive epidemics visited on an errant populace. The moral language surrounding plague in the early modern period (which Daniel Defoe captures in his 1722 *Journal of the Plague Year*) is remarkably similar to the discourse surrounding AIDS in the 1980s and 1990s.

Sontag identifies discourses, borrowed from other domains, which become frameworks for understanding and dealing with a disease like cancer. She draws a trajectory from the militaristic language of late-nineteenth-century bacteriology and the discourse surrounding cancer in the late twentieth century. In the 1880s, when disease-causing bacteria were discovered, they were said to 'invade' or 'infiltrate', and a hundred years later, we are using a similarly literal and authoritative language to describe cancer as 'the enemy on which society wages war' ([1978] 2002: 67). The cancer patient's body is under 'siege': its weakened 'defenses' are bombarded by 'invasive' and colonizing cells ([1978] 2002: 66–8). And so our researchers, health authorities and governments have declared 'a war on cancer' ([1978] 2002: 67). This is more than an exploration of the ways society describes disease and disease sufferers – although that is a major undertaking in itself. Sontag uncovers how deeply the past influences both public and professional reactions to disease, in order to encourage readers to change the way they speak about and conceive of disease, and the way they treat sufferers. Sontag's work has had its detractors, including those who argue that metaphors are a necessary way to make meaningful sense of illness.[23] Nevertheless, Sontag's synthesis of discourse analysis and literary and medical history is an important protest against the damaging consequences of the way we use metaphor to make sense of the things we fear or can't understand. She condemns, perhaps most pointedly, the way metaphors have been used to conflate the patient with the disease. To describe syphilis as 'pollution', to see leprosy as a hideous 'emblem of decay', to see AIDS as 'contamination' is to stigmatize and ostracize ([1978] 2002: 36, 55; [1989]: 109, 149–50). Metaphors may help us make sense of frightening things, but they also cause further harm to those who are already harmed.

III POETRY: WHAT IS IT GOOD FOR?

Since poetry is at the centre of this anthology, it is fitting in this final section to adapt the question posed above – 'what can the medical humanities offer?' – to ask specifically what poetry can do. The easiest answer is that even the simplest of poetic forms can communicate things in ways that prose forms cannot. Consider, for example, this poem:

> Sir Humphry Davy
> Abominated gravy.
> He lived in the odium
> Of having discovered sodium.

As children, our first introduction to Davy may have been through this clerihew (a whimsical, rhyming 4-line poem invented in 1905 by Edmund Clerihew Bentley). But, the comical juxtaposition of words – 'odium/sodium' and 'abominated gravy' – does more than make us remember an elementary science lesson. This is also a parody of the tradition of panegyric, a form typically associated with an uncritical celebration of authority.

---

[23]For instance, see Clow (2001).

Clerihews can encourage us to wonder what lies beneath the simplicity and light humour, as in this one about the philosopher René Descartes and his famous maxim 'Cogito ergo sum', or 'I think, therefore I am':

Did Descartes
Depart
With the thought
'Therefore I'm not'?

Even the lightest of poems can take on the weightiest of theories. Is Bentley's poem about Descartes a statement about the triumph of materialism – the belief that matter is the fundamental substance of human life? Is this a negation of the belief in an eternal, immaterial, intangible human soul, which exists separately from the material body? Is this the early twentieth-century writing back to the seventeenth to say, we no longer believe in the human as divinely made? That modern medical science has shown us that the human is a sum of his or her biological parts? This clever reversal of Descartes' dictum 'I think therefore I am', suggests that once the heart stops pumping and the lungs stop respiring, the 'I' simply ceases to exist – in any form. Perhaps the suggestion is that in his last moments even the great dualist Descartes had a crisis of faith, and thought, 'is this it?'

Of course, in terms of form and content, the selections in this anthology go well beyond the humble clerihew. There are lyric poems that communicate the realities of experiencing disease, aging, recovery, death and loss. There are confessional poems that ask for non-judgemental compassion as they communicate personal experiences with addiction, sexual dysfunction or abortion. There are humorous odes that provide perspective in anxious times and reveal the resilience of the human spirit. Readers will find that parody and satire once mediated our experiences with quacks in the eighteenth century, and continues to do so with respect to bureaucracy, machines and pills in the twenty-first. Free verse that is patterned on the rhythms of regular speech encourages dialogue about difficult subjects where there might otherwise be silence. The prose poem, which is a blend of two forms, mimics the experience of hovering between life and death, hope and despair, even comedy and tragedy. Their fragmentary quality can mirror the sense of disconnection from everyday life that illness, trauma and psychological disturbance can bring. Sometimes, the fragment is all that can be expressed.

Poetic language, which is typically distilled, concentrated and more spare than regular prose, encourages the reader to focus closely on the meanings that inhere in single words. Through the lens of personal lived experience, or imagined experiences, poetry reveals how the perceptions and practices associated with freighted words like *natural* and *normal* or *unnatural* and *abnormal* inscribe the bodies and psyches of individuals. Kwame Dawes's 'Fat Man' is a political poem, but it also describes being physically weighed down by extra weight: medical discourses warning of premature death colour the experience of living with short breath and an awkward waddle. The narrator's search for poetic words and phrases – 'plump existentialism' – is intended to put distance between himself and the word that weighs heaviest: fat. Robert Lowell redefines the word 'life' as 'both the fire and the fuel', but for

William Earnest Henley, 'life' is 'a blunder and a shame'. Death shambles by in Arthur Stringer's poem, but reveals itself to W. H. Auden as 'right and splendid', while Will Carleton's 'Country Doctor' learns that 'Death is master both of Science and of Art'. These are examples of how, in poetry, the single word is brought sharply into focus; poetry distills, redefines and makes words confrontational.

It may be obvious to say that of the literary forms, the rhythm and beat of poetry makes it closest to music, but less obvious is the way this association with sound makes poetry suited to the rhythms of the body. Poetry can mimic the energetic or lethargic pulses of the blood; the rhythmic or the ragged breathing of the lungs. Imagine, too, what happens when verse translates the professional prose of medical experts; the objective prose of textbooks; the sympathetic prose of well-wishers; the plaintive, bewildered, resigned or angry prose of the dying into rhythm, rhyme, meter and line. Poetry then becomes the music of bodies in pain; bodies in recovery; bodies in mourning; and perhaps most importantly, bodies with good stories. This then, is the poetry of 'holding one's own in the face of the multiple threats that are the occasion of suffering', to use Arthur Frank's words (2014: 23).

Finally, if all else fails, and skeptics and non-believers will still insist that 'verse is only for the healthy arty-farties' or that the utility of the arts and humanities is limited or that poetry doesn't do anything, we are content to leave the final words to the physician and poet Dannie Abse:

> Some may argue that poetry is a useless thing, an activity that can rival the counting of the cats of Zanzibar. But whatever else poems do, or do not do, at the very least they profoundly alter the man or woman who wrote them (1998: 364).

REFERENCES

Abse, D. (1998), 'More Than a Green Placebo', *Lancet*, 351: 362–64.

Arnold, M. ([1882] 1974), 'Literature and Science', rpt. *Matthew Arnold: The Complete Prose*, ed. H R. Super, vol. 10, 51–73, Ann Arbor, MI: University of Michigan Press.

Bates, V. and S. Goodman (2014), 'Critical Conversations: Establishing Dialogue in the Medical Humanities', *Medicine, Health and the Arts: Approaches to Medical Humanities*, ed. V. Bates et al., Abingdon and Oxford: Routledge.

Broyard, A. (1992), *Intoxicated by My Illness*, New York: Ballantyne.

Charon, R. (2001), 'Narrative Medicine: A Model for Empathy, Reflection, Profession, and Trust', *Journal of the American Medical Association*, 286: 1897–1902.

Charon R. (2003), 'Two Hemispheres Unite: Medical Humanities Become Narrative Medicine', *Practicing the Medical Humanities: Engaging Physicians and Patients*, ed. R. Carson, C. Burns and T. Cole, 143–56, Hagerstown, MD: University Publishing Group.

Charon, R. (2004), 'Narrative and Medicine', *The New England Journal of Medicine*, 350 (9): 862–64.

Charon, R. (2008), *Narrative Medicine: Honoring the Stories of Illness*, New York: Oxford University Press.

Charon, R. and Montello M, eds. (2002), *Stories Matter: The Role of Narrative in Medical Ethics*, New York: Routledge.

Clow, B. (2001), 'Who's Afraid of Susan Sontag? or, the Myths and Metaphors of Cancer Reconsidered', *Social History of Medicine*, 14 (2): 293–312.

Collini, S. (2013), 'What, Ultimately, for? The Elusive Goal of Cultural Criticism', *Raritan*, 33: 4–26.

Culler, J. (2005), 'In Need of a Name? A Response to Geoffrey Harpham,' *New Literary History*, 36 (1): 37–42.

DasGupta, S. and R. Charon (2004), 'Personal Illness Narratives: Using Reflective Writing to Teach Empathy', *Academic Medicine*, 79: 351–56.

Davy, H. ([1805] 1840), 'Parallels between Art and Science,' *The Collected Works of Sir Humphry Davy,* vol. viii., 306–08, London: Smith, Elder & Co.

Downie, R., R. Hendry, R. Macnaughton, and B. Smith (1997), 'Humanizing Medicine: A Special Study Module', *Medical Education*, 31: 276–80.

Evans, M. and D. Greaves (1999), 'Exploring the Medical Humanities.' *British Medical Journal*, 319: 1216.

Evans, M and D. Greaves (2000), 'Conceptions of Medical Humanities'. *Medical Humanities*, 26: 1–2.

Evans, M. and J. Mcnaughton (2000), 'Should Medical Humanities be a Multidisciplinary or an Interdisciplinary Study?', *Medical Humanities*, 30: 1–4.

Foucault, M. (1980), 'Nietzsche, Genealogy, History,' *Language, Counter-memory, Practice*, ed. Daniel Bouchard, 139–64, Ithaca, NY: Cornell University Press.

Frank, A. (1997), *The Wounded Story Teller: Body, Illness and Ethics*, Chicago: University of Chicago Press.

Frank, A. (2014), 'Being a Good Story: The Humanities as Therapeutic Practice,' *Health Humanities Reader*, ed. T. Jones, D. Wear and L. Friedman, New Brunswick, NJ: Rutgers.

Gillis, C. (2008), 'Medicine and Humanities: Voicing Connections,' *Journal of Medical Humanities*, 29: 5–14.

Goldberg, D. (2012), American Society for Bioethics and Humanities Literature and Medicine Listserv, October 31. litmed@listserv.com.

Groopman, J. (2007), *How Doctors Think*, Boston: Houghton Mifflin.

Harley Warner, J. (2013), 'Humanizing Power of Medical History: Responses to Biomedicine in the 20th-century United States', *Procedia – Social and Behavioral Sciences*, 77: 322–32.

Hartman, G. (2004), 'Narrative and Beyond,' *Literature and Medicine*, 23: 334–45.

Holmes, R. (2008), *The Age of Wonder: How the Romantic Generation Discovered the Terror and Beauty of Science*, London: Harper.

Huxley, T. H. ([1882] 1896), 'On Science and Art in Relation to Education', *Science and Education: Essays*, New York: Appleton.

Jones, A. H. (1984), 'Reflections, Projections, and the Future of Literature-and-Medicine', *Literature and Medicine: A Claim for a Discipline*, ed. D. Wear, M. Kohn and S. Stocker, 29–40, McLean, VA: Society for Health and Human Values.

Jones, D., J. Greene, J. Duffin and J. Harley Warner (2015), 'Making the Case for History in Medical Education', *Journal of the History of Medicine and Allied Sciences*, Epub ahead of publication: doi:10.1093/jhmas/jru026.

Jones, T., D. Wear and L. D. Friedman (2014), 'Introduction', *Health Humanities Reader*, New Brunswick, NJ: Rutgers University Press.

Keats, J. ([1818] 1958), *Letters of John Keats: 1814-1821*, 1 of 2 vols., ed. Hyder Edward Rollins, Cambridge, MA: Harvard University Press.

Keen, S. (2007), *Empathy and the Novel*, Oxford: Oxford University Press.

Kimball, R. (2009), 'The Two Cultures Today', *From Two Cultures to No Culture*, ed. Robert Whelan, 1–30, Trowbridge, Wilts: Civitas.

Leavis, F. R. ([1962] 2013), *The Two Cultures?: The Significance of C. P. Snow*, ed. Stefan Collini, Cambridge: Cambridge University Press.

McDonagh, M. (1945), *Poet Physicians: An Anthology of Medical Poetry*, Springfield, IL: Charles C. Thomas.

Perry, M., N. Maffulli, S. Willson, and D. Morrissey (2011), 'The Effectiveness of Arts-Based Interventions in Medical Education: A Literature Review', *Medical Education*, 45: 141–8.

Rees, G. (2010), 'The Ethical Imperative of Medical Humanities', *Journal of Medical Humanities*, 31: 267–77.

Sacks, O. (2015), 'My Own Life', *The New York Times*, February 19: A25.

Shapiro, J. (2012), 'Whither (Whether) Medical Humanities? The Future of Humanities and Arts in Medical Education', *Journal for Learning Through the Arts*, 8: 1.

Shuttleton, D. (2012), *Smallpox and the Literary Imagination, 1660-1820*, Cambridge: Cambridge University Press.

Sigerist, H. (1939), 'Medical History in the Medical Schools of the United States', *Bulletin of the History of Medicine*, 7: 627–62.

Slingerland, E. and M. Collard (2012), *Creating Consilience: Integrating the Sciences and the Humanities*, Oxford: Oxford University Press.

Smith, R. (1999), 'Editor's choice – Struggling Towards Coherence', *British Medical Journal*, 319: 0a.

Snow, C. P. ([1959] 2012), *The Two Cultures*, ed. Stefan Collini, Cambridge: Cambridge University Press.

Snow, J. (1854),'The Cholera near Golden-square, and at Deptford', *Medical Times Gazette*, 9: 321–22.

Sontag, S. ([1978] 2002), 'Illness as Metaphor,' *Illness as Metaphor and AIDS and Its Metaphors*, London: Penguin.

Sontag, S. ([1989] 2002), 'AIDS and Its Metaphors', *Illness as Metaphor and AIDS and Its Metaphors*, London: Penguin.

Stokes, J. (1980), 'Grief and the Performing Arts: A Brief Experiment in Humanizing Medical Education', *Journal of Medical Education*, 55: 215.

Wagner, C. (2013), *Pathological Bodies: Medicine and Political Culture*, Berkeley, CA: University of California Press.

Wilson, E. O. (1998), *Consilience: The Unity of Knowledge*, New York: Knopf.

CHAPTER ONE

Body as Machine

from *A Farewell to Poetry, with a Long Digression on Anatomy*
Jane Barker (1688)

Farewell, my gentle Friend, kind *Poetry*,
For we no longer must Acquaintance be;
Though sweet and charming to me as thou art,
Yet I must dispossess thee of my Heart.
On new Acquaintance now I must dispense
What I receiv'd from *thy* bright influence.
Wise *Aristotle* and *Hippocrates*,
Galen, and the most Wise *Socrates*;
Æsculapius,[1] whom first I should have nam'd,
And all *Apollo's* younger brood so fam'd,
Are they with whom I must Acquaintance make,
Who will, no doubt, receive me for the sake
Of *Him*, from whom they did expect to see
New Lights to search *Nature's* obscurity.

Now, *Bartholine*,[2] the first of all this Crew,
Does to me Nature's *Architecture* shew;
He tells me how th' Foundation first is laid
Of Earth; how Pillars of strong *Bones* are made;
How th' Walls consist of *carneous* parts within,
The out-side *pinguid*,[3] over-laid with Skin;
The Fretwork, Muscles, Arteries, and Veins,
With their *Implexures*, and how from the Brains
The Nerves descend; and how they do dispense
To ev'ry Member, Motive Pow'r and Sense;
He shews what Windows in this Structure's fix'd,
How tribly Glaz'd, and Curtains drawn betwixt

---

[1]Aristotle (384–322 BC) was a Greek philosopher and scientist. Hippocrates (c. 460–370 BC) is often referred to as 'the father of Western medicine'. Galen of Pergamon (129–c.216 AD) was an important Greek physician, early surgeon and philosopher. The Greek philosopher Socrates (469–399 BC) was one of the founders of Western philosophy. Aesculapius was a god of medicine in ancient Greek myth, representing the healing aspects of the medical arts.
[2]Rasmus Bartholin (1625–98), Danish scientist and physician, was professor at the University of Copenhagen, first in geometry, later in medicine.
[3]Pinguid: fatty.

Them and Earth's objects; all which proves in vain
To keep out *Lust*, and *Innocence* retain:
For 'twas the Eye that first discern'd the food,
As pleasing to itself, then thought it good
To *eat*, as being inform'd it would refine
The half-wise *Soul*, and make it all Divine.
But ah, how dearly *Wisdom's* bought with Sin,
Which shuts out Grace, lets Death and Darkness in!

And because we *precipitated* first,
To Pains and Ignorance are most accurs'd;
Ev'n by our *Counter-parts*, who that they may
Exalt themselves, insultingly will say,
Women know little, and they practise less;
But Pride and Sloth they glory to profess.
But as we were *expatiating* thus,
Walæus and *Harvey*[4] cry'd, Madam, follow us,
They brought me to the first and largest Court
Of all this Building, where as to a *Port*,
All necessaries are brought from far,
For sustentation both in Peace and War:
For *War* this Common-wealth do's oft infest,
Which pillages this part, and storms the rest.

We view'd the Kitchin call'd *Ventriculus*,
Then pass'd we through the space call'd *Pylorus*;
And to the Dining-Room we came at last,
Where the *Lactæans* take their sweet repast.
From thence we through a Drawing-room did pass,
And came where Madam *Jecur*[5] busy was;
Sanguificating the whole Mass of Chyle,
And severing the *Cruoral* parts from bile:
And when she's made it tolerably good,
She pours it forth to mix with other Blood.
This and much more we saw, from thence we went
Into the next Court, by a small *ascent*:
Bless me, said I, what Rarities are here!
A Fountain like a Furnace did appear,
Still boiling o'er, and running out so fast,
That one should think its Efflux could not last;
Yet it sustain'd no loss as I could see,

---

[4]John Walæus (d. 1649), professor of medicine at Leyden, made important discoveries on the circulation of the blood. William Harvey (1578–1657), English physician, described the properties of blood and the circulatory system in detail in his 1628 *De motu cordis* (*On the Motion of the Heart and Blood*).
[5]Madam Jecur: (Latin) 'the liver'.

Which made me think it a strange Prodigy.
Come on, says *Harvey*, don't stand gazing here,
But follow me, and I thy doubts will clear.
Then we began our Journey with the *Blood*,
Trac'd the *Meanders* of its Purple flood.
Thus we through many *Labyrinths* did pass,
In such, I'm sure, Old *Dædalus*[6] ne'er was;
Sometimes i'th' Out-works, sometimes i'th' first Court;
Sometimes i'th' third these winding streams wou'd sport
Themselves; but here methought I needs must stay,
And listen next to what the *Artists* say:
Here's *Cavities*, says one; and here, says he,
Is th' Seat of Fancy, Judgment, Memory:
Here, says another, is the *fertile* Womb,
From whence the Spirits *Animal* do come,
Which are mysteriously *ingender'd* here,
Of Spirits from *Arterious* Blood and Air:
Here, said a third, *Life* made her first approach,
Moving the Wheels of her Triumphant Coach:
Hold there, said *Harvey*, that must be deny'd,
'Twas in the deaf Ear on the *dexter* side.
Then there arose a trivial small dispute,
Which he by Fact and Reason did confute:
Which being ended, we began again
Our former Journey, and forsook the Brain.
And after some small *Traverses* about,
We came to th' place where we at first set out:
Then I perceiv'd how all this *Magick* stood
By th' *Circles* of the *circulating* Blood,
As *Fountains* have their Waters from the Sea,
To which again they do themselves convey.

But here we find great *Lower*[7] by his Art,
Surveying the whole *Structure* of the Heart:
Welcome, said he, sweet Cousin, are you here,
Sister to him whose Worth we all *revere?*
But ah, alas, so cruel was his Fate,
As makes us since almost our Practice hate;
Since we could find out nought in all our Art,
That could prolong the motion of his Heart.

---

[6]In Greek mythology, Dædalus created the Labyrinth on Crete, in which the minotaur was kept.
[7]Richard Lower (1631–91), was a Cornish physician who performed the first blood transfusion experiments in England.

Upon the Sight of an Anatomy
Nahum Tate (1696)

Nay, start not at that *Skeleton*,
'Tis your own Picture which you shun;
Alive it did resemble Thee,
And thou, when dead, like that shalt be:
Converse with it, and you will say,
You cannot better spend the Day;
You little think how you'll admire
The Language of those *Bones* and *Wire*.

The *Tongue* is gone, but yet each Joint
Reads Lectures, and can speak to th' Point.
When all your Moralists are read,
You'll find no Tutors like the Dead.

If in Truth's Paths those *Feet* have trod,
'Tis all one whether bare, or shod:
If us'd to travel to the Door
Of the Afflicted Sick and Poor,
Though to the Dance they were estrang'd,
And ne'er their own rude Motion chang'd;
Those Feet, now wing'd, may upwards fly,
And tread the Palace of the Sky.

Those *Hands*, if ne'er with Murder stain'd,
Nor fill'd with Wealth unjustly gain'd,
Nor greedily at Honours grasped,
But to the *Poor-Man's* Cry unclasped;
It matters not, if in the Mine
They delv'd, or did with Rubies shine.

Here grew the *Lips*, and in that Place,
Where now appears a vacant space,
Was fix'd the *Tongue*, an Organ, still
Employ'd extremely well or ill;
I know not if it could retort,
If vers'd i' th' Language of the Court;
But this I safely can aver,
That if it was no Flatterer;
If it traduc'd no Man's Repute,
But, where it could not Praise, was Mute:
If no false Promises it made,
If it sung Anthems, if it Pray'd,
'Twas a blest *Tongue*, and will prevail
When Wit and Eloquence shall fail.

If Wise as *Socrates*, that *Skull*,
Had ever been 'tis now as dull
As *Mydas's*[8]; or if its Wit
To that of *Mydas* did submit,

'Tis now as full of Plot and Skill,
As is the Head of *Matchiavel*[9]:
Proud Laurels once might shade that Brow,
Where not so much as Hair grows now.

Prime Instances of Nature's Skill,
The *Eyes*, did once those Hollows fill:
Were they quick-fighted, sparkling, clear,
(As those of Hawks and Eagles are,)
Or say they did with Moisture swim,
And were distorted, blear'd, and dim;
Yet if they were from Envy free,
Nor lov'd to gaze on Vanity;
If none with scorn they did behold,
With no lascivious Glances roll'd:
Those Eyes, more bright and piercing grown,
Shall view the Great Creator's Throne;
They shall behold th' *Invisible*,
And on Eternal Glories dwell.

See! not the least Remains appear
To show where Nature plac'd the *Ear*!
Who knows if it were Musical,
Or could not judge of Sounds at all?
Yet if it were to Council bent,
To Caution and Reproof attent,
When the shrill Trump shall rouse the Dead,
And others hear their Sentence read;
That *Ear* shall with these Sounds be blest,
Well done, and, *Enter into Rest*.

On the Dissection of a Body
Anonymous (1770)

Observe this wonderful machine,
View its connection with each part,
Thus furnish'd by the hand unseen,
How far surpassing human art!

---

[8]According to at least one ancient myth, the vain and greedy King Midas, who turned everything he touched into gold, starved when his food and drink also hardened into gold.
[9]Niccolo de Bernardo dei Machiavelli (1469–1527) was a Florentine diplomat and an important Renaissance philosopher.

Should ablest imitators try,
With utmost skill, to form a like,
Could they so charm the curous, eye?
Could they with equal wonder strike?

See how the motion of each part
Upon some other still depends,
When all a mutual aid impart,
Conducing to their various ends.

Whilst we th' amazing frame explore,
More secret wonders still we spy,
Yet there remain ten thousand more
Hid from the microscopic eye.

Here may the stupid Atheist see
Convincing proofs – which all combine
To overthrow his wretched plan,
And speak the Maker's hand divine.

What great emoluments accrue[10]
To those who Nature's laws obey?
From such instructions to her view,
Ye sons of Esculapius[11] say!

Tho' God has call'd the life he lent,
Each vital function dormant laid,
Here we trace Nature's deep intent,
And see how once the springs were play'd.

These tubes convey'd the purple juice,
Which with new strength supply'd the whole;
And here branch'd forth the nerves, whose use
Was to keep converse with the soul.

This silent preacher points us out
The cause of many a latent ill,
Which, heretofore, lay hid in doubt,
Baffling each effort of our skill.

from *The Immortality of the Soul*
William Hay (1794)

Can man celestial motions, and their cause,
Know to describe, and by what stated laws

---

[10]An emolument is a salary, fee or profits.
[11]In ancient Greek myth, Aesculapius was the god of medicine.

Worlds round our sun hold on their course decreed,
And through the void immense the comets speed;
Numberless suns within, beyond our sight,
In ether fix'd, their circling planets light?
And think you not a mind, which even here
Flies through the skies, and through the starry sphere,
From heav'n descended, will her pinions stretch,
And mount again, her native home to reach?

Could this be so, did not the mind retain
A force innate, free from material stain?
Of her own acts by herself conscious made,
She uses not, nor needs, the body's aid.
Her choice, refusal, love, aversion,
Her hopes, fears, joys, and griefs, are all her own.
By her own strength she things compares, and finds
How to divide them into diff'rent kinds:
By slow degrees gleans the dismember'd spoils
Of scatter'd truth, and nicely reconciles;
Causes extracts; and a foundation lays
In one fair building arts on arts to raise;
To science tends, exerting ev'ry pow'r,
Mounting to scale her most exalted tow'r;
And thence the chain of causes view in one,
Let down to earth from the almighty throne.
Then sinks into herself; with mental eyes
There sees ideas of things, and how they rise;
Sees from what source swift cogitation flows;
All but her frame, and that almost, she knows.
Corporeal virtue this? can a machine
Perceive what feeds it, or its powers within?
All body's mere machine; impell'd alone
By outward force, not inward and its own.

To the Automaton Chess Player[12]
Hannah F. Gould (1829)

Thou wond'rous cause of speculation –
Of deep research and cogitation,
Of many a head, and many a nation –
While all in vain
Have tried their wits to answer whether
In silver, gold, steel, silk, or leather,

---

[12]The chess playing machine 'The Turk', invented by Wolfgang von Kempelen (1734–1804).

Or human parts, or all together,
Consists thy brain!

When first I view'd thine awful face,
Rising above that ample case
Which gives thy cloven foot a place,
Thy double shoe,
I marvell'd whether I had seen
Old Nick[13] himself, or a machine,
Or something fix'd midway between
The distant two!

A sudden shuddering seized my frame;
With feeling that defies a name,
Of wonder, horror, doubt and shame,
The *tout ensemble.*
I deem'd thee form'd with power and will;
My hair rose up – my blood stood still,
And curdled with a fearful chill,
Which made me tremble.

I thought if, e'en within thy glove,
Thy cold and fleshless hand should move
To rest on me, the touch would prove
Far worse than death; –
That I should be transform'd, and see
Thousands, and thousands, gaze on me,
A living, moving thing, like thee,
Devoid of breath.

When busy, curious, learn'd, and wise,
Regard thee with inquiring eyes
To find wherein thy mystery lies,
On thy stiff neck,
Turning thy head with grave precision,
Their optic light and mental vision
Alike defying, with decision,
Thou giv'st them '*check*!'

Some say a little man resides
Between thy narrow, bony sides,
And round the world within thee rides:
Absurd the notion!
For what's the human thing 'twould lurk
In thine unfeeling breast, Sir Turk,

---

[13]Old Nick: the devil.

Performing thus, thine inward work,
And outward motion?

Some whisper that thou'rt him who fell
From heaven's high courts, down, down to dwell
In that deep place of sulphury smell
And lurid flame.
Thy keeper, then, deserves a pension
For seeking out this wise invention,
To hold thee harmless, in detention,
Close at thy game.

Now, though all Europe has confest
That in thy master Maelzel's[14] breast
Hidden, thy secret still must rest,
Yet, 'twere great pity,
With all our intellectual sight,
That none should view thy nature right –
But thou must leave in fog and night
Our keen-eyed city.

Then just confide in me, and show,
Or tell how things within thee go,
Speak in my ear so quick and low
None else shall know it.
But, mark me! if I should discover
Without thine aid, thy secret mover,
With thee for ever all is over;
I'll quickly blow it!

from *I Sing the Body Electric*
Walt Whitman (1867)

I sing the Body electric;
The armies of those I love engirth me, and I engirth them;
They will not let me off till I go with them, respond to them,
And discorrupt them, and charge them full with the charge of the Soul.

Was it doubted that those who corrupt their own bodies conceal themselves?
And if those who defile the living are as bad as they who defile the dead?
And if the body does not do as much as the Soul?
And if the body were not the Soul, what is the Soul?

---

[14]Johann Nepomuk Maelzel (1772–1838) was a German inventor, showman and maker of musical automatons. In 1805 he purchased von Kempelen's fraudulent chess playing machine and toured it in America.

The love of the Body of man or woman balks account – the body itself balks
    account;
That of the male is perfect, and that of the female is perfect.

The expression of the face balks account;
But the expression of a well-made man appears not only in his face;
It is in his limbs and joints also, it is curiously in the joints of his hips and wrists;
It is in his walk, the carriage of his neck, the flex of his waist and knees – dress
    does not hide him;
The strong, sweet, supple quality he has, strikes through the cotton and flannel;
To see him pass conveys as much as the best poem, perhaps more;
You linger to see his back, and the back of his neck and shoulder-side.

   ...

A man's Body at auction;
I help the auctioneer – the sloven does not half know his business.

Gentlemen, look on this wonder!
Whatever the bids of the bidders, they cannot be high enough for it;
For it the globe lay preparing quintillions of years, without one animal or plant;
For it the revolving cycles truly and steadily roll'd.

In this head the all-baffling brain;
In it and below it, the makings of heroes.

Examine these limbs, red, black, or white – they are so cunning in tendon and
    nerve;
They shall be stript, that you may see them.

Exquisite senses, life-lit eyes, pluck, volition,
Flakes of breast-muscle, pliant back-bone and neck, flesh not flabby, good sized
    arms and legs,
And wonders within there yet.

Within there runs blood,
The same old blood!
The same red-running blood!
There swells and jets a heart – there all passions, desires, reachings, aspirations;
Do you think they are not there because they are not express'd in parlors and
    lecture rooms?. . .

If any thing is sacred, the human body is sacred,
And the glory and sweet of a man, is the token of manhood untainted;
And in man or woman, a clean, strong, firm-fibred body, is beautiful as the most
    beautiful face.

Have you seen the fool that corrupted his own live body? or the fool that
    corrupted her own live body?
For they do not conceal themselves, and cannot conceal themselves.

O my Body! I dare not desert the likes of you in other men and women, nor the
    likes of the parts of you;
I believe the likes of you are to stand or fall with the likes of the Soul, (and that
    they are the Soul);
I believe the likes of you shall stand or fall with my poems – and that they are
    poems,
Man's, woman's, child's, youth's, wife's, husband's, mother's, father's, young
    man's, young woman's poems;
Head, neck, hair, ears, drop and tympan of the ears,
Eyes, eye-fringes, iris of the eye, eye-brows, and the waking or sleeping of the lids,
Mouth, tongue, lips, teeth, roof of the mouth, jaws, and the jaw-hinges,
Nose, nostrils of the nose, and the partition,
Cheeks, temples, forehead, chin, throat, back of the neck, neck-slue,
Strong shoulders, manly beard, scapula, hind-shoulders, and the ample side-
    round of the chest,
Upper-arm, arm-pit, elbow-socket, lower-arm, arm-sinews, arm-bones,
Wrist and wrist-joints, hand, palm, knuckles, thumb, fore-finger, finger-balls,
    finger-joints, finger-nails,
Broad breast-front, curling hair of the breast, breast-bone, breast-side,
Ribs, belly, backbone, joints of the back-bone,
Hips, hip-sockets, hip-strength, inward and outward round, man-balls,
    man-root,
Strong set of thighs, well carrying the trunk above,
Leg-fibres, knee, knee-pan, upper-leg, under-leg,
Ankles, instep, foot-ball, toes, toe-joints, the heel;
All attitudes, all the shapeliness, all the belongings of my or your body, or of any
    one's body, male or female,
The lung-sponges, the stomach-sac, the bowels sweet and clean,
The brain in its folds inside the skull-frame,
Sympathies, heart-valves, palate-valves, sexuality, maternity,
Womanhood, and all that is a woman – and the man that comes from woman,
The womb, the teats, nipples, breast-milk, tears, laughter, weeping, love-looks,
    love-perturbations and risings,
The voice, articulation, language, whispering, shouting aloud,
Food, drink, pulse, digestion, sweat, sleep, walking, swimming,
Poise on the hips, leaping, reclining, embracing, arm-curving and tightening,
The continual changes of the flex of the mouth, and around the eyes,
The skin, the sun-burnt shade, freckles, hair,
The curious sympathy one feels, when feeling with the hand the naked meat of
    the body,
The circling rivers, the breath, and breathing it in and out,
The beauty of the waist, and thence of the hips, and thence downward toward
    the knees,
The thin red jellies within you, or within me – the bones, and the marrow in the
    bones,

The exquisite realization of health;
O I say, these are not the parts and poems of the Body only, but of the Soul,
O I say now these are the Soul!

from *The Birth and Death of Pain*
Silas Weir Mitchell (1896)[15]

The Birth of Pain! Let centuries roll away;
Come back with me to nature's primal day.
What mighty forces pledged the dust to life!
What awful will decreed its silent strife,
Till through vast ages rose on hill and plain
Life's saddest voice, the birthright wail of pain!
The keener sense and ever-growing mind
Served but to add a torment twice refined,
As life, more tender as it grew more sweet,
The cruel links of sorrow found complete
When yearning love, to conscious pity grown,
Felt the mad pain-thrills that were not its own.

What will implacable, beyond our ken,
Set this stern fiat for the tribes of men?
This none shall 'scape who share our human fates:
One stern democracy of anguish waits
By poor men's cots, within the rich man's gates.
What purpose hath it? Nay, thy quest is vain:
Earth hath no answer. If the baffled brain
Cries, 'tis to warn, to punish! – ah, refrain.
When writhes the child beneath the surgeon's hand,
What soul shall hope that pain to understand?
Lo! Science falters o'er the hopeless task,
And Love and Faith in vain an answer ask,
When thrilling nerves demand what good is wrought
Where torture clogs the very source of thought.

Lo! Mercy, ever broadening down the years,
Seeks but to count a lessening sum of tears.
The rack is gone; the torture-chamber lies
A sorry show for shuddering tourist eyes.
How useless pain both Church and State have learned
Since the last witch or patient martyr burned.
Yet still, forever, he who strove to gain

---

[15]The poem was read on 16 October 1896, at the commemoration of the fiftieth anniversary of the first public demonstration of surgical anæsthesia in the Massachusetts General Hospital, Boston.

By swift despatch a shorter lease for pain
Saw the grim theatre, and 'neath his knife
Felt the keen torture in the quivering life.
A word for him who, silent, grave, serene,
The thought-stirred actor on that tragic scene,
Recorded pity through the hand of skill,
Heard not a cry, but, ever conscious, still
In mercy merciless, swift, bold, intent,
Felt the slow moment that in torture went
While 'neath his touch, as none to-day has seen,
In anguish shook life's agonized machine.
The task is o'er; the precious blood is stayed;
But double price the hour of tension paid.
A pitying hand is on the sufferer's brow –
'Thank God, 'tis over!' Few who face me now
Recall this memory. Let the curtain fall;
Far gladder days shall know this storied hall!

Though Science, patient as the fruitful years,
Still taught our art to close some fount of tears,
Yet who that served this sacred home of pain
Could e'er have dreamed one scarce-imagined gain,
Or hoped a day would bring his feartful art
No need to steel the ever-kindly heart?

Auto-Facial-Construction
Mina Loy (1919)

The face is our most potent symbol of personality.

The adolescent has facial contours in harmony with the condition of his soul. Day by day the new interests and activities of modern life are prolonging the youth of our souls, and day by day we are becoming more aware of the necessity for our faces to express that youthfulness, for the sake of psychic logic. Different systems of beauty culture have compromised our inherent right not only to be ourselves but to look like ourselves by producing a facial contour in middle age which does duty as a 'well preserved appearance'. This preservation of partially distorted muscles is, at best, merely a pleasing parody of youth. That subtle element of the ludicrous inherent in facial transformation by time is the signpost of discouragement pointing along the path of the evolution of personality. For to what end is our experience of life if deprived of a fitting esthetic revelation in our faces? Once distorted muscle causes a fundamental disharmony in self-expression, for no matter how well gowned or groomed men or women may be, how exquisitely the complexion is cared for, or how beautiful the expression of the eyes, if the original form of the face (intrinsic symbol of personality) has been effaced in muscular transformation, they have lost the power to communicate their true personalities to others and all expression of sentiment is veiled in pathos. Years of specialized interest in physiognomy as an artist have brought me to an understanding of the human face which has made it possible for me to find the basic principle of facial integrity, its conservation, and, when necessary, its reconstruction.

I will instruct men or women who are intelligent and for the briefest period, patient, to become masters of their facial destiny. I understand the skull with its muscular sheath as a sphere whose superficies can be voluntarily energized. And the foundations of beauty as embedded in the three interconnected zones of energy encircling this sphere: the centers of control being at the base of the skull and the highest point of the cranium. Control, through the identity of your Conscious Will with these centers and zones, can be perfectly attained through my system, which does not include any form of cutaneous hygiene (the care of the skin being left to the skin specialists) except insofar as the stimulus to circulation it induces is of primary importance in the conservation of all the tissues. Through Auto-Facial-Construction the attachments of the muscles to the bones are revitalized, as also the gums, and the original facial contours are permanently preserved as a structure which can be relied upon without anxiety as to the ravages of time a structure which Complexion Culture enhances in beauty instead of attempting to disguise.

This means renascence for the society woman, the actor, the actress, the man of public career, for everybody who desires it. The initiation to this esoteric anatomical science is expensive, but economical in result; for it places at the disposal of individuals a permanent principle for the independent conservation of beauty to which, once it is mastered, they have constant and natural resource.

Healing
D. H. Lawrence (1932)

> I am not a mechanism, an assembly of various sections.
> And it is not because the mechanism is working wrongly, that I am ill.
> I am ill because of wounds to the soul, to the deep emotional self
> and the wounds to the soul take a long, long time, only time can help
> and patience, and a certain difficult repentance
> long, difficult repentance, realization of life's mistake, and the freeing oneself
> from the endless repetition of the mistake
> which mankind at large has chosen to sanctify.

Epidermal Macabre
Theodore Roethke (1941)

> Indelicate is he who loathes
> The aspect of his fleshy clothes, –
> The flying fabric stitched on bone,
> The vesture of the skeleton,
> The garment neither fur nor hair,
> The cloak of evil and despair,

The veil long violated by
Caresses of the hand and eye.
Yet such is my unseemliness:
I hate my epidermal dress,
The savage blood's obscenity,
The rags of my anatomy,
And willingly would I dispense
With false accoutrements of sense,
To sleep immodestly, a most
Incarnadine and carnal ghost.

Ode to the Liver
Pablo Neruda (1956)[16]

Modest,
organized
friend,
underground
worker,
let me give you
the wing of my song,
the thrust
of the air,
the soaring
of my ode:
it is born
of your invisible
machinery,
it flies
from your tireless
confined mill,
delicate
powerful
entrail,
ever alive and dark.

While
the heart resounds and attracts
the music of the mandolin,
there, inside,
you filter
and apportion,
you separate

---

[16]Trans. Oriana Josseau Kalant.

and divide,
you multiply
and lubricate,
you raise
and gather
the threads and the grams
of life, the final
distillate,
the intimate essences.

Submerged
viscous,
measurer
of the blood,
you live
full of hands
and full of eyes,
measuring and transferring
in your hidden
alchemical
chamber.
Yellow
is the matrix
of your red hydraulic flow,
diver
of the most perilous
depths of man,
there forever hidden,
everlasting,
in the factory,
noiseless.
And every feeling
or impulse
grew in your machinery,
received some drop
of your tireless
elaboration,
to love you added
fire or melancholy,
let one tiny cell
be in error
or one fiber be worn
in your labor
and the pilot flies into the wrong sky,
the tenor collapses in a wheeze,

the astronomer loses a planet.

Up above, how
the bewitching eyes of the rose
and the lips
of the matinal carnation
sparkle!
How the maiden
in the river laughs!
And down below,
the filter and the balance,
the delicate chemistry
of the liver,
the storehouse
of the subtle changes:
no one
sees or celebrates it,
but, when it ages
or its mortar wastes away,
the eyes of the rose are gone,
the teeth of the carnation wilted
and the maiden silent in the river.

Austere portion
or the whole
of myself,
grandfather
of the heart,
generator
of energy:
I sing to you
and I fear you
as though you were judge,
meter,
implacable indicator,
and if I can not
surrender myself in shackles to austerity,
if the surfeit of
delicacies,
or the hereditary wine of my country
dared
to disturb my health
or the equilibrium of my poetry,
from you,
dark monarch,

giver of syrups and of poisons,
regulator of salts,
from you I hope for justice:
I love life: Do not betray me! Work on!
Do not arrest my song.

Paralytic
Sylvia Plath (1963)

It happens. Will it go on? –
My mind a rock,
No fingers to grip, no tongue,
My god the iron lung[17]

That loves me, pumps
My two
Dust bags in and out,
Will not

Let me relapse
While the day outside glides by like ticker tape.
The night brings violets,
Tapestries of eyes,

Lights,
The soft anonymous
Talkers: 'You all right?'
The starched, inaccessible breast.

Dead egg, I lie
Whole
On a whole world I cannot touch,
At the white, tight

Drum of my sleeping couch
Photographs visit me –
My wife, dead and flat, in furs,
Mouth full of pearls,

Two girls
As flat as she, who whisper 'We're your daughters.'
The still waters
Wrap my lips,

Eyes, nose and ears,

---

[17]Iron lung: a negative pressure ventilator, used to enable a patient to breathe when the patient's muscle control is lost.

A clear
Cellophane I cannot crack.
On my bare back

I smile, a buddha, all
Wants, desire
Falling from me like rings
Hugging their lights.

The claw
Of the magnolia,
Drunk on its own scents,
Asks nothing of life

What the Heart is Like
Miroslav Holub (1963)[18]

Officially the heart
is oblong, muscular,
and filled with longing.

But anyone who has painted the heart knows
that it is also

spiked like a star
and sometimes bedraggled
like a stray dog at night
and sometimes powerful
like an archangel's drum.

And sometimes cube-shaped
like a draughtsman's dream
and sometimes gaily round
like a ball in a net.

And sometimes like a thin line
and sometimes like an explosion.

And in it is
only a river,
a weir
and at most one little fish
by no means golden.

More like a grey
jealous
loach.

---

[18]Trans. Ewald Osers.

It certainly isn't noticeable
at first sight.

Anyone who has painted the heart knows
that first he had to
discard his spectacles,
his mirror,
throw away his fine-point pencil
and carbon paper

and for a long while
walk
outside.

Brief Reflection on the Word Pain
Miroslav Holub (1971)[19]

Wittgenstein[20] says: the words 'it hurts' have replaced
        tears and cries of pain. The word 'Pain'
        does not describe the expression of pain but replaces it.
        Thus it creates a new behaviour pattern
        in the case of pain.

The word enters between us and the pain
        like a pretence of silence.
        It is a silencing. it is a needle
        unpicking the stitch
        between blood and clay.

The word is the first small step
        to freedom
        from oneself.

In case others
        are present.

Watchmaker God[21]
Robert Lowell (1973)

Say life is the one-way trip, the one-way flight,
say this without hysterical undertones –

---

[19]Trans. Ewald Osers.
[20]Ludwig Wittgenstein (1889–1951) was an Austrian-British philosopher of logic, mathematics, mind and language.
[21]The 'watchmaker god' theory is a belief in the intelligent design of the universe, supported by Creationists. Darwinian evolution offers a counterargument.

then you could say you stood in the cold light of science,
seeing as you are seen, espoused to fact.
Strange, life is both the fire and fuel; and we,
the animals and objects, must be here
without striking a spark of evidence
that anything that ever stopped living
ever falls back to living when life stops.
There's a pale romance to the watchmaker God
of Descartes[22] and Paley[23]; He drafted and installed
us in the Apparatus. He loved to tinker;
but having perfected what He had to do,
stood shrouded in his loneliness.

In the Waiting Room
Elizabeth Bishop (1976)

In Worcester, Massachusetts,
I went with Aunt Consuelo
to keep her dentist's appointment
and sat and waited for her
in the dentist's waiting room.
It was winter. It got dark
early. The waiting room
was full of grown-up people,
arctics and overcoats,
lamps and magazines.
My aunt was inside
what seemed like a long time
and while I waited I read
the *National Geographic*
(I could read) and carefully
studied the photographs:
the inside of a volcano,
black, and full of ashes;
then it was spilling over
in rivulets of fire.
Osa and Martin Johnson
dressed in riding breeches,
laced boots, and pith helmets.

---

[22]Réne Descartes (1596–1650) was an influential French philosopher and mathematician, who viewed the cosmos as a great timepiece, wound by the great watchmaker God.
[23]William Paley (1743–1805) was an English clergyman, philosopher and utilitarian, who used the 'watchmaker god' analogy to argue for the existence of God in his work *Natural Theology or Evidences of the Existence and Attributes of the Deity*.

A dead man slung on a pole
– 'Long Pig', the caption said.
Babies with pointed heads
wound round and round with string;
black, naked women with necks
wound round and round with wire
like the necks of light bulbs.
Their breasts were horrifying.
I read it right straight through.
I was too shy to stop.
And then I looked at the cover:
the yellow margins, the date.
Suddenly, from inside,
came an *oh!* of pain
– Aunt Consuelo's voice –
not very loud or long.
I wasn't at all surprised;
even then I knew she was
a foolish, timid woman.
I might have been embarrassed,
but wasn't. What took me
completely by surprise
was that it was *me:*
my voice, in my mouth.
Without thinking at all
I was my foolish aunt,
I – we – were falling, falling,
our eyes glued to the cover
of the *National Geographic,*
February, 1918.

I said to myself: three days
and you'll be seven years old.
I was saying it to stop
the sensation of falling off
the round, turning world,
into cold, blue-black space.
But I felt: you are an *I,*
you are an *Elizabeth,*
you are one of *them.*
Why should you be one, too?
I scarcely dared to look
to see what it was I was.
I gave a sidelong glance
– I couldn't look any higher –

at shadowy gray knees,
trousers and skirts and boots
and different pairs of hands
lying under the lamps.
I knew that nothing stranger
had ever happened, that nothing
stranger could ever happen.

Why should I be my aunt,
or me, or anyone?
What similarities –
boots, hands, the family voice
I felt in my throat, or even
the *National Geographic*
and those awful hanging breasts –
held us all together
or made us all just one?
How – I didn't know any
word for it – how 'unlikely' …
How had I come to be here,
like them, and overhear
a cry of pain that could have
got loud and worse but hadn't?

The waiting room was bright
and too hot. It was sliding
beneath a big black wave,
another, and another.

Then I was back in it.
The War was on. Outside,
in Worcester, Massachusetts,
were night and slush and cold,
and it was still the fifth
of February, 1918.

Circulation
Raymond Carver (1986)

By the time I came around to feeling pain
and woke up, moonlight
flooded the room. My arm lay paralyzed,
propped up like an old anchor under
your back. You were in a dream,
you said later, where you'd arrived
early for the dance. But after

a moment's anxiety you were okay
because it was really a sidewalk
sale, and the shoes you were wearing,
or not wearing, were fine for that.

*

'Help me,' I said. And tried to hoist
my arm. But it just lay there, aching,
unable to rise on its own. Even after
you said, 'What is it? What's wrong?'
it stayed put – deaf, unmoved
by any expression of fear or amazement.
We shouted at it, and grew afraid
when it didn't answer. 'It's gone to sleep,'
I said, and hearing those words
knew how absurd this was. But
I couldn't laugh. Somehow,
between the two of us, we managed
to raise it. *This can't be my arm*
is what I kept thinking as
we thumped it, squeezed it, and
prodded it back to life. Shook it
until that stinging went away.

We said a few words to each other.
I don't remember what. Whatever
reassuring things people
who love each other say to each other
given the hour and such odd
circumstance. I do remember
you remarked how it was light
enough in the room that you could see
circles under my eyes.
You said I needed more regular sleep,
and I agreed. Each of us went
to the bathroom, and climbed back into bed
on our respective sides.
Pulled the covers up. 'Good night,'
you said, for the second time that night.
And fell asleep. Maybe
into that same dream, or else another.

*

I lay until daybreak, holding
both arms fast across my chest.
Working my fingers now and then.

While my thoughts kept circling
around and around, but always going back
where they'd started from.
That one inescapable fact: even while
we undertake this trip,
there's another, far more bizarre,
we still have to make.

The Anatomy of the Hand
Ronald Wallace (1987)

Consider, she says, all the things
you could not do without hands.
And while she's appraising
the buttons and stays,
the feeding and hygiene,
the doorknobs and levers and drawers,
I'm watching handfuls of words fall away
into the lackluster cadaver bin
with all the amputated phrases:
grasp, snatch, hold, caress, and fondle,
touch, finger, fist, punch, and feel,
squeeze, clutch, grip, slap, and tickle,
heaped up with the glad hands,
the high hands, the upper hands,
the in hands, and out of hands,
even hands, under hands...

Meanwhile, the hands,
stiff on their meaty limbs,
yellow and waxen,
the skinned tendons splayed back
to display the conjunction
of nerve end and jointure,
tensor and flexor,
phalange and digit,
the synovial sheaths,
the cutaneous circulation,
the horned fingernails
ordinary as corn,
the crabbed fingers bending
to fend off or fondle,
reaching up from their silvery tray,
say nothing.

She's talking with her hands,
she who would be
the perpetual wallflower –
studious, friendless, lost
in her glasses and splotchy complexion,
her mumble and stringy hair,
her pimples and shapeless frame –
while her hands,
delicate in their precision,
flash in the air, flutter and rush,
bloom and maneuver and swim through
the endless movements
of navicular, lunate, triangular, and pisiform,
her carpal diagrams and charts.

I imagine late hours at the anatomy lab,
alone with the hands
reaching up toward her, cradled
as if she were reading what's left
of their palms, or casually doing
their nails, or just holding on,
her own hands glistening with
acetic acid or sweat
to loosen the movement,
the last one asked to dance,
gently stroking the hands,
attentive to every nerve end and fiber,
every involuntary signal and twitch,
the hands, reaching, stretching,
the hands in her lap turning, dancing,
the hands saying nothing
in a language all their own.

The Woman Who Could Not Live With Her Faulty Heart
Margaret Atwood (1987)

I do not mean the symbol
of love, a candy shape
to decorate cakes with,
the heart that is supposed
to belong or break;

I mean this lump of muscle
that contracts like a flayed biceps,
purple-blue, with its skin of suet,

its skin of gristle, this isolate,
this caved hermit, unshelled
turtle, this one lungful of blood,
no happy plateful.

All hearts float in their own
deep oceans of no light,
wetblack and glimmering,
their four mouths gulping like fish.
Hearts are said to pound:
this is to be expected, the heart's
regular struggle against being drowned.

But most hearts say, I want, I want,
I want, I want. My heart
is more duplicitous,
though no twin as I once thought.
It says, I want, I don't want, I
want, and then a pause.
It forces me to listen,

and at night it is the infra-red
third eye that remains open
while the other two are sleeping
but refuses to say what it has seen.

It is a constant pestering
in my ears, a caught moth, limping drum,
a child's fist beating
itself against the bedsprings:
I want, I don't want.
How can one live with such a heart?

Long ago I gave up singing
to it, it will never be satisfied or lulled.
One night I will say to it:
Heart, be still,
and it will.

A Story about the Body
Robert Haas (1989)

The young composer, working that summer at an artist's colony, had watched her
for a week. She was Japanese, a painter, almost sixty, and he thought he was in
love with her. He loved her work, and her work was like the way she moved her
body, used her hands, looked at him directly when she made amused or considered
answers to his questions. One night, walking back from a concert, they came to her

door and she turned to him and said, 'I think you would like to have me. I would like that too, but I must tell you I have had a double mastectomy,' and when he didn't understand, 'I've lost both my breasts.' The radiance that he had carried around in his belly and chest cavity – like music – withered very quickly, and he made himself look at her when he said, 'I'm sorry. I don't think I could.' He walked back to his own cabin through the pines, and in the morning he found a small blue bowl on the porch outside his door. It looked to be full of rose petals, but he found when he picked it up that the rose petals were on top; the rest of the bowl – she must have swept them from the corners of her studio – was full of dead bees.

Frankenstein's Monster
Marvin Bell (1990)

'BIGGER THAN LIFE'

Bigger than the best, but not the best,
who can take history by the throat
and squeeze the steam from the new bread,
turn glass to sand, and grind the gears
of planets to oil and oil to water,
until the earth is rid of that Creator
who dared to make a thing without a soul.

I walked because of Science and a scientist.
I stood because he had it in his thought
that life should come from what is dead,
should turn time back and dry your tears.
I, who was made from brick and mortar,
meant to be inferior, was greater.
Given the parts, I assumed the role.

I am the dark body that cannot rest
free from an hysterical note,
made as I was to symbolize your dread.
Through the magnifying lens of fear
you watch me in your son and by your daughter.
While you disperse in every dark theatre
in streams of light, inside you I am whole.

Carnal Knowledge
Dannie Abse (1990)

1.
You, student, whistling those elusive bits
of Schubert when phut, phut, phut, throbbed the sky
of London. Listen: the servo-engine cut
and the silence was not the desired silence

between the two movements of music. Then
Finale, the Aldwych echo of crunch
and the urgent ambulances loaded
with the fresh dead. You, young, whistled again,
entered King's, climbed the stone-murky steps
to the high and brilliant Dissecting Room
where nameless others, naked on the slabs,
reclined in disgraceful silences – twenty
amazing sculptures waiting to be vandalised.

2.
You, corpse, I pried into your bloodless meat
without the morbid curiosity of Vesalius,[24]
did not care that the great Galen[25] was wrong,
Avicenna[26] mistaken, that they had described
the approximate structure of pigs and monkeys
rather than the human body. With scalpel
I dug deep into your stale formaldehyde
unaware of Pope Boniface's decree
but, as instructed, violated you –
the reek of you in my eyes, my nostrils,
clothes, in the kisses of my girlfriends.
You, anonymous. Who were you, mister?
Your thin mouth could not reply, 'Absent, sir,'
or utter with inquisitionary rage.
Your neck exposed, muscles, nerves, vessels,
a mere coloured plate in some anatomy book;
your right hand, too, dissected, never belonged
it seemed to someone once shockingly alive,
never held surely, another hand in greeting
or tenderness, never clenched a fist in anger,
never took up a pen to sign an authentic name.
You, dead man, Thing, each day, each week,
each month, you slowly decreasing Thing
visibly losing Divine proportions,
you residue, mere trunk of a man's body,
you, X, legless, armless, headless Thing
that I dissected so casually.
Then went downstairs to drink wartime coffee.

---

[24]Andreas Vesalius (1514–64) was an anatomist, physician and author of one of the most influential books on human anatomy, *De humani corporis fabrica (On the Fabric of the Human Body)*.
[25]Galen of Pergamon (129–c.216 AD) was the most renowned Greek physician, surgeon and philosopher of antiquity.
[26]Avicenna, Latinate form of Ibn-Sīnā (c.980–1037) was a Perisan philosopher of the Islamic Golden Age, often described as the father of early modern medicine.

3.
When the hospital priest, Father Jerome,
remarked, 'The Devil made the lower parts
of a man's body, God the upper,'
I said, 'Father, it's the other way round.'
So, the Anatomy Course over, Jerome,
thanatologist,[27] did not invite me
to the Special Service for the Twenty Dead,
did not say to me, 'Come for the relatives' sake.'
(Surprise, surprise, that they had relatives
those lifeless-size, innominate creatures.)

Other students accepted, joined in the fake chanting,
organ solemnity, cobwebbed theatre.
And that's all it would have been,
a ceremony propitious and routine,
an obligation forgotten soon enough
had not the strict priest with premeditated rage
called out the Register of the Twenty Dead –
each non-cephalic carcass gloatingly identified
with a local habitation and a name
till one by one, made culpable, the students cried.

4.
I did not learn the name of my intimate,
the twentieth sculpture, the one next to the door.
No matter. Now all these years later
I know those twenty sculptures were but one,
the same one duplicated. You.
I hear not Father Jerome but St Jerome cry,
'No, John will be John, Mary will be Mary,'
as if the dead would have ears to hear
the Register on Judgement Day.
Look, on gravestones many names.
There should be one only. Yours.
No, not even one since you have no name.
In the newspapers' memorial columns
many names. A joke.
On the canvases of masterpieces
the same figure always in disguise. Yours.
Even in the portraits of the old anchorite
fingering a dry skull you are half concealed
lest onlookers should turn away blinded.
In certain music, too, with its sound of loss,

---

[27]Thanatology is the biological, forensic, and cultural study of death.

in that Schubert Quintet, for instance,
you are there in the Adagio,
playing the third cello that cannot be heard.
You are there and there and there, nameless,
and here I am older by far and nearer,
perplexed, trying to recall what you looked like
before I dissected your face – you, threat,
molesting presence, and I in a white coat
your enemy, in a purple one, your nuncio,
writing this while a winter twig, not you,
scrapes, scrapes the windowpane.
Soon I shall climb the stairs. Gratefully,
I shall wind up the usual clock at bedtime
(the steam vanishing from the bathroom mirror)
with my hand, my living hand.

Anatomy Lesson
Peter Porter (1992)

So long since passing through the epidermis
We may forget the outer casements of
This curious pale: we are in an echo-theatre
Where the central dynamo continues purring
In inviolate light. Here are the power points,
Their names and functions, the famished trades
Which must prevail. So much has been revealed
And yet we cannot sight the seed of terror
Planted here. Watered in dreams, it grows
To harvest size in pure hallucination
And hangs another world behind the eyes.
Then the great factory reappears – a wreck
With ribs deep in sand, a woman's body
Booby-trapped, pleasure gardens fringed
By poisoned plants. The words in latin on
The labels are disguises for our ignorance,
The hired cassettes purr culture-speak – 'just one
Consequence of an evolutionary leg-up',
'Without this fear we never would have
Outsoared the plants and animals' ... they send us
To the distant tower where words are made,
Where data are transformed by tribal wish.
Destroy this living library, it won't
Be Alexandria burning to the water,
Merely a setback to an integer.
Finally the knowledge is absorbed
In all description and all mystery,

The code of copulation and amplexus.[28]
We close the body up and move to more
Conjectural cavities: we seek at last
The nervous gardens and the plains of Hell,
The parenthetic walls of Paradise.

Artificial Blood
Matthew Sweeney (1992)

As the artificial blood that saved him
was Japanese, he went to live in Japan.
And of course he found the raw fish
the best for his patched-up heart.
The doctors were reassuring too,
even if they spoke a stretched English
and couldn't laugh. He kept in touch
with his golfer son – golf was played
throughout Japan; perhaps one day
his son would visit with sake ...
Some nights he'd walk to a noodle bar
and point, then eat. He'd hurry
past the geisha parlours, and maybe
he'd stop at a phone, then stay outside
till he was too tired to remember
those walks on the Malvern Hills
he'd taken too seldom. Too long ago
when his son was little, his wife alive,
before his heart operation,
before the white, thin artificial blood
entered his body and led him to Japan.

Unsystematic Anatomy (after Rabelais)
Ian Bamforth (1996)

The vault of his cranium was an ordinary day shouting from the door
and his forehead was a drawer of objections
and his pineal was a big bellows
and his irises were Geminids[29] on a bush evening
and his eardrums were tight skeins of geese
And the auricle of his ear a leaf stroked by Kafka in 1910

---

[28]Amplexus refers to the mating position of frogs and toads, in which the male clasps the female around her back.
[29]Geminids: a form of meteor shower.

and his uvula was Benny Lynch's[30] punchbag
and his saliva was a come-on
and his tongue was the negotiation of sweat-bath rituals.
His gullet was snake's knowledge
and his thyroid was the shield over Patroclus[31]
and his recurrent laryngeal nerve was a prize-winning dissection
and his trachea was a ladder to the gods.
His spinal cord was all the news in sixty seconds.
His diaphragm was a bivouac on Cul Mor[32]
and his lungs were the creature from the lagoon
and his liver was sitting all alone
and his gallbladder was the prodigal returning
and his mesentery was enough said about Boolahoola
and his spleen was the history of Belgium
and his stomach was pots and pans
and his small intestine the scarf that strangled Isadora Duncan.[33]
His vena cava was the Third Man[34]
and his mitral valve was a fond attachment
and his aorta was the Twenty-Third Psalm sung in the Hebrides
and his heart was an artichoke.
His kidneys were Pliny[35] on recycling
and his ureters were double bungee jumpers reclining
and his bladder was a seat at the Citz[36] watching the Chalk Circle[37]
and his spermatic cords were a strung violin
and his penis was done on a dare.
His hips were titanium-vanadium, where the angel touched,
and his perineum was a canvas big top
and his pelvis was Lear's fool
and his femurs were a dream of being next in command
and his calves were pay first, touch later
and one foot was a Lisbon lion
and the other took a while.
His memory was laminar germ theory
and his commonsense was seasick in the heart of Europe
and his imagination was an open cast

---

[30]Benny Lynch (1913–46) was a Scottish professional flyweight boxer.
[31]Patroclus, in Homer's *Iliad*, was comrade in arms to Achilles.
[32]Cùl Mòr is a twin summited mountain and high point in Inverpolly, Scotland.
[33]Isadora Duncan (1877–1927) was an American dancer, who died in an automobile accident in Nice, France, when her silk scarf became entangled in the car's wheels and axle, breaking her neck.
[34]*The Third Man* (1949) is a classic of British film noir.
[35]Pliny (23–79 AD) was a Roman author, naturalist, philosopher and army commander.
[36]The Citz (1969–2003), shortened form of The Glasgow Citizens Theatre Company.
[37]The German playwright Bertolt Brecht reworked Li Qianfu's verse play and crime drama *Circle of Chalk* or *The Chalk Circle* (Yuan dynasty, 1259–1368), into *The Caucasian Chalk Circle* (1944).

and his thoughts were English composition and rhetoric
and his conscience was a lease on a bird cage in the Walled City
and his appetite was Boswell's inkhorn
and his hope was one for the road
and his undertakings were Daedalus and Icarus in the maze
and his will was the Cape of Good Hope
and his desire was the wounds of possibility
and his judgement was Solomon's treatises on deep tongues
and his compassion was undergrowth
and his discretion was beached, between herring and seaweed
and his reason sat down to turn itself in

in the gap between the boyhood burning of his ears
and finally arriving as himself.

What the Body Told
Rafael Campo (1996)

Not long ago, I studied medicine.
It was terrible, what the body told.
I'd look inside another person's mouth,
And see the desolation of the world.
I'd see his genitals and think of sin.

Because my body speaks the stranger's language,
I've never understood those nods and stares.
My parents held me in their arms, and still
I think I've disappointed them; they care
And stare, they nod, they make their pilgrimage

To somewhere distant in my heart, they cry.
I look inside their other-person's mouths
And see the wet interior of souls.
It's warm and red in there – like love, with teeth.
I've studied medicine until I cried

All night. Through certain books, a truth unfolds.
Anatomy and physiology,
The tiny sensing organs of the tongue –
Each nameless cell contributing its needs.
It was fabulous, what the body told.

Heart
David Scott (1998)

I thought of other significant hearts:
Christ's, which in the Greek

would throw itself out;
Shelley's saved from fire and water
brought back to Bournemouth.
Now this child's. The doctor's hand
went far either side of it.
The pink tubes of the stethoscope
divined an unfamiliar sluicing.
Something in nature was too tight.
Something in Greek had gone wrong,
and although it made the old phrases
new – 'take heart', 'with all my heart'
for three days we put them aside
until the valve, tough as tripe, came tight.

Calcium
Deryn Rees-Jones (1998)

Because I love the very bones of you,
and you are somehow rooted in my bone,
I'll tell you of the seven years

by which the skeleton renews itself,
so that we have the chance to be
a person, now and then, who's

something other than ourselves;
and how the body, if deficient,
will bleed the calcium it needs –

for heart, for liver, spleen –
from bone, which incidentally,
I might add, is not the thorough

structure that you might
suppose, but living tissue which
the doctors say a woman of my age

should nurture mindfully with fruit,
weightbearing exercise, and supplements
to halt the dangers of a fracture when I'm old;

and because I love you I will also tell
how stripped of skin the papery bone
is worthy of inscription, could hold

a detailed record of a navy or a store of grain,
and how, if it's preserved
according to the pharaohs,

wrapped in bandages of coca leaf, tobacco,
it will survive long after all our books,
and even words are weightless;

and perhaps because the heaviness of your head,
the way I love the slow, sweet sense of you,
the easiness by which you're stilled,

how the fleshy structures that your skeleton,
your skull maintain, are easily interrogated,
it reminds me how our hands,

clasped for a moment, now, amount
to everything I have; how even your smile
as it breaks me up, has the quality of ice,

the long lines of loneliness
like a lifetime ploughed across a palm,
the permanence of snow.

Small Intestine
Brian McCabe (1999)

I don't know much about my duodenum:
only that it is part of my small intestine
between my stomach and my jejunum,
and that its name means the intestine
of twelve fingers' length – twelve, not ten,
as if the duodenum is unwilling
to be gauged by human hands.

All I know of my jejunum is that
it is part of my small intestine
between my duodenum and my ileum
and that its name means empty –
from the belief that it is empty after death.
I would like to think that my jejunum
will not disgrace itself
and after death will maintain
an emptiness worthy of its name.

On the subject of my ileum I know
next to nothing, but that it is
the part of my small intestine
between my jejunum and my caecum
and that insects have one too.
Tunnel from jejunum to caecum,

bridge between insect and man.
If only every part of me
showed such versatility.

My caecum, as you may have guessed,
is something of a mystery to me:
all I know is that this poor, blind pouch
marks the start of my large intestine
and is, strictly speaking,
outwith the scope of this poem.

Small intestine with your four strange gods
duodenum, jejunum, ileum, caecum.

Forgive me.

Donor
Brian McCabe (1999)

I signed a form giving my consent.
So technically I am the donor.

The papers have had a field day.
The Sun called me Son of Frankenstein.
The Independent freaked me out in another way
with its 'haunting ethical questions.'

The question that haunted me
was this: if I survive – who will I be?
I have, and I'm still who I am, but
it's as if a stranger has become me.

Sometimes when I touch myself
I want to tell him I'm sorry.
When he goes to the bathroom
I want to look the other way.

I tell myself: the donor
was the brain-dead head
whose body I have inherited.
Maybe one day we'll be intimate.

Something his wife said scared me.
She said: 'In you, my John lives on.'
We smiled for the cameras
both afraid of rejection.

My lawyers have advised me
that she does have a case.

Twin Found in Man's Chest
Jo Shapcott (2002)

It is birth: at the first breath how curiously
the tissues of the lungs flower
with the sudden inrush of blood.

A paragraph marked AP (Moscow)
tells of a mid-life driver from Baku:
probing beneath his ribs they found
'A thick-walled, many-chambered cyst
lodged in a lobe of the left lung.'

Inside it, packed as neat as a baby bee,
was the embryo of that man's unborn twin.
Imagine the first drama in the womb:
one clump of bioplasts edging towards brother,

opening jaw-buds (fratricide? speech?
reflex?), snuffing the little fish
right down – his cell-mate, just like that –
inside his lung. I'm drawn
to cross examine Mr. Kilner Jar –

hey Tutankhamun, what (I ask)
goes coiling through your ventricles
to nest inside the cleanness of your cortex.

Post-Mortem
Michael Symmons Roberts (2002)

This is my body, me on the slab,
lying in the sun which burns
as if to melt the etched frost
from the man-tall windows.

In this swelter, how can flies
resist the game, the deep red
sweetmeats in the cavern of me,
vascular stamens of a Venus trap?

My three skin-petals gape,
one from each shoulder to waist,
and one up from my chest,
which covers nose and mouth.

She wears a mask too,
a plastic face-shield, gloves,
blue shiny gown; armour of life
against the seeds of where I've been.

She feels ice-spores of marble
in my pulse-less arms.
She pictures, on my tight shut eyes,
the exile's distant glaze.

She heaves huge jars down from a shelf,
unscrews one, lifts my gut coil
from its marinade of formalin,
gently shakes the drips onto the floor.

She weighs it on a grocer's scales
and slips it into me. It's cold,
but her assistant settles it
and stitches it in place.

Liver, stomach, lungs, each cradled,
slid and sewn; painstaking work.
They lift my sawn ribs like a lid,
plant the heart, and close its cage.

They take out the wood brick
that propped my shoulder-blades
and arched me open. I sink onto
the metal slab as though I'm sighing.

My viscera complete, they fold in
all three petals, seal with thread
the Y-shaped wound.
I am all of a piece, but lifeless.

My skin sticks to the stainless steel.
They hose me down, under and over,
yanking me up with a leg or an arm
to drench me, peel me from the slab.

Water gutters over earth-brown tiles
and chokes into a central drain.
She scissors free my mouth and eyes
from stitched serenity.

She kisses – passionless –
my paper lips
and waits for my first gasp,
then gestures to a mustard-coloured door:

'It has been longer than you think',
she says, *'In the next room you will find*
some simple clothes and food. You will
be hungry. Leave us now.'

The Straight and Narrow
Simon Armitage (2002)

When the tall and bearded careers advisor
set up his stall and his slide-projector

something clicked. There on the silver screen,
like a photograph of the human soul,

the X-ray plate of the ten-year-old girl
who swallowed a toy. Shadows and shapes,

mercury-tinted lungs and a tin-foil heart,
alloy organs and tubes, but bottom left,

the caught-on-camera lightning strike
of the metal car: like a neon bone,

some classic roadster with an open top
and a man at the wheel in goggles and cap,

motoring on through deep, internal dark.
The clouds opened up; we were leaving the past,

drawn by a star that had risen inside us,
some as astronauts and some as taxi-drivers.

De Humani Corporis Fabrica[38]
John Burnside (2005)

I know the names of almost
nothing

                not the bone
between my elbow and my wrist
that sometimes aches
from breaking

                years ago

                        and not
the plumb line
from the pelvis
to the knee

less ache than hum
                        where
in my nineteenth year
a blade slit through nerves

---

[38]Andreas Vesalius's *On the Fabric of the Human Body* (1543) is a canonical text of human anatomy.

and nicked a vein

leaving the walls intact
                          the valves
still working
so the blood kept flooding out
till Eleanor
              a nurse on evening shift

opened the wound
and made me whole again.

I have no words
for chambers in the heart
the smaller bones
                    the seat of gravity

or else I know the names
but not the function:
ganglia
        the mental foramen
the hypothalamus
                  the duodenum.

Once
      in our old school library
                                I took
a book down from the shelf
and opened it to stripped flesh
                                and the cords
of muscle
          ribbed and charred
like something barbecued

the colours wrong
                  the single eye exposed:
a window into primal emptiness.

I sat for hours
                amazed
                        and horrified
as if I had been asked to paraphrase
this body with the body I possessed:
hydraulics for a soul
                      cheese-wire for nerves
a ruff of butcher's meat
                          in place of thought.

I've read how Michelangelo would buy

a stolen corpse
            to study
                    in the dark
the movement of a joint
                    or how a face
articulates the workings of the heart

how Stubbs[39] would peel
the cold hide from a horse
and peer into the dark machinery
of savage grace

but I have never learned
                        nor wished to learn
how bodies work
                other than when they move
and breathe
            corporis fabrica

is less to me than how a shudder starts
and runs along the arm
                    towards the wings
that flex and curl
between the shoulder blades

– so I will lie beside you here
                        unnamed
until my hands recover from your skin

a history of tides
                a flock of birds
the love that answers love
                    when bodies meet

and map themselves anew
                    cell after cell
touch after glancing touch
                    the living flesh

revealing and erasing what it knows
on secret charts
            of watermark
                    and vellum.

---

[39]George Stubbs (1724–1806) was an English painter, best known for his paintings of horses.

Dissections
C. K. Williams (2006)

Not only have the skin and flesh and parts of the skeleton
of one of the anatomical effigies in the *Musée de l'Homme*[40]
been excised, stripped away, so that you don't just look at,
but through the thing – pink lungs, red kidneys and heart,
tangles of yellowish nerves he seems snarled in, like a net;

not only are his eyes without eyelids, and so shallowly
embedded beneath the blade of the brow, that they seem,
with no shadow to modulate them, flung open in pain or fear;
and not only is his gaze so frenziedly focused that he seems to be
receiving everything, even our regard scraping across him as *blare*;

not only that, but when I looked more closely, I saw he was *real*,
that he'd been constructed, reconstructed, on an actual skeleton:
the nerves and organs were wire and plaster, but the armature,
the staring skull, the spine and ribs, were varnished, oxidizing bone;
someone was there, his personhood discernible, a self, a soul.

I felt embarrassed, as though I'd intruded on someone's loneliness,
or grief, and then, I don't know why, it came to me to pray,
though I don't pray, I've unlearned how, to whom, or what,
what fiction, what illusion, or, it wouldn't matter, what true thing,
as mostly I've forgotten how to weep ... Only mostly, though,

sometimes I can sense the tears in there, and sometimes, yes,
they come, though rarely for a reason I'd have thought –
a cello's voice will catch in mine, a swerve in a poem, and once,
a death, someone I hardly knew, but I found myself sobbing, sobbing,
for everyone I had known who'd died, and some who almost had.

In the next display hall, evolution: half, the quarter creatures,
Australopithecus, Pithecanthropus, Cro-Magnon,[41]
sidle diffidently along their rocky winding path towards us.
Flint and fire, science and song, and all of it coming to this,
this unhealable self in myself who knows what I should know.

Anusol®[42]
Alan Buckley (2009)

Although she dropped by without warning, conversation
was easy, until she came back from the bathroom. I felt

---

[40]Museum of Anthropology, Paris, France.
[41]These are extinct genera of hominids.
[42]Anusol is a brand of medications used to treat hemorrhoids (piles).

the air heavier, thickened with embarrassment. Later,

I saw the tube where I'd left it, perched on the edge
of the tub: that blunt, un-English name, the manufacturer –
Canadian – unaware of our sensitivities. Please understand:

we are born uncomfortable. We must apologise for these
bodies that block up our narrow streets, that brush
and bump in Underground trains. We have smoked them

brown as kippers, stuffed them with pig fat until they drip,
soaked them in cheap gin; and yet they persist, refuse
to go away. We wish they would show some decency

and do what they do behind closed doors. We want
to be left on our own, with only our monkey-house minds
for company, the chatter and scream of our thoughts.

Supra-Ventricular Tachycardia[43]
Jean Sprackland (2013)

Shocking to learn the heart's element is not love
but electricity. It's bathed in signals.
the wet circuits spark, the armature vibrates.

A beautiful piece of wiring the syncytium[44]:
all the cells of the heart connected by bridges,
and the electric shiver sprinting across.

But my excitable cells don't wait for the messenger.
They jump at rumour and guesswork. So the trip
and thud, the voltage spike –

and all I can do is stop and wait
and listen to the fibrillation,
my own system arcing and shorting.

This heart is what I carry. It's what carries me.
This twitching fist of gristle, this hurt machine,
this rigged ship in a bottle.

---

[43]Supra-ventricular tachycardia refers to abnormal electrical activity of the heart, which presents as a rapid heart rhythm.
[44]Syncytium cells are interconnected and synchronized electrically in an action potential, as seen in heart muscle cells and other smooth muscle cells.

Écorché[45]
Andy Brown (2014)

> *Plaster cast crucifixion of the body of James Legg,*
> *Chelsea pensioner, hanged for murder, 1801,*
> *by Thomas Banks, Royal Academy.*

They made me to settle an artists' debate –
my seventy-three-year-old body deposed
from the hangman's gibbet and nailed to a cross
to put the Academics' minds at rest:

the sculptor Banks, the painters Cosway, West.[46]
Gentlemen! Let me help you put it straight:
most paintings of the Crucifixion mask
gross inaccuracies ... *physically*, of course.

Captain William Lamb was my undoing;
Lamb who wouldn't meet me in a duel;
Lamb, that 'tyrannical tempered man'
who shunned my guns. I shot *him* in the chest.

I confess: I was melancholy. I was dejected.
I woke like a person surprised from sleep
when matron arrived with my tincture.
The surgeon Joseph Carpue[47] cut *me* down

to put the artists' theory to the test.
He took my body from the hanging place,
then winched me up until my muscles slumped
into the proper pose of crucifixion.

There I hung until my carcass cooled
and when I'd cooled, he flayed me so that Banks
could make his cast. (West said he'd never *seen*
the human hand till then.) And here I hang, still,

in the exact way of our Saviour – this mock
James Legg – survivor of the noose, the knife,
the cross – where curious Anatomy meets Art,
where Religion meets Justice, and firm proof.

---

[45]*Écorché*: a flayed figure, which shows the muscles of the body with the skin and fat removed.
[46]Thomas Joseph Banks (1735–1805) was an important British sculptor. Richard Cosway RA (1742–1821) was a leading English portrait painter of the Regency era, noted for his miniatures. Benjamin West (1738–1820) was an Anglo-American painter and second president of the Royal Academy in London.
[47]Joseph Constantine Carpue (1764–1846) was an English surgeon known for performing the first rhinoplastic (nasal) surgery in England, as well as for his pioneering medical experiments with electricity.

MEDICAL WRITING:

Characteristics of Men, Manners, Opinions, Times
Anthony Ashley Cooper, 3rd Earl of Shaftesbury (1711)

There are certain humours in mankind, which of necessity must have vent. The human mind and body are both of them naturally subject to commotions: and as there are strange ferments in the blood, which in many bodies occasion an extraordinary discharge; so in reason too, there are heterogeneous particles which must be thrown off by fermentation. Should physicians endeavour absolutely to allay those ferments of the body, and strike in the Humours which discover themselves in such eruptions, they might, instead of making a cure, bid fair perhaps to raise a plague, and turn a spring-ague or an autumn-surfeit into an epidemical malignant fever. They are certainly as ill physicians in the body-politick, who would needs be tampering with these mental eruptions; and under the specious pretence of healing this itch of superstition, and saving souls from the contagion of enthusiasm, should set all nature in an uproar, and turn a few innocent carbuncles into an inflammation and mortal gangrene.

An Enquiry Concerning Human Understanding
David Hume (1748; 1777 ed.)

It may be said, that we are every moment conscious of internal power; while we feel, that, by the simple command of our will, we can move the organs of our body, or direct the faculties of our mind. An act of volition produces motion in our limbs, or raises a new idea in our imagination. This influence of the will we know by consciousness. Hence we acquire the idea of power or energy; and are certain, that we ourselves and all other intelligent beings are possessed of power. This idea, then, is an idea of reflection, since it arises from reflecting on the operations of our own mind, and on the command which is exercised by will, both over the organs of the body and faculties of the soul.

We shall proceed to examine this pretension; and first with regard to the influence of volition over the organs of the body. This influence, we may observe, is a fact, which, like all other natural events, can be known only by experience, and can never be foreseen from any apparent energy or power in the cause, which connects it with the effect, and renders the one an infallible consequence of the other. The motion of our body follows upon the command of our will. Of this we are every moment conscious. But the means, by which this is effected; the energy, by which the will performs so extraordinary an operation; of this we are so far from being immediately conscious, that it must for ever escape our most diligent enquiry.

For *first*; is there any principle in all nature more mysterious than the union of soul with body; by which a supposed spiritual substance acquires such an influence over a material one, that the most refined thought is able to actuate the grossest matter? Were we empowered, by a secret wish, to remove mountains, or control the planets in their orbit; this extensive authority would not be more extraordinary, nor more beyond our comprehension. But if by consciousness we perceived any power or energy in the will, we must know this power; we must know its connexion with the effect; we must know the secret union of soul and body, and the nature of both these substances; by which the one is able to operate, in so many instances, upon the other.

Secondly, we are not able to move all the organs of the body with a like authority; though we cannot assign any reason besides experience, for so remarkable a difference between one and the other. Why has the will an influence over the tongue and fingers, not over the heart or liver? This question would never embarrass us, were we conscious of a power in the former case, not in the latter. We should then perceive, independent of experience, why the authority of will over the organs of the body is circumscribed within such particular limits. Being in that case fully acquainted with the power or force, by which it operates, we should also know why its influence reaches precisely to such boundaries, and no farther.

A man, suddenly struck with a palsy in the leg or arm, or who had newly lost those members, frequently endeavours, at first, to move them, and employ them in their usual offices. Here he is as much conscious of power to command such limbs, as a man in perfect health is conscious of power to actuate any member which remains in its natural state and condition. But consciousness never deceives. Consequently, neither in the one case nor in the other, are we ever conscious of any power. We learn the influence of our will from experience alone. And experience only teaches us how one event constantly follows another; without instructing us in the secret connexion, which binds them together, and renders them inseparable.

Thirdly, we learn from anatomy, that the immediate object of power in voluntary motion, is not the member itself which is moved, but certain muscles, and nerves, and animal spirits, and, perhaps, something still more minute and more unknown, through which the motion is successively propagated, ere it reach the member itself whose motion is the immediate object of volition. Can there be a more certain proof, that the power, by which this whole operation is performed, so far from being directly and fully known by an inward sentiment or consciousness, is, to the last degree, mysterious and unintelligible? Here the mind wills a certain event: Immediately another event, unknown to ourselves, and totally different from the one intended, is produced: This event produces another, equally unknown: Till at last, through a long succession, the desired event is produced. But if the original power were felt, it must be known: Were it known, its effect must also be known; since all power is relative to its effect. And *vice versa*, if the effect be not known, the power cannot be known nor felt. How indeed can we be conscious of a power to move our limbs, when we have no such power; but only that to move certain animal spirits, which, though they produce at last the motion of our limbs, yet operate in such a manner as is wholly beyond our comprehension?

We may, therefore, conclude from the whole, I hope, without any temerity, though with assurance; that our idea of power is not copied from any sentiment or consciousness of power within ourselves, when we give rise to animal motion, or apply our limbs to their proper use and office. That their motion follows the command of the will is a matter of common experience, like other natural events:

But the power or energy by which this is effected, like that in other natural events, is unknown and inconceivable.

...

A peasant can give no better reason for the stopping of any clock or watch than to say that it does not commonly go right: But an artist easily perceives, that the same force in the spring or pendulum has always the same influence on the wheels; but fails of its usual effect, perhaps by reason of a grain of dust, which puts a stop to the whole movement. From the observation of several parallel instances, philosophers form a maxim, that the connexion between all causes and effects is equally necessary, and that its seeming uncertainty in some instances proceeds from the secret opposition of contrary causes.

Thus for instance, in the human body, when the usual symptoms of health or sickness disappoint our expectation; when medicines operate not with their wonted powers; when irregular events follow from any particular cause; the philosopher and physician are not surprized at the matter, nor are ever tempted to deny, in general, the necessity and uniformity of those principles, by which the animal economy is conducted. They know that a human body is a mighty complicated machine: That many secret powers lurk in it, which are altogether beyond our comprehension: That to us it must often appear very uncertain in its operations: And that therefore the irregular events, which outwardly discover themselves, can be no proof, that the laws of nature are not observed with the greatest regularity in its internal operations and government.

Man a Machine
Julian Offray de la Mettrie (1749)

Man is a machine so compound, that it is impossible to form at first a clear idea thereof, and consequently to define it. This is the reason, that all the enquiries the philosophers have made *a priori*, that is, by endeavouring to raise themselves on the wings of the understanding, have proved ineffectual. Thus it is only *a posteriori*,[48] or as it were by disentangling the soul from the organs of the body, that we can, I do not say, discover with evidence the nature of man, but obtain the greatest degree of probability the subject will admit of.

...

The body and soul seem to fall asleep together. In proportion as the motion of the blood grows calm a soft soothing sense of peace and tranquillity spreads itself over the whole machine; the soul finds itself sweetly weighed down with slumber, and sinks with the fibres of the brain: it becomes thus paralitic as it were, by degrees, together with all the muscles of the body. The latter are no longer able to support the head; the head itself can no longer bear the weight of thought; the soul is during sleep, as if it had no existence.

---

[48]A priori: propositions known independent of any experience; *a posteriori*: knowledge based on reasoning from experience or past events, rather than by making assumptions or predictions.

If the circulation goes on with too great rapidity; the soul cannot sleep. If the soul be thrown into too great an agitation, the blood loses its calm, and rushes through the veins with a noise that sometimes may be distinctly heard: such are the two reciprocal causes of insomnia. A frightful dream makes the heart beat double, and tears us from the sweet necessity of rest, as effectually as a lively pain, or pressing want. In a word, as the sole cessation of the functions of the soul produces sleep, man is subject even during some walking moments (when in reality the soul is no more than half awake) to certain sorts of revery or slumbers of the soul, which are very frequent, and sufficiently prove that the soul does not wait for the body to fall asleep. For if it does not entirely sleep, how little does it want of it? Since it is impossible for her to recollect one object, to which she gave attention, amidst that innumerable crowd of confused ideas, which as so many vanishing clouds had filled up, if I may so say, the atmosphere of the brain.

...

The human body is a machine that winds up its own springs.

Signs of the Times
Thomas Carlyle (1829)

Nay, our whole Metaphysics itself, from Locke's[49] time downward, has been physical; not a spiritual philosophy, but a material one. The singular estimation in which his Essay was so long held as a scientific work (an estimation grounded, indeed, on the estimable character of the man) will one day be thought a curious indication of the spirit of these times. His whole doctrine is mechanical, in its aim and origin, in its method and its results. It is not a philosophy of the mind: it is a mere discussion concerning the origin of our consciousness, or ideas, or whatever else they are called; a genetic history of what we see *in* the mind. The grand secrets of Necessity and Freewill, of the Mind's vital or non-vital dependence on Matter, of our mysterious relations to Time and Space, to God, to the Universe, are not, in the faintest degree touched on in these inquiries; and seem not to have the smallest connexion with them.

The last class of our Scotch Metaphysicians had a dim notion that much of this was wrong; but they knew not how to right it. The school of Reid[50] had also from the first taken a mechanical course, not seeing any other. The singular conclusions at which Hume,[51] setting out from their admitted premises, was arriving, brought this school into being; they let loose Instinct, as an undiscriminating ban-dog, to guard them against these conclusions; – they tugged lustily at the logical chain by which Hume was so coldly towing them and the world into bottomless abysses

---

[49]John Locke (1632–1704) was an English philosopher, physician and early empiricist, the founder of Liberalism, a key figure of Enlightenment, and author of *An Essay Concerning Human Understanding* (1689).
[50]Thomas Reid (1710–96) was a religiously trained Scottish philosopher, a key figure in the Scottish Enlightenment and critic of David Hume.
[51]David Hume (1711–76) was a Scottish historian, philosopher, economist, diplomat and essayist known for his radical philosophical empiricism and skepticism. See pp. 70–2.

of Atheism and Fatalism. But the chain somehow snapped between them; and the issue has been that nobody now cares about either, any more than about Hartley's, Darwin's, or Priestley's[52] contemporaneous doings in England. Hartley's vibrations and vibratiuncles, one would think, were material and mechanical enough; but our Continental neighbours have gone still farther. One of their philosophers has lately discovered, that 'as the liver secretes bile, so does the brain secrete thought'; which astonishing discovery Dr Cabanis,[53] more lately still, in his *Rapports du Physique et du Morale de l'Homme*, has pushed into its minutest developments. The metaphysical philosophy of this last inquirer is certainly no shadowy or unsubstantial one. He fairly lays open our moral structure with his dissecting-knives and real metal probes; and exhibits it to the inspection of mankind, by Leeuwenhoek[54] microscopes, and inflation with the anatomical blowpipe. Thought, he is inclined to hold, is still secreted by the brain; but then Poetry and Religion (and it is really worth knowing) are 'a product of the smaller intestines!' We have the greatest admiration for this learned doctor: with what scientific stoicism he walks through the land of wonders, unwondering; like a wise man through some huge, gaudy, imposing Vauxhall, whose fire-works, cascades and symphonies, the vulgar may enjoy and believe in – but where he finds nothing real but the saltpetre, pasteboard and catgut. His book may be regarded as the ultimatum of mechanical metaphysics in our time; a remarkable realisation of what in Martinus Scriblerus[55] was still only an idea, that 'as the jack had a meat-roasting quality, so had the body a thinking quality,' upon the strength of which the Nurembergers were to build a wood-and-leather man, 'who should reason as well as most country parsons.' Vaucanson[56] did indeed make a wooden duck, that seemed to eat and digest; but that bold scheme of the Nurembergers remained for a more modern virtuoso.

Lectures on the Principles of Surgery
John Hunter (1839)

Animal matter is endowed with a principle called, in common language, life. This principle is, perhaps, conceived of with more difficulty than any other in nature, which arises from its being more complex in its effects than any other; and it is therefore no wonder that it is the least understood. But although life may appear very compounded in its effects in a complicated animal like man, it is as simple in

---

[52]David Hartley (1705–57) was an English philosopher and founder of the Associationist school of psychology. Erasmus Darwin (1731–1802), grandfather to Charles Darwin, was a physician, philosopher and poet. See pp. 394–97. Joseph Priestley (1733–1804) was a scientist, theologian and political philosopher. All these figures could be described as rationalists and materialists.

[53]Pierre Jean George Cabanis (1757–1808) was a French physiologist, freemason and materialist philosopher.

[54]Antonie Philips van Leeuwenhoek (1632–1723) was a Dutch tradesman and scientist, known as the 'father of microbiology' and renowned for his work on the improvement of the microscope.

[55]The *Memoirs of Martinus Scriblerus* is an unfinished satire by the members of the eighteenth-century Scriblerus Club of satirists.

[56]Jacques de Vaucanson (1709–82) was a French inventor and artist who created automata, including his famous mechanical digesting duck.

him as in the most simple animal, and is reducible to one simple property in every animal.

I have observed that animal matter may be in two states; in one it is endowed with the living principle, in the other it is deprived of it. From this it appears that the principle called life cannot arise from the peculiar modification of matter, because the same modification exists where this principle is no more. The matter abstracted from life appears at all times to be the same, as far as our senses and experiments carry us. If life arose out of this peculiar modification, it would not be destroyed until the modification was destroyed, either by spontaneous changes, as fermentation, or by some chemical processes; and were it destroyed by the last, it might sometimes be restored again by another process. Life, then, appears to be something superadded to this peculiar modification of matter; or this modification of matter is so arranged that the principle of life arises out of the arrangement, and this peculiar disposition of parts may be destroyed, and still the modification, from which it is called animal matter, remain the same. If the latter be the true explanation, this arrangement of parts, on which life should depend, would not be that position of parts necessary to the formation of a whole part or organ, for that is probably a mechanical, or at least organical, arrangement, but just a peculiar arrangement of the most simple particles, giving rise to a principle of preservation; so that matter so arranged could not undergo any destructive change till this arrangement were destroyed, which is death. This simple principle of life can with difficulty be conceived; but to show that matter may take on new properties without being altered in itself as to the species of matter, it may be not improper to illustrate this idea by such acquirements in other matter. Perhaps magnetism affords us the best illustration we can give of this. Iron appears at all times the same, whether endued with this property or not; magnetism does not seem to depend on the formation of any of its parts. A bar of iron without magnetism may be considered like animal matter without life; set it upright and it acquires a new property, of attraction and repulsion, at its different ends. Now is this any substance added; or is it a certain change which takes place in the arrangement of the particles of iron giving it this property? If we take a piece of glass, it is transparent; we break it into a thousand pieces and it becomes white. Whiteness is not a new matter added to it, but a property arising from its being composed of a number of small pieces.

It was not sufficient that animal matter should be endowed with this first principle, the principle of preservation, it was necessary that it should have action or motion within itself. This does not necessarily arise out of the arrangement for preservation; on the other hand, the arrangement for preservation, which is life, becomes the *principle* of action, not the power of action, for the power of action is one step further. The *power of action* must arise from a particular position of those living parts for before action can take place the matter must be arranged with this view. This is generally effected by the union of two or more living parts, so united as to allow of motion on each other, which motion the principle of action is capable of effecting when so disposed. A number of these simple acting parts, united, make a muscular fibre; when a number of these are put together they form a muscle, which, joined with other kinds of animal matter, as tendon, ligament, composes what may be called an organ. Thus, too, by the arrangement of the living particles, the other organs of the body are formed, their various dispositions and actions depending on the nature of the arrangement, for action is not confined to muscle, the nerves also have action arising from the arrangement of their living particles.

The principle of life has been compared to the spring of a watch, or the moving powers of other machinery; but its mode of existence is entirely different. In a machine the power is only the cause of the first action or movement, and thereby becomes the remote cause of the second, third, etc.; but this is not the case with an animal; animal matter has a principle of action in every part, independent of the others, and whenever the action of one part (which is always the effect of the living principle,) becomes the cause of an action in another, it is by stimulating the living principle of that other part, the action in the second part being as much the effect of the living principle of that part as the action of the first was of the living principle in it. The living principle, then, is the immediate cause of action in every part; it is therefore essential to every part, and is as much the property of it as gravity is of every particle of matter composing the whole. Every individual particle of the animal matter, then, is possessed of life, and the least imaginable part which we can separate is as much alive as the whole.

Border Lines of Knowledge in Some Provinces of Medical Science
Oliver Wendell Holmes (1861)

'Every animal presents itself as a sum of vital unities, every one of which manifests all the characteristics of life.'[57]

The *mechanism* is as clear, as unquestionable, as absolutely settled and universally accepted, as the order of movement of the heavenly bodies, which we compute backward to the days of the observatories on the plains of Shinar, and on the faith of which we regulate the movements of war and trade by the predictions of our ephemeris.

The *mechanism*, and that is all. We see the workman and the tools, but the skill that guides the work and the power that performs it are as invisible as ever. I fear that not every listener took the significance of those pregnant words in the passage I quoted from John Bell, – *'thinking to discover its properties in its form.'*[58] We have discovered the working bee in this great hive of organization. We have detected the cell in the very act of forming itself from a nucleus, of transforming itself into various tissues, of selecting the elements of various secretions. But why one cell becomes nerve and another muscle, why one selects bile and another fat, we can no more pretend to tell, than why one grape sucks out of the soil the generous juice which princes hoard in their cellars, and another the wine which it takes three men to drink, – one to pour it down, another to swallow it, and a third to hold him while it is going down. Certain analogies between this selecting power and the phenomena

---

[57]This is quoted from Virchow, *Cellular Pathology* (see pp. 77–9).
[58]John Bell (1763–1820) was a Scottish anatomist and surgeon.

of endosmosis in the elective affinities of chemistry we can find, but the problem of force remains here, as everywhere, unsolved and insolvable.

Do we gain anything by attempting to get rid of the idea of a special vital force because we find certain mutually convertible relations between forces in the body and out of it? I think not, any more than we should gain by getting rid of the idea and expression Magnetism[59] because of its correlation with electricity. We may concede the unity of all forms of force, but we cannot overlook the fixed differences of its manifestations according to the conditions under which it acts. It is a mistake, however, to think the mystery is greater in an organized body than in any other. We see a stone fall or a crystal form, and there is nothing stranger left to wonder at, for we have seen the Infinite in action.

Cellular Pathology
Rudolf Virchow (1863)[60]

The present reform in medicine, of which you have all been witnesses, essentially had its rise in new anatomical observations, and the exposition also, which I have to make to you, will therefore principally be based upon anatomical demonstrations. But for me it would not be sufficient to take, as has been the custom during the last ten years, pathological anatomy alone as the groundwork of my views; we must add thereto those facts of general anatomy also, to which the actual state of medical science is due. The history of medicine teaches us, if we will only take a somewhat comprehensive survey of it, that at all times permanent advances have been marked by anatomical innovations, and that every more important epoch has been directly ushered in by a series of important discoveries concerning the structure of the body. So it was in those old times, when the observations of the Alexandrian school, based for the first time upon the anatomy of man, prepared the way for the system of Galen[61]; so it was, too, in the Middle Ages, when Vesalius[62] laid the foundations of anatomy, and therewith began the real reformation of medicine; so, lastly, was it at the commencement of this century, when Bichat[63] developed the principles of general anatomy. What Schwann,[64] however, has done for histology, has as yet been but in a very slight degree built up and developed for pathology, and it may be said that nothing has penetrated less deeply into the minds of all than the cell-theory in its intimate connection with pathology.

---

[59]Animal magnetism, or mesmerism, was a popular nineteenth-century belief that living beings exerted an invisible natural force, which practitioners could harness for healing.

[60]Trans. Frank Chance.

[61]The theories of Galen of Pergamon (129–c.216 AD) dominated Western medical science until the early modern era.

[62]Andreas Vesalius (1514–64) was an anatomist, physician and author of De humani corporis fabrica (On the Fabric of the Human Body), often referred to as the founding work of modern human anatomy.

[63]Marie François Xavier Bichat (1771–1802) was a French anatomist and physiologist, known as the founder of modern histology (the microscopic study of tissues; microscopic anatomy).

[64]Theodor Schwann (1810–82) was a German physiologist who developed cell theory, coined the term 'metabolism', and discovered pepsin and Schwann cells, which insulate nerve fibers.

If we consider the extraordinary influence which Bichat in his time exercised upon the state of medical opinion, it is indeed astonishing that such a relatively long period should have elapsed since Schwann made his great discoveries, without the real importance of the new facts having been duly appreciated. This has certainly been essentially due to the great incompleteness of our knowledge with regard to the intimate structure of our tissues which has continued to exist until quite recently, and, as we are sorry to be obliged to confess, still even now prevails with regard to many points of histology to such a degree, that we scarcely know in favour of what view to decide.

Especial difficulty has been found in answering the question, from what parts of the body action really proceeds – what parts are active, what passive; and yet it is already quite possible to come to a definitive conclusion upon this point, even in the case of parts the structure of which is still disputed. The chief point in this application of histology to pathology is to obtain a recognition of the fact, that the cell is really the ultimate morphological element in which there is any manifestation of life, and that we must not transfer the seat of real action to any point beyond the cell. Before you, I shall have no particular reason to justify myself, if in this respect I make quite a special reservation in favour of life. In the course of these lectures you will be able to convince yourselves that it is almost impossible for any one to entertain more mechanical ideas in particular instances than I am wont to do, when called upon to interpret the individual processes of life. But I think that we must look upon this as certain, that, however much of the more delicate interchange of matter, which takes place within a cell, may not concern the material structure as a whole, yet the real action does proceed from the structure as such, and that the living element only maintains its activity as long as it really presents itself to us as an independent whole.

...

The nucleus and membrane, recur with great constancy, and ... by their combination a simple element is obtained, which, throughout the whole series of living vegetable and animal forms, however different they may be externally, however much their internal composition may be subjected to change, presents us with a structure of quite a peculiar conformation, as a definite basis for all the phenomena of life. According to my ideas, this is the only possible starting-point for all biological doctrines. If a definite correspondence in elementary form pervades the whole series of all living things, and if in this series something else which might be placed in the stead of the cell be in vain sought for, then must every more highly developed organism, whether vegetable or animal, necessarily, above all, be regarded as a progressive total, made up of larger or smaller number of similar or dissimilar cells. Just as a tree constitutes a mass arranged in a definite manner, in which, in every single part, in the leaves as in the root, in the trunk as in the blossom, cells are discovered to be the ultimate elements, so is it also with the forms of animal life. Every animal presents itself as a sum of vital unities, every one of which manifests all the characteristics of life. The characteristics and unity of life cannot be limited to any one particular spot in a highly developed organism (for example, to the brain of man), but are to be found only in the definite, constantly recurring structure, which every individual element displays. Hence it follows that the structural composition of a body of considerable size, a so-called individual, always represents a kind of social arrangement of parts, an arrangement of a social kind, in which a number of individual existences are mutually dependent, but in such a way, that every element has its own special action, and, even though it derive its stimulus to activity from other parts, yet alone effects the actual performance of its duties.

On the Physical Basis of Life
T. H. Huxley (1869)

In order to make the title of this discourse generally intelligible, I have translated the term 'Protoplasm' which is the scientific name of the substance of which I am about to speak, by the words 'the physical basis of life.' I suppose that, to many, the idea that there is such a thing as a physical basis, or matter, of life may be novel – so widely spread is the conception of life as a something which works through matter, but is independent of it; and even those who are aware that matter and life are inseparably connected, may not be prepared for the conclusion plainly suggested by the phrase 'the physical basis or matter of life', that there is some one kind of matter which is common to all living beings, and that their endless diversities are bound together by a physical, as well as an ideal, unity. In fact, when first apprehended, such a doctrine as this appears almost shocking to common sense. What, truly, can seem to be more obviously different from one another in faculty, in form, and in substance, than the various kinds of living beings? What community of faculty can there be between the brightly-colored lichen, which so nearly resembles a mere mineral incrustation of the bare rock on which it grows, and the painter, to whom it is instinct with beauty, or the botanist, whom it feeds with knowledge?

Again, think of the microscopic fungus – a mere infinitesimal ovoid particle, which finds space and duration enough to multiply into countless millions in the body of a living fly; and then of the wealth of foliage, the luxuriance of flower and fruit, which lies between this bald sketch of a plant and the giant pine of California, towering to the dimensions of a cathedral spire, or the Indian fig, which covers acres with its profound shadow, and endures while nations and empires come and go around its vast circumference? Or, turning to the other half of the world of life, picture to yourselves the great Finner whale, hugest of beasts that live, or have lived, disporting his eighty or ninety feet of bone, muscle and blubber, with easy roll, among waves in which the stoutest ship that ever left dockyard would founder hopelessly; and contrast him with the invisible animalcules – mere gelatinous specks, multitudes of which could, in fact, dance upon the point of a needle with the same ease as the angels of the schoolmen could, in imagination. With these images before your minds, you may well ask what community of form, or structure, is there between the animalcule and the whale, or between the fungus and the fig-tree? And, *a fortiori*[65] between all four?

---

[65]*a fortiori*: 'with stronger reason'.

Finally, if we regard substance, or material composition, what hidden bond can connect the flower which a girl wears in her hair and the blood which courses through her youthful veins; or, what is there in common between the dense and resisting mass of the oak, or the strong fabric of the tortoise, and those broad disks of glassy jelly which may be seen pulsating through the waters of a calm sea, but which drain away to mere films in the hand which raises them out of their element? Such objections as these must, I think, arise in the mind of every one who ponders, for the first time, upon the conception of a single physical basis of life underlying all the diversities of vital existence; but I propose to demonstrate to you that, notwithstanding these apparent difficulties, a threefold unity – namely, a unity of power or faculty, a unity of form, and a unity of substantial composition – does pervade the whole living world. No very abstruse argumentation is needed, in the first place, to prove that the powers, or faculties, of all kinds of living matter, diverse as they may be in degree, are substantially similar in kind.

Goethe has condensed a survey of all the powers of mankind into the well-known epigram: *Warum treibt sich das Volk so und schreit? Es will sich emfthren Kinder zeugen, und sie nahren so gut es vermag. Weiter bringt es kein Mensch, stell' er sich, wie er auch will.*[66]

In physiological language this means, that all the multifarious and complicated activities of man are comprehensible under three categories. Either they are immediately directed towards the maintenance and development of the body, or they effect transitory changes in the relative positions of parts of the body, or they tend towards the continuance of the species. Even those manifestations of intellect, of feeling, and of will, which we rightly name the higher faculties, are not excluded from this classification, inasmuch as to every one but the subject of them, they are known only as transitory changes in the relative positions of parts of the body. Speech, gesture, and every other form of human action are, in the long run, resolvable into muscular contraction, and muscular contraction is but a transitory change in the relative positions of the parts of a muscle. But the scheme, which is large enough to embrace the activities of the highest form of life, covers all those of the lower creatures.

'Religion and Neurology' from *The Varieties of Religious Experience*
William James (1902)

We are surely all familiar in a general way with this method [providing medical explanations] of discrediting states of mind for which we have an antipathy. We all use it to some degree in criticizing persons whose states of mind we regard as overstrained. But when other people criticize our own more exalted soul-flights by calling them 'nothing but' expressions of our organic disposition, we feel outraged and hurt, for we know that, whatever be our organism's peculiarities, our mental

---

[66]Johann Wolfgang von Goethe (1749–1832) was a German Romantic poet, lyricist, writer and statesman. His epigram reads: 'Why are the people yelling in such agitation? They want to nourish themselves, beget children and feed them as well as they can. Beyond that, no one can go, no matter how hard they may try.'

states have their substantive value as revelations of the living truth; and we wish that all this medical materialism could be made to hold its tongue.

Medical materialism seems indeed a good appellation for the too simple-minded system of thought which we are considering. Medical materialism finishes up Saint Paul by calling his vision on the road to Damascus a discharging lesion of the occipital cortex, he being an epileptic. It snuffs out Saint Teresa as an hysteric, Saint Francis of Assisi as an hereditary degenerate. George Fox's[67] discontent with the shams of his age, and his pining for spiritual veracity, it treats as a symptom of a disordered colon. Carlyle's[68] organ-tones of misery it accounts for by a gastro-duodenal catarrh. All such mental overtensions, it says, are, when you come to the bottom of the matter, mere affairs of diathesis (auto-intoxications most probably), due to the perverted action of various glands which physiology will yet discover. And medical materialism then thinks that the spiritual authority of all such personages is successfully undermined.

Let us ourselves look at the matter in the largest possible way. Modern psychology, finding definite psycho-physical connections to hold good, assumes as a convenient hypothesis that the dependence of mental states upon bodily conditions must be thoroughgoing and complete. If we adopt the assumption, then of course what medical materialism insists on must be true in a general way, if not in every detail: Saint Paul certainly had once an epileptoid, if not an epileptic seizure; George Fox was an hereditary degenerate; Carlyle was undoubtedly auto-intoxicated by some organ or other, no matter which – and the rest.

But now, I ask you, how can such an existential account of facts of mental history decide in one way or another upon their spiritual significance? According to the general postulate of psychology just referred to, there is not a single one of our states of mind, high or low, healthy or morbid, that has not some organic process as its condition. Scientific theories are organically conditioned just as much as religious emotions are; and if we only knew the facts intimately enough, we should doubtless see 'the liver' determining the dicta of the sturdy atheist as decisively as it does those of the Methodist under conviction anxious about his soul. When it alters in one way the blood that percolates it, we get the methodist, when in another way, we get the atheist form of mind. So of all our raptures and our drynesses, our longings and pantings, our questions and beliefs. They are equally organically founded, be they religious or of non-religious content.

To plead the organic causation of a religious state of mind, then, in refutation of its claim to possess superior spiritual value, is quite illogical and arbitrary, unless one has already worked out in advance some psycho-physical theory connecting spiritual values in general with determinate sorts of physiological change. Otherwise none of our thoughts and feelings, not even our scientific doctrines, not even our *dis*-beliefs,

---

[67]George Fox (1624–91) was an English Dissenter and founder of the religious Society of Friends, commonly known as the Quakers.
[68]Thomas Carlyle (1795–1881) was a Scottish philosopher, essayist and historian, who deplored medical materialism. See the extract from *Signs of the Times* earlier in this section.

could retain any value as revelations of the truth, for every one of them without exception flows from the state of its possessor's body at the time.

It is needless to say that medical materialism draws in point of fact no such sweeping skeptical conclusion. It is sure, just as every simple man is sure, that some states of mind are inwardly superior to others, and reveal to us more truth, and in this it simply makes use of an ordinary spiritual judgment. It has no physiological theory of the production of these its favorite states, by which it may accredit them; and its attempt to discredit the states which it dislikes, by vaguely associating them with nerves and liver, and connecting them with names connoting bodily affliction, is altogether illogical and inconsistent.

CHAPTER TWO

Nerves, Mind and Brain

from *The Spleen*
Anne Finch (1701)

What art thou, *Spleen*, which ev'ry thing dost ape?
Thou *Proteus*[1] to abus'd Mankind,
Who never yet thy real Cause could find,
Or fix thee to remain in one continued Shape.
Still varying thy perplexing Form,
Now a Dead Sea thou'lt represent,
A Calm of stupid Discontent,
Then, dashing on the Rocks wilt rage into a Storm.
Trembling sometimes thou dost appear,
Dissolv'd into a Panic Fear;
On Sleep intruding dost thy Shadows spread,
Thy gloomy Terrors round the silent Bed,
And crowd with boding Dreams the Melancholy Head:
Or, when the Midnight Hour is told,
And drooping Lids thou still dost waking hold,
Thy fond Delusions cheat the Eyes,
Before them antic Spectres dance,
Unusual Fires their pointed Heads advance,
And airy Phantoms rise.
Such was the monstrous *Vision* seen,
When *Brutus*[2] (now beneath his Cares opprest,
And all *Rome's* Fortunes rolling in his Breast,
Before *Philippi's*[3] latest Field,
Before his Fate did to *Octavius* lead)
Was vanquish'd by the *Spleen*.

Falsely, the Mortal Part we blame
Of our deprest and pond'rous Frame,

---

[1]In Greek mythology, Proteus is a sea-god or god of rivers, symbolic of constant change.
[2]Marcus Junius Brutus (85–42 BC) was a Roman politician, best known for his part in the assassination of Julius Caesar.
[3]The Battle of Philippi (Macedonia, 42 BC) was the final battle in the Wars of the Second Triumvirate between the forces of Mark Antony and Octavian, and the forces of Caesar's assassins – Marcus Junius Brutus and Gaius Cassius Longinus.

Which, till the First degrading Sin
Let Thee, its dull Attendant, in,
Still with the Other did comply,
Nor clogg'd the Active Soul, dispos'd to fly,
And range the Mansions of its native Sky.

Nor, whilst in his own Heaven he dwelt,
Whilst Man his Paradise possest,
His fertile Garden in the fragrant East,
And all united Odours smelt,
No armed Sweets, until thy Reign,
Could shock the Sense, or in the Face
A flushed, unhandsome Colour place.
Now the *Jonquille* o'ercomes the feeble Brain;
We faint beneath the Aromatic Pain,
Till some offensive Scent thy Pow'rs appease,
And Pleasure we resign for short, and nauseous Ease. ...

Whilst *Touch* not, *Taste* not, what is freely giv'n,
Is but thy niggard Voice, disgracing bounteous Heav'n.
From Speech restrain'd, by thy Deceits abus'd,
To Deserts banish'd, or in Cells reclus'd,
Mistaken Vot'ries to the Pow'rs Divine,
Whilst they a purer Sacrifice design,
Do but the *Spleen* obey, and worship at thy Shrine.
In vain to chase thee ev'ry Art we try,
In vain all Remedies apply,
In vain the *Indian* Leaf infuse,
Or the parch'd *Eastern* Berry bruise;
Some pass, in vain, those Bounds, and nobler Liquors use.
Now Harmony, in vain, we bring,
Inspire the Flute, and touch the String.
From Harmony no help is had;
Music but soothes thee, if too sweetly sad,
And if too light, but turns thee gayly Mad.

Tho' the Physicians greatest Gains,
Altho' his growing Wealth he sees
Daily increas'd by Ladies Fees,
Yet dost thou baffle all his studious Pains.
Not skilful *Lower*[4] thy Source could find,
Or thro' the well-dissected Body trace
The secret, the mysterious ways,
By which thou dost surprise, and prey upon the Mind.

---

[4]Richard Lower (1631–91) was a renowned Cornish anatomist, who performed the first recorded successful blood transfusion on two dogs (1665).

Tho' in the Search, too deep for Humane Thought,
With unsuccessful Toil he wrought,
'Til thinking Thee to've catch'd, Himself by thee was caught,
Retain'd thy Pris'ner, thy acknowleg'd Slave,
And sunk beneath thy Chain to a lamented Grave.

from *The Spleen*
Matthew Green (1737)

First know, my friend, I do not mean
To write a treatise on the spleen;
Nor to prescribe, when nerves convulse,
Nor mend th'alarum watch, your pulse:
If I am right, your question lay,
What course I take to drive away
The day-mare spleen, by whose false pleas
Men prove mere suicides in ease;
And how I do myself demean
In stormy world to live serene.

When by its magick lanthorn spleen
With frightful figures spread life's scene,
And threatning prospects urg'd my fears,
A stranger to the luck of heirs;
Reason, some quiet to restore,
Show'd part was substance, shadow more;
With spleen's dead weight tho' heavy grown,
In life's rough tide I sunk not down,
But swam, till fortune threw a rope
Buoyant on bladders fill'd with hope.

I always choose the plainest food
To mend viscidity of blood.
Hail! water-gruel, healing power,
Of easy access to the poor;
Thy help love's confessors implore,
And doctors secretly adore:
To thee I fly, by thee dilute,
Through veins my blood doth quicker shoot;
And by swift current throws off clean
Prolific particles of spleen.

I never sick by drinking grow,
Nor keep myself a cup too low:
And seldom Cloe's lodgings haunt,
Thrifty of spirits, which I want.

Hunting I reckon very good
To brace the nerves, and stir the blood;
But after no field-honours itch,
Achiev'd by leaping hedge and ditch.
While spleen lies soft relax'd in bed,
Or o'er coal-fires inclines the head,
Hygea's[5] sons with hound and horn,
And jovial cry awake the morn:
These see her from her dusky plight,
Smear'd by th' embraces of the night,
With roral[6] wash redeem her face,
And prove herself of Titan's race,
And mounting in loose robes the skies,
Shed light and fragrance, as she flies.
Then horse and hound fierce joy display,
Exulting at the Hark-away,
And in pursuit o'er tainted ground
From lungs robust field-notes resound.
Then, as St. George the dragon slew,
Spleen pierc'd, trod down, and dying view,
While all the spirits are on wing,
And woods, and hills, and valleys ring.

A Receipt to Cure the Vapors
Lady Mary Wortley Montagu (1748)

Why will Delia thus retire,
  And idly languish life away?
While the sighing crowd admire,
  'Tis too soon for hartshorn tea:

All those dismal looks and fretting
  Cannot Damon's[7] life restore;
Long ago the worms have eat him,
  You can never see him more.

Once again consult your toilette,
  In the glass your face review:
So much weeping soon will spoil it,
  And no spring your charms renew.

---

[5]In Greek and Roman mythology, Hygea (also Hygiea), the daughter of the god of medicine, Asclepius and Epione, was the goddess/personification of health, cleanliness and hygiene.
[6]Roral: dew.
[7]Both Delia and Damon are conventional poetic names.

I, like you, was born a woman,
    Well I know what vapors mean:
The disease, alas! is common;
    Single, we have all the spleen.

All the morals that they tell us,
    Never cured the sorrow yet:
Chuse, among the pretty fellows,
    One of honor, youth, and wit.

Prithee hear him every morning
    At least an hour or two;
Once again at night returning –
    I believe the dose will do.

Lines Written During a Period of Insanity
William Cowper (1773)

Hatred and vengeance, my eternal portion,
Scarce can endure delay of execution,
Wait with impatient readiness to seize my
    Soul in a moment.

Damned below Judas; more abhorred than he was,
Who for a few pence sold his holy Master.
Twice-betrayed, Jesus me, the last delinquent,
    Deems the profanest.

Man disavows, and Deity disowns me;
Hell might afford my miseries a shelter;
Therefore Hell keeps her ever-hungry mouths all
    Bolted against me.

Hard lot! encompassed with a thousand dangers;
Weary, faint, trembling with a thousand terrors;
I'm called, if vanquished, to receive a sentence
    Worse than Abiram's.[8]

Him the vindictive rod of angry justice
Sent quick and howling to the centre headlong;
I, fed with judgement, in a fleshy tomb, am
    Buried above ground.

---

[8]In the Bible, Abiram was the son of Eliab who, along with his brother Dathan, joined Korah in the conspiracy against Moses and Aaron. He and all the conspirators, with their families and possessions, were swallowed up by the ground (Numbers 16:1–40; 26:9–11; Psalms 106:17).

Ode on Melancholy
John Keats (1820)

No, no, go not to Lethe,[9] neither twist
Wolf's-bane,[10] tight-rooted, for its poisonous wine;
Nor suffer thy pale forehead to be kiss'd
By nightshade,[11] ruby grape of Proserpine[12];
Make not your rosary of yew-berries,
Nor let the beetle, nor the death-moth be
Your mournful Psyche,[13] nor the downy owl
A partner in your sorrow's mysteries;
For shade to shade will come too drowsily,
And drown the wakeful anguish of the soul.

But when the melancholy fit shall fall
Sudden from heaven like a weeping cloud,
That fosters the droop-headed flowers all,
And hides the green hill in an April shroud;
Then glut thy sorrow on a morning rose,
Or on the rainbow of the salt sand-wave,
Or on the wealth of globed peonies;
Or if thy mistress some rich anger shows,
Emprison her soft hand, and let her rave,
And feed deep, deep upon her peerless eyes.

She dwells with Beauty – Beauty that must die;
And Joy, whose hand is ever at his lips
Bidding adieu; and aching Pleasure nigh,
Turning to poison while the bee-mouth sips:
Ay, in the very temple of Delight
Veil'd Melancholy has her sovran shrine,
Though seen of none save him whose strenuous tongue
Can burst Joy's grape against his palate fine;
His soul shall taste the sadness of her might,
And be among her cloudy trophies hung.

---

[9]In Greek mythology, Lethe was one of the five rivers of the underworld, and was associated with forgetfulness and oblivion.
[10]Wolfsbane is a highly poisonous, flowering plant from which opiates were extracted.
[11]Some of the family of nightshade plants have sedative properties.
[12]Proserpine was the Roman goddess of springtime.
[13]Here, Psyche refers to the soul, often symbolized by a moth that flies out of the mouth at death.

The Maniac's Funeral
Charles Dibdin (1825)

The portal open'd wide – where madness sits,
'Bays to the moon,' or churns, in moody fits –
A coffin came; age made the bearers slow;
One weeping woman all the train of woe!
Her pace and port like somewhat without breath;
Life's shadow walking in the vale of death.
The widow's weeds, all neat, though scant and poor,
Girt her thin, tottering, frame; her face, obscure,
Close-curtain'd by a hood; a 'kerchief old,
But white, of modest decency that told,
Clench'd in her hand, oft hast'ning to her eyes,
Publish'd her tears; her labouring breast with sighs
Seem'd struggling; down she hung her wretched head,
And seem'd half dying, while she mourn'd the dead!
Mourn'd? – 'twas a maniac to the grave they bore;
And, sure, 'twas blessing that his life was o'er;
Joy should have hail'd it – joy? – the widow's tear
Gush'd for past days, when every hour was dear;
For their first love, and joys for ever flown –
And then, with horror, to his mind o'erthrown
Quick flew her thoughts, and half-o'erturn'd her own.
She saw him wooing her consenting smile;
Then heard him raving with demoniac bile –
Saw him a corpse, his madness all forgot,
Felt all her loss, and shudder'd at her lot:
A widow, desolate! – while life was his,
Hope to returning reason look'd, and bliss;
Each false remission of his mental strife
Rous'd fear to fortitude, gave hope new life;
And scarce a starting tear – for tears would start –
Could gush, ere check'd by Hope's officious art.

But, *now* – all's past! herself alone remains;
No kindly care her sinking heart sustains;
Dank, frigid, certainty has hope revers'd,
And fear has flown, and death has done his worst:
Herself, alone! her tears, entreating, fall
To Death, to take herself, and finish all!

The Fear of Madness
Lucretia Maria Davidson (1831)[14]

There is a something which I dread;
It is a dark, a fearful thing;
It steals along with withering tread,
Or sweeps on wild destruction's wing.

That thought comes o'er me in the hour
Of grief, of sickness, or of sadness;
'Tis not the dread of death, – 'tis more –
It is the dread of madness.

Oh! may these throbbing pulses pause,
Forgetful of their feverish course;
May this hot brain, which, burning, glows
With all a fiery whirlpool's force,

Be cold, and motionless, and still,
A tenant of its lowly bed;
But let not dark delirium steal –
....

The Stammerer's Complaint
Martin Tupper (1838)

Ah! think it not a light calamity
To be denied free converse with my kind,
To be debarred from man's true attribute,
The proper glorious privilege of Speech.
Hast ever seen an eagle chain'd to earth?
A restless panther in his cage immured?
A swift trout by the wily fisher checked?
A wild bird hopeless strain its broken wing?
Hast ever felt, at the dark dead of night,
Some undefined and horrid incubus
Press down the very soul – and paralyse
The limbs in their imaginary flight
From shadowy terrors in unhallowed sleep?
Hast ever known the sudden icy chill
Of dreary disappointment, as it dashes
The sweet cup of anticipated bliss
From the parched lips of long-enduring hope?
Then thou canst picture – aye, in sober truth,

---

[14]These lines, expressing fears of insanity, were written while confined to bed in the last stage of consumption. This, Davidson's last poem, is unfinished.

In real, unexaggerated truth –
The constant, galling, festering chain that binds
Captive my mute interpreter of thought;
The seal of lead enstamp'd upon my lips,
The load of iron on my labouring chest,
The mocking demon that at every step
Haunts me – and spurs me on – to burst with silence!
Oh! tis a sore affliction to restrain,
From mere necessity, the glowing thought;
To feel the fluent cataract of speech
Check'd by some wintry spell, and frozen up,
Just as it leapeth from the precipice!
To be the butt of wordy captious fools,
And see the sneering self-complacent smile
Of victory on their lips, when I might prove,
(But for some little word I dare not utter,)
That innate truth is not a specious lie:
To hear foul slander blast an honour'd name,
Yet breathe no fact to drive the fiend away:
To mark neglected virtue in the dust,
Yet have no word to pity or console:

To feel just indignation swell my breast,
Yet know the fountain of my wrath is sealed:
To see my fellow-mortals hurrying on
Down the steep cliff of crime, down to perdition,
Yet have no voice to warn – no voice to win!
'Tis to be mortified in every point,
Baffled at every turn of life, for want
Of that most common privilege of man,
The merest drag of gorged society,
Words – windy words.

And is it not in truth,
A poison'd sting in every social joy,
A thorn that rankles in the writhing flesh,
A drop of gall in each domestic sweet,
An irritating petty misery,
That I can never look on one I love,
And speak the fullness of my burning thoughts?
That I can never with unmingled joy
Meet a long-loved and long-expected friend,
Because I feel, but cannot vent my feelings –
Because I know I ought – but must not speak,
Because I mark his quick impatient eye
Striving in kindness to anticipate

The word of welcome, strangled in its birth!
Is it not sorrow, while I truly love
Sweet social converse, to be forced to shun
The happy circle, from a nervous sense,
An agonizing poignant consciousness
That I must stand aloof, nor mingle with
The wise and good, in rational argument,
The young in brilliant quickness of reply,
Friendship's ingenuous interchange of mind,
Affection's open-hearted sympathies,
But feel myself an isolated being,
A very wilderness of widow'd thought!

Aye, 'tis a bitter thing – and not less bitter
Because it is not reckoned in the ills,
'The thousand natural shocks that flesh is heir to;'
Yet the full ocean is but countless drops,
And misery is an aggregate of tears,
And life, replete with small annoyances,
Is but one long protracted scene of sorrow.

I scarce would wonder, if a godless man,
(I name not him whose hope is heavenward),
A man, whom lying vanities hath scath'd
And harden'd from all fear – if such an one
By this tyrannical Argus[15] goaded on
Were to be wearied of his very life,
And daily, hourly foiled in social converse,
By the slow simmering of disappointment
Become a sour'd and apathetic being,
Were to feel rapture at the approach of death,
And long for his dark hope – annihilation.

The Camera Obscura[16]
John Addington Symonds (1880)

Inside the skull the wakeful brain,
Attuned at birth to joy and pain,

---

[15]In Greek mythology, Argus Panoptes, or Argos (meaning 'all seeing'), is the name of the hundred-eyed giant.
[16]A *Camera Obscura* (Latin: 'dark chamber') is an optical device and precursor to the camera. Light passes through a hole in a box, striking a surface on which it is reproduced, upside down, but with colour and perspective preserved.

Dwells for a lifetime; even as one
Who in a closed tower sees the sun
Cast faint-hued shadows, dim or clear,
Upon the darkened disc: now near,
Now far, they flit; while he, within,
Surveys the world he may not win:
Whate'er he sees, he notes; for nought
Escapes the net of living thought;
And what he notes, he tells again
To last and build the brains of men.
Shades are we; and of shades we weave
A trifling pleasant make-believe;
Then pass into the shadowy night,
Where formless shades blindfold the light.

Neurasthenia[17]
A. Mary F. Robinson (1888)

I watch the happier people of the house
Come in and out, and talk, and go their ways;
I sit and gaze at them; I cannot rouse
My heavy mind to share their busy days.

I watch them glide, like skaters on a stream,
Across the brilliant surface of the world.
But I am underneath: they do not dream
How deep below the eddying flood is whirl'd.

They cannot come to me, nor I to them;
But, if a mightier arm could reach and save,
Should I forget the tide I had to stem?
Should I, like these, ignore the abysmal wave?

Yes! in the radiant air how could I know
How black it is, how fast it is, below?

Much Madness is Divinest Sense
Emily Dickinson (1890)

Much madness is divinest sense
To a discerning eye;

---

[17]Neurasthenia is a condition characterized by lassitude, fatigue, headache and irritability, associated chiefly with emotional disturbance.

Much sense the starkest madness.
'Tis the majority
In this, as all, prevails.
Assent, and you are sane;
Demur, – you're straightway dangerous,
And handled with a chain.

Melancholy
Edward Thomas (1915)

The rain and wind, the rain and wind, raved endlessly.
On me the Summer storm, and fever, and melancholy
Wrought magic, so that if I feared the solitude
Far more I feared all company: too sharp, too rude,
Had been the wisest or the dearest human voice.
What I desired I knew not, but whate'er my choice
Vain it must be, I knew. Yet naught did my despair
But sweeten the strange sweetness, while through the wild air
All day long I heard a distant cuckoo calling
And, soft as dulcimers, sounds of near water falling,
And, softer, and remote as if in history,
Rumours of what had touched my friends, my foes, or me.

On the Asylum Road
Charlotte Mew (1916)

Theirs is the house whose windows – every pane –
Are made of darkly stained or clouded glass:
Sometimes you come upon them in the lane,
The saddest crowd that you will ever pass.

But still we merry town or village folk
Throw to their scattered stare a kindly grin,
And think no shame to stop and crack a joke
With the incarnate wages of man's sin.

None but ourselves in our long gallery we meet,
The moor-hen stepping from her reeds with dainty feet,
The hare-bell bowing on his stem,
Dance not with us; their pulses beat
To fainter music; nor do we to them
Make their life sweet.

The gayest crowd that they will ever pass
Are we to brother-shadows in the lane:
Our windows, too, are clouded glass
To them, yes, every pane!

Mental Cases
Wilfred Owen (1917)

Who are these? Why sit they here in twilight?
Wherefore rock they, purgatorial shadows,
Drooping tongues from jaws that slob their relish,
Baring teeth that leer like skulls' tongues wicked?
Stroke on stroke of pain – but what slow panic,
Gouged these chasms round their fretted sockets?
Ever from their hair and through their hands' palms
Misery swelters. Surely we have perished
Sleeping, and walk hell; but who these hellish?

– These are men whose minds the Dead have ravished.
Memory fingers in their hair of murders,
Multitudinous murders they once witnessed.
Wading sloughs of flesh these helpless wander,
Treading blood from lungs that had loved laughter.
Always they must see these things and hear them,
Batter of guns and shatter of flying muscles,
Carnage incomparable and human squander
Rucked too thick for these men's extrication.

Therefore still their eyeballs shrink tormented
Back into their brains, because on their sense
Sunlight seems a bloodsmear; night comes blood-black;
Dawn breaks open like a wound that bleeds afresh.
– Thus their heads wear this hilarious, hideous,
Awful falseness of set-smiling corpses.
– Thus their hands are plucking at each other;
Picking at the rope-knots of their scourging;
Snatching after us who smote them, brother,
Pawing us who dealt them war and madness.

Hysteria
T. S. Eliot (1917)

As she laughed I was aware of becoming involved in her laughter and being part of it, until her teeth were only accidental stars with a talent for squad-drill. I was drawn in by short gasps, inhaled at each momentary recovery, lost finally in the dark caverns of her throat, bruised by the ripple of unseen muscles. An elderly waiter with trembling hands was hurriedly spreading a pink and white checked cloth over the rusty green iron table, saying: 'If the lady and gentleman wish to take their tea in the garden, if the lady and gentleman wish to take their tea in the garden ...' I decided that if the shaking of her breasts could be stopped, some of the fragments of the afternoon might be collected, and I concentrated my attention with careful subtlety to this end.

Lines Upon Leaving a Sanitarium
Theodor Roethke (1937)

Self-contemplation is a curse
That makes an old confusion worse.

Recumbency is unrefined
And leads to errors in the mind.

Long gazing at the ceiling will
In time induce a mental ill.

The mirror tells some truth, but not
Enough to merit constant thought.

He who himself begins to loathe
Grows sick in flesh and spirit both.

Dissection is a virtue when
It operates on other men.

The Halls of Bedlam
Robert Graves (1938)

Forewarned of madness:
In three days' time at dusk
The fit masters him.

How to endure those days?
(Forewarned is foremad)
– 'Normally, normally.'

He will gossip with children,
Argue with elders,
Check the cash account.

'I shall go mad that day –'
The gossip, the argument,
The neat marginal entry.

His case is not uncommon,
The doctors pronounce;
But prescribe no cure.

To be mad is not easy,
Will earn him no more
Than a niche in the news.

Then to-morrow, children,
To-morrow or the next day
He resigns from the firm.

His boyhood's ambition
Was to become an artist –
Like any City man's.

To the walls and halls of Bedlam
The artist is welcome –
Bold brush and full palette.

Through the cell's grating
He will watch his children
To and from school.

'Suffer the little children
To come unto me
With their Florentine hair!'

A very special story
For their very special friends –
They burst in the telling:

Of an evil thing, armed,
Tap-tapping on the door,
Tap-tapping on the floor,
'On the third day at dusk.'

Father in his shirt-sleeves
Flourishing a hatchet –
Run, children, run!

No one could stop him,
No one understood;
And in the evening papers...

(Imminent genius,
Troubles at the office,
Normally, normally,
As if already mad.)

Evening in the Sanitarium
Louise Bogan (1941)

The free evening fades, outside the windows fastened with decorative iron grilles.
The lamps are lighted; the shades drawn; the nurses are watching a little.
It is the hour of the complicated knitting on the safe bone needles;
Of the games of anagrams and bridge;
The deadly game of chess; the book held up like a mask.

The period of the wildest weeping, the fiercest delusion, is over.
The women rest their tired half-healed hearts; they are almost well.
Some of them will stay almost well always:
The blunt-faced woman whose thinking dissolved
Under academic discipline; the manic-depressive girl
Now leveling off; one paranoiac afflicted with jealousy.
Another with persecution. Some alleviation has been possible.

O fortunate bride, who never again will become elated after childbirth!
O lucky older wife, who has been cured of feeling unwanted!
To the suburban railway station you will return, return,
To meet forever Jim home on the 5:35.
You will be again as normal and selfish and heartless as anybody else.

There is life left: the piano says it with its octave smile.
The soft carpets pad the thump and splinter of the suicide to be.
Everything will be splendid: the grandmother will not drink habitually.
The fruit salad will bloom on the plate like a bouquet
And the garden produce the blue-ribbon aquilegia.
The cats will be glad; the fathers feel justified; the mothers relieved.
The sons and husbands will no longer need to pay the bills.
Childhoods will be put away, the obscene nightmare abated.

At the ends of the corridors the baths are running.
Mrs. C. again feels the shadow of the obsessive idea.
Miss R. looks at the mantel-piece, which must mean something.

Dolor
Theodore Roethke (1943)

I have known the inexorable sadness of pencils,
Neat in their boxes, dolor of pad and paper weight,
All the misery of manilla folders and mucilage,
Desolation in immaculate public places,
Lonely reception room, lavatory, switchboard,
The unalterable pathos of basin and pitcher,
Ritual of multigraph, paper-clip, comma,
Endless duplication of lives and objects.
And I have seen dust from the walls of institutions,
Finer than flour, alive, more dangerous than silica,
Sift, almost invisible, through long afternoons of tedium,
Dropping a fine film on nails and delicate eyebrows,
Glazing the pale hair, the duplicate grey standard faces.

Waking in the Blue
Robert Lowell (1959)

The night attendant, a B.U. sophomore,[18]
rouses from the mare's-nest of his drowsy head
propped on *The Meaning of Meaning*.[19]
He catwalks down our corridor.
Azure day

---

[18]A second year Boston University undergraduate.
[19]A 1923 study of language by C. K. Odgen and I. A. Richards.

makes my agonized blue window bleaker.
Crows maunder on the petrified fairway.
Absence! My hearts grows tense
as though a harpoon were sparring for the kill.
(This is the house for the 'mentally ill.')

What use is my sense of humor?
I grin at Stanley, now sunk in his sixties,
once a Harvard all-American fullback,
(if such were possible!)
still hoarding the build of a boy in his twenties,
as he soaks, a ramrod
with a muscle of a seal
in his long tub,
vaguely urinous from the Victorian plumbing.
A kingly granite profile in a crimson gold-cap,
worn all day, all night,
he thinks only of his figure,
of slimming on sherbet and ginger ale –
more cut off from words than a seal.

This is the way day breaks in Bowditch Hall at McLean's;
the hooded night lights bring out 'Bobbie',
Porcellian '29,[20]
a replica of Louis XVI
without the wig –
redolent and roly-poly as a sperm whale,
as he swashbuckles about in his birthday suit
and horses at chairs.

These victorious figures of bravado ossified young.

In between the limits of day,
hours and hours go by under the crew haircuts
and slightly too little nonsensical bachelor twinkle
of the Roman Catholic attendants.
(There are no Mayflower[21]
screwballs in the Catholic Church.)

After a hearty New England breakfast,
I weigh two hundred pounds

---

[20]The Porcellian Club, Harvard University, was a men-only 'final club', founded by a group of thirty students who wanted to avoid dining hall food by roasting their own pigs. 'Bobbie' is Louis Agassiz Shaw II, son of a wealthy and influential Boston family. He confessed to strangling the family maid, Delia Holland, in April 1964. Judged to be unfit to stand trial due to reasons of insanity, he was committed instead to McLean Hospital, a private psychiatric institution, where he lived at Upham Memorial Hall for twenty-three years.
[21]The *Mayflower* ship transported English pilgrims from Plymouth to New England in 1620. The comment here refers to class conflict: Catholics attend Boston University and Mayflowers, 'Boston Brahmin', or old money Protestants, attend Harvard.

this morning. Cock of the walk,
I strut in my turtle-necked French sailor's jersey
before the metal shaving mirrors,
and see the shaky future grow familiar
in the pinched, indigenous faces
of these thoroughbred mental cases,
twice my age and half my weight.
We are all old-timers,
each of us holds a locked razor.

Counting the Mad
Donald Justice (1959)

This one was put in a jacket,
This one was sent home,
This one was given bread and meat
But would eat none,
And this one cried No No No No
All day long.

This one looked at the window
As though it were a wall,
This one saw things that were not there,
This one things that were,
And this one cried No No No No
All day long.

This one thought himself a bird,
This one a dog,
And this one thought himself a man,
An ordinary man,
And cried and cried No No No No
All day long.

Noon Walk on the Asylum Lawn
Anne Sexton (1960)

The summer sun ray
shifts through a suspicious tree.
though I walk through the valley of the shadow
It sucks the air
and looks around for me.

The grass speaks.
I hear green chanting all day.
I will fear no evil, fear no evil
The blades extend
and reach my way.

The sky breaks.
It sags and breathes upon my face.
in the presence of mine enemies, mine enemies
The world is full of enemies.
There is no safe place.

You, Doctor Martin
Anne Sexton (1960)

You, Doctor Martin, walk
from breakfast to madness. Late August,
I speed through the antiseptic tunnel
where the moving dead still talk
of pushing their bones against the thrust
of cure. And I am queen of this summer hotel
or the laughing bee on a stalk

of death. We stand in broken
lines and wait while they unlock
the doors and count us at the frozen gates
of dinner. The shibboleth is spoken
and we move to gravy in our smock
of smiles. We chew in rows, our plates
scratch and whine like chalk

in school. There are no knives
for cutting your throat. I make
moccasins all morning. At first my hands
kept empty, unraveled for the lives
they used to work. Now I learn to take
them back, each angry finger that demands
I mend what another will break

tomorrow. Of course, I love you;
you lean above the plastic sky,
god of our block, prince of all the foxes.
The breaking crowns are new
that Jack wore.
Your third eye
moves among us and lights the separate boxes
where we sleep or cry.

What large children we are
here. All over I grow most tall
in the best ward. Your business is people,
you call at the madhouse, an oracular
eye in our nest. Out in the hall

the intercom pages you. You twist in the pull
of the foxy children who fall

like floods of life in frost.
And we are magic talking to itself,
noisy and alone. I am queen of all my sins
forgotten. Am I still lost?
Once I was beautiful. Now I am myself,
counting this row and that row of moccasins
waiting on the silent shelf.

I Was Reading A Scientific Article
Margaret Atwood (1965)

They have photographed the brain
and here is the picture, it is full of
branches as I always suspected,

each time you arrive the electricity
of seeing you is a huge
tree lumbering through my skull, the roots waving.

It is an earth, its fibres wrap
things buried, your forgotten words
are graved in my head, an intricate

red blue and pink prehensile chemistry
veined like a leaf
network, or is it a seascape
with corals and shining tentacles.

I touch you, I am created in you
somewhere as a complex
filament of light.

You rest on me and my shoulder holds

your heavy unbelievable
skull, crowded with radiant
suns, a new planet, the people
submerged in you, a lost civilization
I can never excavate:

my hands trace the contours of a total
universe, its different
colours, flowers, its undiscovered
animals, violent or serene

its other air
its claws

its paradise rivers

from *Twenty Words: Twenty Days: A Sketchbook and a Morula*
Gael Turnbull (1965)

and at

approximately 4:45 p.m. a child brought in to the
hospital that had tripped, struck her head –

not much

more than dazed at first, then slowly lapsing, until
rapidly depressed, the breathing almost arrested –

'linear fracture of the skull in the left temporo-parietal area'

    a decision, and with decision –
to

surgery, each of us in place, to accomplish what must be –
    an incision –
at 5:17 p.m. the fault exposed, a

torn artery ligated, a clot removed, the brain free to
expand –
    without words or only of trivia –

bonded by

our intent and intent upon it –

made explicit though

unspoken –
    an obligation assuaged, as discovered –
and a unison –

Maalox Bland Diet Prescribed
Michael S. Harper (1973)

MAALOX BLAND DIET PRESCRIBED;
GI SERIES CONDUCTED, NEGATIVE;
30-DAY CONVALESCENT LEAVE;
AWOL 90 DAYS; SUBJECT RETURN ARMY HOSPITAL;
BACKPAY, AWOL CHARGE DISMISSED;

SUBJECT AGREED TO PSYCHIATRIC EXAM;
DIVISION CHIEF PSYCHIATRIST ASSIGNED
DUE TO SUBJECT'S OUTSTANDING RECORD.

DIAGNOSIS: 'POST-VIETNAM ADJUSTMENT DE-
PRESSION PROBLEM.'

from *Essay on Psychiatrists*
Robert Pinsky (1975)

I. Invocation

It's crazy to think one could describe them –
Calling on reason, fantasy, memory, eyes and ears –
As though they were all alike any more

Than sweeps, opticians, poets or masseurs.
Moreover, they are for more than one reason
Difficult to speak of seriously and freely,

And I have never (even this is difficult to say
Plainly, without foolishness or irony)
Consulted one for professional help, though it happens

Many or most of my friends have – and that,
Perhaps, is why it seems urgent to try to speak
Sensibly about them, about the psychiatrists.

II. Some Terms

'Shrink' is a misnomer. The religious
Analogy is all wrong, too, and the old,
Half-forgotten jokes about Viennese accents

And beards hardly apply to the good-looking woman
In boots and a knit dress, or the man
Seen buying the *Sunday Times* in mutton-chop

Whiskers and expensive running shoes.
In a way I suspect that even the terms 'doctor'
And 'therapist' are misnomers; the patient

Is not necessarily 'sick'. And one assumes
That no small part of the psychiatrist's
Role is just that: to point out misnomers.

VI. Their Seriousness, With Further Comparisons

In a certain sense, they are not serious.
That is, they are serious – useful, deeply helpful,
Concerned – only in the way that the pilots of huge

Planes, radiologists, and master mechanics can,
At their best, be serious. But however profound
The psychiatrists may be, they are not serious the way

A painter may be serious beyond pictures, or a businessman
May be serious beyond property and cash – or even
The way scholars and surgeons are serious, each rapt

In his work's final cause, contingent upon nothing:
Beyond work; persons; recoveries. And this is fitting:
Who would want to fly with a pilot who was *serious*

About getting to the destination safely? Terrifying idea –
That a pilot could over-extend, perhaps try to fly

Too well, or suffer from Pilot's Block; of course,

It may be that (just as they must not drink liquor
Before a flight) they undergo regular, required check-ups
With a psychiatrist, to prevent such things from happening.

The Euphemisms
Peter Reading (1981)

Crackers, Potty, Loony, Bonkers,
Nutty, Screwy, Ga-Ga, Dull,
Strange, Do-Lally, Dopey, Silly,
Touched, A Bit M., Up the Pole,

Zany, Crazy, Dotty, Batty,
Round the Bend, Remedial, Slow,
Cranky, Turned, Moonstruck, Quixotic,
Odd, Beside Oneself, Loco,

Rambling, Giddy, Flighty, Crackbrained,
Soft, Bewildered, Off One's Head,
Wandering, Wild, Bereft of Reason,
Daft, Distracted, Unhingèd;

attributes of Simple Simons,
Asses, Owls, Donkeys, Mules,
Nincompoops, Wiseacres, Boobies,
Noodles, Numskulls, Gawks, Tomfools,

Addle/Silly/Chuckle/Dunder/
Sap/Bone/Block/Thick/Muddle/Crack-
Heads, The E.S.N., The Balmy,
Silly Billies, Dunces, Jack-

Asses, Dullards, Merry Andrews,
Mooncalves, at least one MP,
Vauxhall Workers (and Execs), Clods,
Paisleyites, Twerps, Plaid Cymru ...

from The Day Room
Kit Wright (1983)

3.

Joan's mouth is a crematorium.
Six years after her husband died
It burns and bleeds and weeps, she cannot beat
His flaring ashes down with her tongue.

All in the mind, and pain
(What was said? What left unsaid?)
A child of the mind
That eats the mother.

The widow is burned alive.

4.

Where cigarettes are the entire economy
Domestic policy is locker-love.
Pink stones to arm the military,
White coats for the judiciary,
One hall in hell for all of the above.

6.

Our road's a green carbolic corridor
Off which on certain days the sun
Ripens in small groves. In one

I find her crying because she had lost her lipstick
And, so she said, her bones.
The sun poured down.

We found the lipstick, couldn't find the bones.

8.

Pat threw herself away
From babies, from
A seventh floor. Foetus-coiled
She sleeps all day
On two sun-coloured plastic chairs,
Snug by the mother-warmth
Of the radiator.

12.

Many streets in the hospital,
'The largest of any kind
In Europe' when it was built and many
Minds within the mind.

'The shifting population
Of a grid-iron city.'
Pathetic co-operations and courtesies,
Hunger and pity.

This is your holy mountain,
Your shallow grave.
When nothing's left this is what's left
To save.

Ode to Psychoanalysis
Martin Bell (1988)

I.

I said to Doctor Hackenbush
During abortive analysis,
'I hate the word, Love.'
I meant parents' unhelpful concern,
I meant they had to bring me up
To work hard and do without money
Just as they had:
I had to be neat and industrious
And flatter any bosses around
With my modest ability to cope.

II.

My penis was dangerous, dangerous, dangerous,
Messy and dangerous,
In danger of being cut off.

(My God, the ducks were quacking for it,
And cocks ran round and round without their heads,
My grandmother's cat chased a rabbit's tail on a string.)

My bladder was sadder and madder and badder
When I used to wet the bed.
I remember a cold rubber sheet underneath.
(Dear waters, please, bring back the Flood).

My bowels were a sheer embarrassment,
Holding back in white-faced spite,
And then erupting generosity,
A richness on a social afternoon...

III.

I didn't get very far, acting it out
With Doctor Hackenbush.
I developed, he said,
'A massive negative transference,'
So the analysis was cut off
After I hadn't paid him
For over two months –
He took two-fifths of my wages.
(His name wasn't Hackenbush anyway).
I still wanted to kill Stalin[22]
After that. But I felt I'd let Freud[23] down.

---

[22] Josef Stalin (1878–1953) was leader of the Soviet Union, from the mid-1920s until his death in 1953.
[23] Sigmund Freud (1856–1939) was an Austrian neurologist and founder of psychoanalysis.

The cook would not run the State,
And the State wouldn't wither away,
And psychoanalysis
Was very expensive indeed:
Postpone, for the time being,
The New Jerusalem.

IV.
So here I am, in the middle of several paths,
More or less where I've always been
Having survived war and intensive masturbation
Getting away with murder, maybe
But suffering Hell because I'm always overdrawn
At the bank whose manager hovers
Clacking revengeful shears.

Hey there! Nobodaddy![24]
That's *my* flaming sword...

Bath Night
Hugo Williams (1990)

A nurse kneels on the floor of the bath house
pulling loose Jim's protective underclothes.
'Washing you,' she murmurs,
touching the marks left by the laces.
'Remember now. Washing you.'

Jim stands up very straight and tall,
his eyes screwed shut.
His toes grip the edge of the bath mat.
'Washing you,' he repeats after her.
'Remember washing you.'

The nurse picks up Jim in her arms
and lets him slip out of the towel
into the disinfected water. His wasted legs
loom to the surface like slender birch trunks.
His feet stand up like pale stalks.

He wheels at anchor now, in his element,
and sometimes he floats free of the dry world
in that narrow white boat
that is going nowhere, wreathed in steam.

---

[24]In the work of the English poet, William Blake, Nobodaddy was a satirical conflation of mythical, retributive, paternal gods.

And sometimes he remembers her.

'Washing you,' he murmurs, as the green water
laps his body. 'Remember washing you.'
His eyes are screwed shut.
His arms are folded across his chest
as if he is flying into himself.

Parkinson's Disease[25]
Galway Kinnell (1994)

While spoon-feeding him with one hand
she holds his hand with her other hand,
or rather lets it rest on top of his,
which is permanently clenched shut.
When he turns his head away, she reaches
around and puts in the spoonful blind.
He will not accept the next morsel
until he has completely chewed this one.
His bright squint tells her she finds
the shrimp she has just put in delicious.
Next to the voice and touch of those we love,
food may be our last pleasure on earth –
a man on death row takes his T-bone
in small bites and swishes each sip
of the jug wine around in his mouth,
tomorrow will be too late for them to jolt
this supper out of him. She strokes
his head very slowly, as if to cheer up
each separate discomfited hair sticking up
from its root in his stricken brain.
Standing behind him, she presses
her cheek to his, kisses his jowl,
and his eyes seem to stop seeing
and do nothing but emit light.
Could heaven be a time, after we are dead,
of remembering the knowledge
flesh had from flesh? The flesh
of his face is hard, perhaps
from years spent facing down others
until they fell back, and harder
from years of being himself faced down
and falling back in his turn, and harder still

---

[25]Parkinson's Disease is a degenerative disorder of the central nervous system.

from all the while frowning
and beaming and worrying and shouting
and probably letting go in rages.
His face softens into a kind
of quizzical wince, as if one
of the other animals were working at
getting the knack of the human smile.
When picking up a cookie he uses
both thumbtips to grip it
and push it against an index finger
to secure it so that he can lift it.
She takes him then to the bathroom,
where she lowers his pants and removes
the wet diaper and holds the spout of the bottle
to his old penis until he pisses all he can,
then puts on the fresh diaper and pulls up his pants.
When they come out, she is facing him,
walking backwards in front of him
and holding his hands, pulling him
when he stops, reminding him to step
when he forgets and starts to pitch forward.
She is leading her old father into the future
as far as they can go, and she is walking
him back into her childhood, where she stood
in bare feet on the toes of his shoes
and they foxtrotted on this same rug.
I watch them closely: she could be teaching him
the last steps that one day she may teach me.
At this moment, he glints and shines,
as if it will be only a small dislocation
for him to pass from this paradise into the next.

The Tender Place
Ted Hughes (1995)

Your temples, where the hair crowded in,
Were the tender place. Once to check
I dropped a file across the electrodes
Of a twelve-volt battery – it exploded
Like a grenade. Somebody wired you up.
Somebody pushed the lever. They crashed
The thunderbolt into your skull.
In their bleached coats, with blenched faces,
They hovered again
To see how you were, in your straps.

Whether your teeth were still whole.
The hand on the calibrated lever
Again feeling nothing
Except feeling nothing pushed to feel
Some squirm of sensation. Terror
Was the cloud of you
Waiting for these lightnings. I saw
An oak limb sheared at a bang.
You your Daddy's leg. How many seizures
Did you suffer this god to grab you
By the roots of the hair? The reports
Escaped back into clouds. What went up
Vaporized? Where lightning rods wept copper
And the nerve threw off its skin
Like a burning child
Scampering out of the bomb-flash. They dropped you
A rigid bent bit of wire
Across the Boston City grid. The lights
In the Senate House dipped
As your voice dived inwards
Right through the bolt-hole basement.
Came up, years later,
Over-exposed, like an X-ray –
Brain-map still dark-patched
With the scorched-earth scars
Of your retreat. And your words,
Faces reversed from the light,
Holding in their entrails.

Duke
Bob Hicok (1995)

He was hit back of the head for a haul of $15,
a Diner's Club Card and picture of his daughter in a helmet
on a horse tethered to a pole that centered
its revolving universe. Pacing the halls, he'd ask

for a blow job he didn't want. The ward's new visitors
didn't know this request was all the injury
had left him to say, and would be shamed or pissed,
a few hitting him as he stood with his mouth

slightly open and large frame leaning in. His wife
divorced him for good and blameless reasons. He would not
be coming home to share his thoughts on film and weather,
or remembering her any longer than it took to leave a room.

He liked ham. Kept newspapers in drawers and under his bed,
each unread page hand-pressed flat. And when it snowed
he leaned into one of the sealed, unbreakable windows,
a cheek to the cool glass as he held his fingers

over his mouth and moaned low and constant like the sound
of a boat on the far side of a lake. When he died
they cut him open to see how his habits had been rewired
and so tightly looped. Having known him they were afraid

of what can happen when you cross the lot to the office
or pull up to a light and thump the wheel as you might
any hour. If you stare at the dyed
and beautiful cross sections of a brain, it's natural

to wonder how we extract the taste of coffee
or sense of a note accurately found and held on an oboe
from this bramble. On Duke's slides they circled
the regions of blight which explain

why almost all behavior we recognize as human was lost,
but not why a man who'd curl into a ball
like a caterpillar when barely touched, could only ask
for sex, for intimacy, for the very thing

he could least accept and lived twelve years without,
no embrace or caress, no kiss on the lips before sleep,
until he died in the lounge looking out on winter sky
that seemed eager to snow all day but didn't.

The Coma[26]
C. K. Williams (1997)

'My character wound,' he'd written so shortly before, 'my flaw,' and now he
    was dying,
his heart, his anguished heart stopping, maiming his brain, then being started
    again;
'my loneliness,' in his childish square cursive, 'I've been discarded but I've
    earned it,
I'd like to grow fainter and fainter then disappear; my arrogant, inauthentic
    false self.'

'My weak, hopeless, incompetent reparations,' he'd written in his lone-lines
    and despair,
'there's so much I'm afraid of facing, my jealousy, my inertia; roots are tearing
    from my brain.'

---

[26]In memory of S. J. Marks.

And now, as he lay in his coma, I thought I could hear him again, 'I'm
    insensitive, ineffectual,
I seethe with impatience,' hear him driving himself with the shattered bolt of his
    mind deeper,

'It's my fault, my arrogant doubt, my rage,' but I hoped, imagining him now
    waking downwards,
hoped he'd believe for once in the virtues his ruined past had never let him
    believe in,
his gifts for sympathy, kindness, compassion; in the ever-ascending downwards
    of dying,
I hoped he'd know that his passion to be goodness had made him good-ness,
    like a child;

not 'my malaise, my destructive neurosis': let him have known for him-self his
    purity and his warmth;
not 'my crippled, hateful disdain': let have come to him, in his last lift away
    from himself,
his having wanted to heal the world he'd found so wounded in himself; let him
    have known,
though his sorrow wouldn't have wanted him to, that, in his love and affliction,
    he had.

Alzheimer's[27]
Bob Hicok (1998)

Chairs move by themselves, and books.
Grandchildren visit, stand
new and nameless, their faces' puzzles
missing pieces. She's like a fish

in deep ocean, its body made of light.
She floats through rooms, through
my eyes, an old woman bereft
of chronicle, the parable of her life.

And though she's almost a child
there's still blood between us:
I passed through her to arrive.
So I protect her from knives,

stairs, from the street that calls
as rivers do, a summons to walk away,
to follow. And dress her,
demonstrate how buttons work,

---

[27]Alzheimer's disease is a chronic neurodegenerative disease, accounting for 60–70 per cent of all cases of
dementia.

when she sometimes looks up
and says my name, the sound arriving
like the trill of a bird so rare
it's rumoured no longer to exist.

The Nerve Doctors
Thomas Lux (2001)

Here they come by the busload, the nerve doctors.
Some journey overland
(many die on mountain passes),
some take the river routes, some fly
(after dosing on Veronal),
some just send their brains
or disciples, a few walk all night
across salt plains. They continue
to arrive – every hotel room
two to a bed in nerve doctors,
three deep at the bar of every saloon,
and still they disembark
for the convention,
their big meeting. It's election year
and all the nerve doctors are here – there's a group
from China, and that huddle
over there, they came by train
from Omaha, Nebraska, USA.
The three from France seem to be in psychic pain.
The nerve doctors stand in small aggregations,
nodding, rocking on the balls
of their feet, consulting (each one says
when another finishes a sentence, *I have listened*) about
the election, and about who
the next nerve doctors' president will be,
and where – since it is his choice – the next
nerve doctors' convention
shall be held.

from Lou-Lou
Selima Hill (2004)

In A Hedge JULY 25th

This hedge
is like a nice airy tent
where I can take my overdose
in peace,

hidden from the prying eyes of those
who've chosen not to kill themselves today;
who walk about the streets as if it's easy,
as if they were *born*
to wear big shoes and clothes.
Well, I prefer to sit it out down here,
letting ants play havoc with my hair
before the nurses
turned it into a sort of perfumed hat.
They thought it would cheer me up but it hasn't.
It's like having something alive on top of my head...
in the dusk the tall bony trees
glare at me as if I should be going...

Having it out with Melancholy
Jane Kenyon (2005)

> '*If many remedies are prescribed for an illness,
> you may be certain that the illness has no cure.*'
> A. P. Checkhov, *The Cherry Orchard*

1. From The Nursery

When I was born, you waited
behind a pile of linen in the nursery,
and when we were alone, you lay down
on top of me, pressing
the bile of desolation into every pore.

And from that day on
everything under the sun and moon
made me sad – even the yellow
wooden beads that slid and spun
along a spindle on my crib.

You taught me to exist without gratitude.
You ruined my manners toward God:
'We're here simply to wait for death;
the pleasures of earth are overrated.'

I only appeared to belong to my mother,
to live among blocks and cotton undershirts
with snaps; among red tin lunch boxes
and report cards in ugly brown slipcases.
I was already yours – the anti-urge,
the mutilator of souls.

2. Bottles

Elavil, Ludiomil, Doxepin,
Norpramin, Prozac, Lithium, Xanax,
Wellbutrin, Parnate, Nardil, Zoloft.
The coated ones smell sweet or have
no smell; the powdery ones smell
like the chemistry lab at school
that made me hold my breath.

3. Suggestion From A Friend

You wouldn't be so depressed
if you really believed in God.

4. Often

Often I go to bed as soon after dinner
as seems adult
(I mean I try to wait for dark)
in order to push away
from the massive pain in sleep's
frail wicker coracle.

5. Once There Was Light

Once, in my early thirties, I saw
that I was a speck of light in the great
river of light that undulates through time.

I was floating with the whole
human family. We were all colors – those
who are living now, those who have died,
those who are not yet born. For a few

moments I floated, completely calm,
and I no longer hated having to exist.

Like a crow who smells hot blood
you came flying to pull me out
of the glowing stream.
'I'll hold you up. I never let my dear
ones drown!' After that, I wept for days.

6. In And Out

The dog searches until he finds me
upstairs, lies down with a clatter
of elbows, puts his head on my foot.

Sometimes the sound of his breathing
saves my life – in and out, in
and out; a pause, a long sigh...

7. Pardon

A piece of burned meat
wears my clothes, speaks
in my voice, dispatches obligations
haltingly, or not at all.
It is tired of trying
to be stouthearted, tired
beyond measure.

We move on to the monoamine
oxidase inhibitors. Day and night
I feel as if I had drunk six cups
of coffee, but the pain stops
abruptly. With the wonder
and bitterness of someone pardoned
for a crime she did not commit
I come back to marriage and friends,
to pink fringed hollyhocks; come back
to my desk, books, and chair.

8. *Credo*

Pharmaceutical wonders are at work
but I believe only in this moment
of well-being. Unholy ghost,
you are certain to come again.

Coarse, mean, you'll put your feet
on the coffee table, lean back,
and turn me into someone who can't
take the trouble to speak; someone
who can't sleep, or who does nothing
but sleep; can't read, or call
for an appointment for help.

There is nothing I can do
against your coming.
When I awake, I am still with thee.

9. Wood Thrush

High on Nardil and June light
I wake at four,

waiting greedily for the first
note of the wood thrush. Easeful air
presses through the screen
with the wild, complex song
of the bird, and I am overcome

by ordinary contentment.
What hurt me so terribly
all my life until this moment?
How I love the small, swiftly
beating heart of the bird
singing in the great maples;
its bright, unequivocal eye.

Tinnitus[28]
John McAuliffe (2010)

My father's tinnitus is like the hiss off a water cooler,
only louder. And it doesn't just stop like, say, a hand-dryer – the worst is
it comes and goes. Or you shine a light on it
and it looks permanent as the sea,

a tideless sea that won't go away. The masker
he's been prescribed *is* a machine, an arc of white noise
that blacks out a lot
but can't absorb the interference totally

any more than you or I – taking the air,
stirring milk into coffee, daydreaming through the six o'clock news,
trying to sleep on a wet night –
can simply switch off what's always there, a particular memory

nagging away, the erosive splash off a little river
wearing through the road, say, on the Connor Pass,[29]
a day out, through which he'd accelerate
in the flash, orange Capri.[30]

Public Speaking
Andy Brown (2013)

My father was a man of very few words
and, curiously, a well-versed public speaker.

---

[28]Tinnitus is the perception of sound within the human ear when no external sound is present.
[29]The Connor Pass, Dingle Peninsula, Ireland, is the highest mountain pass in Ireland, with a narrow, winding road.
[30]The Ford Capri is a fastback coupé.

He began every speech with the same old joke:
Unaccustomed as I am to public speaking...

before launching into his theme, after dinner
to the Board, a lunch at the Club,
at weddings, birthdays, parties, funerals,
he'd take the stand and roll the old line out.

My father was an orator, self-taught.
His dog-eared copy of *Teach Yourself...*
sits in his scant library – he never was
a letters man and often was quiet at home

or, when on the phone, found chatting hard.
But publicly he wasn't shy. I think of him
the days before a speech, mugging up
on helpful tips from *Teach Yourself:*

*Practice and rehearse your speech at home
or where you'll surely be at ease, in front
of a mirror, your family, or friends...*
this duly noted, circumscribed in pencil.

Appear relaxed, even when you're not...
he's jotted in the margins of
a well-thumbed page on *Building Your Rapport,*
which also recommends to tell a joke:

Unaccustomed as I am to public speaking...

After the brain disease[31] began to make
greater strangers of his mind and tongue,
we picked-up only garbled fogs of sound.
Squeeze my hand, we used to say, *if you can hear us dad,*

then wait in silence for the pressure.
We watched him disappear until he reached
the farthest point and, though I can't recall
his final words, his marginalia will serve:

*Address your speech to the person farthest away
to ensure your voice is loud enough to be heard.*

---

[31]Amyotrophic lateral sclerosis (ALS, also: Lou Gehrig's disease, Charcot's disease, and motor neurone disease), is characterized by stiff, twitching, wasting muscles, which results in difficulty speaking, swallowing and breathing.

MEDICAL WRITING:

The English Malady
George Cheyne (1733)

The title I have chosen for this treatise is a reproach universally thrown on this island by foreigners, and all our neighbours on the continent, by whom nervous distempers, spleen, vapours, and lowness of spirits are in derision called the English Malady. And I wish there were not so good grounds for this reflection. The moisture of our air, the variableness of our weather, (from the situation amidst the ocean), the rankness and fertility of our soil, the richness and heaviness of our food, the wealth and abundance of the inhabitants (from their universal trade), the inactivity and sedentary occupations of the better sort (among whom this evil mostly rages) and the humour[32] of living in great, populous and consequently unhealthy towns, have brought forth a class and set of distempers, with atrocious and frightful symptoms, scarce known to our ancestors, and never rising to such fatal heights, nor afflicting such numbers in any other known nation. These nervous disorders being computed to make almost one third of the complaints of the people of condition in England.

Observations on the Nature, Causes and Cure of those Disorders which have been commonly called Nervous, Hypochondriac, or Hysteric
Robert Whyte (1765)

Nothing makes more sudden, or more surprising changes in the body, than the several passions of the mind. These, however, act solely by the mediation of the brain, and, in a strong light, show its sympathy with every part of the system.

Such is the constitution of the animal frame, that certain ideas or affections excited in the mind, are always accompanied with corresponding motions or feelings in the body; and these are owing to some change made in the brain and nerves, by the mind or *sentient principle*[33]: but what that change is, or how it produces those effects, we know not: as little can we tell, why shame should raise a heat and redness in the face, while fear is attended with a paleness. These and many other effects of the different passions must be referred to the original constitution of our frame, or the laws of union between the soul and body.

But although, in these matters, we must confess our ignorance, yet, from what we certainly know of the action of the nerves, we can easily see, that a change in them may occasion many of those effects which are produced by the passions.

As the force of the heart, and the regularity with which it contracts, depend, in a great measure, on the state of its nerves, so does the action of the arterial system, in carrying on the circulation; and particularly those alternate contractions, with which

---

[32]Humour: the condition, or characteristic of.
[33]Author's note: By the *sentient principle,* I understand the mind or soul in man, and that principle in brutes which resembles it.

the minuter vessels are continually agitated, and to which the motion of the fluids in them is, in a great measure, owing.

The other muscles of the body are often, by an uncommon exertion of the nervous power, affected either with alternate convulsive motions, or a continued spasm. It is reasonable, therefore, to think, that the heart and vascular system may suffer in the same manner; and that, when the influence of the nerves is much weakened, or in some measure suspended, the vessels will be relaxed, the circulation will become languid, and an universal debility will ensue.

The increased force of the heart, and sometimes indeed of the whole muscles of the body, from great anger or rage, is to be ascribed to a stronger exertion of the nervous power; while the trembling and debility produced by fear, arise from a contrary cause.

The palpitation of the heart from terror, seems to proceed from the blood returning to it, in too great a quantity, in consequence of a sudden spasm or contraction of the veins. It is also, in part, occasioned by the heart being rendered more irritable, or being otherwise disturbed by the violent agitation of the nervous system.

The redness and glow of the face from a sense of shame, are most probably owing to an increased motion of the small arteries of that part; for the florid colour and sudden warmth, seem to be more the consequences of a quicker motion of the blood in these vessels, than a stagnation of it from any compression or spasm of the veins, which would produce but a livid redness and less heat. Besides, we know, that a greater degree of redness is, instantly, brought on the eyes, and, in a short time, on the skin, by an increased motion of their small Vessels, upon the application of acrid substances to them.

Some grow pale upon anger, which effect may be owing to a spasm, or continued contraction of the small arteries of the face, by which the motion of the blood in them will be retarded.

The paleness from fear may arise from a different cause, *viz.* a deficiency of the nervous *power:* Hence, though the small vessels are not affected with any spasm, as in anger; yet they are, in a great measure, deprived of their alternate contractions, to which the motion of the blood in them is principally owing. But the more than usual flow of the blood towards the heart, occasioned by terror, seems to show, that the veins, at least, are suddenly contracted.

The diminution of perspiration attending such passions as affect us with sadness, may be owing to the impaired force of the heart and arteries: and the *diarrhea* from fear, may be a consequence of obstructed perspiration, or of that debility and relaxation, which fear, or grief, is observed to bring on the alimentary canal.

The increased secretion of tears from grief, and the great flux of limpid urine, which is often occasioned by fear or vexation, are owing to an increased motion, excited by these passions, in the small arteries and excretory ducts of the lachrymal glands and kidneys.

The dull look of the eyes in grief, and their lively appearance from joy, depend upon a diminution or increase of the motion of the fluids through the small vessels of that organ, particularly of the *cornea,* in consequence of their vibratory motions being lessened or augmented, by the change which those different passions produce in their nerves.

It would be easy, upon the same principles, to account for various other effects produced by the passions; but what is already said, will be sufficient for showing in what manner we can reason upon this subject.

Mind and Brain
Thomas Laycock (1860)

'The Differences in the Constitutions of the Sexes: The Constitution of Woman'

I have already hinted at the differences which arise in the two sexes, in consequence of that law of physiological division of labour, in virtue of which two distinct organisms are required for the maintenance of the species. Now, while it is certain that many of the peculiarities of woman depend wholly upon her social relations, and these, again, upon the functions of the generative glands, it is equally certain that the evolution of them is due to a primordial difference in the force of evolution in her as compared with man ...

'Differences in Sexes as to the Nervous System'

It is, however, in the emotional development of her nervous system that we have the most striking differences. Woman, as compared with man, is of the nervous temperament. Her nervous system is therefore more easily acted upon by all impressions, and more liable to all diseases of excitement. Her sedentary habits, and the less perfect condition of her blood when resident in towns, greatly increases this natural sensibility or affectibility of her nervous system; and when both are combined with the erethistic[34] influence of the generative glands on the nerve-centres, the varied morbid states of the cœnæsthesis,[35] grouped under the term 'Hysteria', result. Now men, no doubt, are sometimes hysterical; but it will be found that in these apparently exceptional instances, the general causes are really those of hysteria proper.

Men are more liable to that form of insanity which is associated with general paralysis. Its frequency in women is stated very variously by writers, but all recognize that it is comparatively rare in them. The nature and causes of this disease have been much discussed, and are still undetermined by the majority of those few physicians who have inquired into its pathology.

The Fallacies of Memory
Frances Power Cobbe (1866)

In the details of History, the characteristic anecdotes, the striking speeches, the whole character of remarkable men, we find ourselves constantly more and more driven, first to question, and then to rescind the judgment and testimony of the past. In judicial inquiries, we constantly find that the most experienced lawyers are the

---

[34]Erethism is excessive sensitivity or stimulation in an organ, particularly sexual organs.
[35]Cœnæsthesis or vital sense, is the general sensation of one's own body.

most completely satisfied of the unreliability of a large part of the evidence given concerning ordinary events; and of the double doubtfulness attaching to the evidence which relates to events witnessed under strong excitement. In private life we find the vast majority of our past days a blank in recollection, and of the scenes, the persons, the transactions of which we suppose ourselves to have a true remembrance, we rarely test any single point, by memoranda, photographs, collateral testimony, or in any other way, without finding we have erred if not essentially in the main features of the case, yet in details which, according to circumstances, might become precisely the important points of our testimony. Surely, in the face of these facts, it is idle to go on acting as if lapses of memory were exceptional, and the accurate use of the faculty a thing to be expected and calculated upon. Surely, it is time we should change our gratuitous confidence in this most deceptive faculty for a very cautious distrust of its allegations, whenever we lack time or opportunity to verify them.

It would be an invaluable service to mankind, we believe, were it possible to offer such a philosophy of memory as might serve for the basis of scientific analysis of the faculty, and a method of distinguishing its false from its true exercise. To the framing of such a philosophy, the writer of this brief essay can make no pretension; nor to the remotest suggestions, helping to throw more light than has been already shed by psychological writers upon the nature and laws of this department of our mental organization. One observation only we presume to make on this most obscure subject, and that observation will only tend to correct a misleading metaphor, commonly applied to memory, and serving much to keep up the prevalent false estimate of its veracity. Memory is forever likened by poets and rhetoricians to an engraved tablet, treasured in the recesses of mind, and liable only to obliteration by the slow abrasion of time, or the dissolving heat of madness. We venture to affirm that such a simile is not in the remotest degree applicable to the real phenomena of the case, and that memory is neither an impression made, once for all, like an engraving on a tablet, nor yet safe for an hour from obliteration or modification, after being formed. Rather is memory a finger mark traced on shifting sand, ever exposed to obliteration when left unrenewed, and if renewed, then modified, and made not the same, but a fresh and different mark. Beyond the first time of recalling a place or event, it is rare (we maintain), to remember again actually the place or the event. We remember not the things themselves, but the joint recollection of them, and then the second and the third, always the latest recollection of them.

...

By this theory of memory, we obtain an available hypothesis, to account for the notorious but marvellous fact, that liars come in time to believe their own falsehoods. The warping of the original trace of the story, albeit voluntary and conscious, has, equally with unconscious dereliction, effected the end of obliterating the primary mark, and substituting a false one, which has assumed the place of a remembrance. Without conscious falsehood, the same thing happens also occasionally when we realize strongly by imagination some circumstance which never happened, or happened to another person.

A most truthful woman asserted that a certain adventure had befallen her; it had really befallen her child, but the child repeating it often to her, she had realized it so vividly that it seemed her own experience. Another mother asserted that the horses depicted in Rosa Bonheurs great picture were as large as life.[36] Her little boy had asked whether they could be ridden on, and her maternal imagination had stopped with that of her child. A very common way in which the same mendacious effect is produced, is by the habit of speculating on what would have happened had certain contingencies been otherwise than they were. We begin by saying: It might have happened so and so, till having realized in fancy that hypothetical case more vividly than we remember the real one, we suddenly and unconsciously substitute the fancy for the fact.

Principles of Mental Physiology
William B. Carpenter (1875)

The state of Mania is usually characterized by the combination of complete derangement of the Intellectual powers, with passionate excitement upon every point which in the least degree affects the Feelings. There is, however, a considerable amount of variety in the symptoms of Mania, depending upon differences in the relative degree of *intellectual* and of *emotional* disturbance. For there may be such a derangement of the former, as gives rise to complete incoherence in the succession of ideas, so that the reasoning power is altogether suspended; and yet there may be at the same time an entire absence of emotional excitement, so that the condition of the mind is closely allied to that of Dreaming or of rambling Delirium.

On the other hand, the intellectual powers may be themselves but little disturbed, the trains of thought being coherent, and the reasoning processes correctly performed; but there may be such a state of general emotional excitability, that nothing is *felt* as it should be, and the most violent passion may be aroused and sustained by the most trivial incidents, or by the wrong ideas which are formed by the mind as a consequence of their misinterpretation.

Between these two opposite states, and that in which the disturbance affects at the same time the intellectual and the emotional part of the mental nature, there is a complete succession of transitional links; but, underlying all phases of this condition (these often passing into each other in the same individual), there is one constant element, namely, the deficiency of Volitional control over the succession of thought and feeling. This deficiency appears to be a primary element in those forms which, essentially consist in Intellectual disturbance; whilst in those of which Emotional excitement is the prominent feature, it results apparently from the overpowering mastery that is exercised over the Will, by the states of uncontrollable passion which succeed each other with little or no interval. It seems probable, however, from the phenomena of Intoxication, that the very same agency which is the cause of undue emotional excitability, also tends to produce an absolute diminution in the power of volitional control.

It is chiefly (but not solely) in those cases in which the Cerebral power has been weakened by a succession of attacks of Mania, Epilepsy, or some other disorder which consists in a perverted action of the whole organ, that we find the intellectual

---

[36]Rosa Bonheurs' painting *The Horse Fair* (1852–55).

powers specially and permanently disordered; the succession of thought becoming incoherent, and the perception of those relations of ideas on which all reasoning processes depend, being more or less completely obscured. The failure usually shows itself *first* in the power of volitional direction, and especially in the faculty of recollection.

...

There may, however, be no primary disorder of the Intellectual faculties; and the Insanity may essentially consist in a tendency to disordered emotional excitement; which affects the course of thought, and consequently of action, without disturbing the reasoning processes in any other way than by supplying wrong materials to them. Now the Emotional disturbance may be either general or special: that is, there may be a derangement of feeling upon almost every subject, matters previously indifferent becoming invested with strong pleasurable or painful interest, things which were previously repulsive being greedily sought, and those which were previously the most attractive being in like manner repelled; or, on the other hand, there may be a peculiar intensification of some one class of feelings or impulses, which thus acquire a settled domination over the whole character, and cause every idea with which they connect themselves to be presented to the mind under an erroneous aspect.

Lectures on the Diseases of the Nervous System, delivered at La Salpêtrière Jean-Martin Charcot (1877)

I must be allowed once more to declare my firm belief that the wide intervention of the anatomical and physiological sciences in the affairs of medicine is an essential condition to progress; a statement which, by frequent repetition, has verily by this time become almost a platitude. But the point that I wish specially to insist on is this; in order that the intervention of these sciences may be legitimate, and really fruitful, it should take place under conditions which should never be forgotten. Allow me to recall to your minds the opinion which that most illustrious physiologist, Claude Bernard,[37] thus expressed: '*Pathology*,' said he, '*should not he subordinated to physiology. Quite the reverse. Set up first the medical problem which arises from the observation of a malady, and afterwards seek for a physiological explanation. To act otherwise would be to risk overlooking the patient, and distorting the malady.*' These are excellent words, which I have ventured to quote verbatim, because they are absolutely significant. They enable us to clearly understand that the whole domain of pathology appertains strictly to the physician, who alone can cultivate it and make it fruitful, and that it necessarily remains closed to the physiologist who, systematically confined within the precincts of his laboratory, disdains the teaching of the hospital ward.

The method most suitable to the exploration of the vast domains of pathology can be described as the *nosological*.[38] It is, in fact, the traditional method, for it is

---

[37]Claude Bernard (1813–78) was a French physiologist and one of the first to suggest the use of blind experiments to ensure the objectivity of scientific observations.

[38]Author's note: Nosological refers to the nomenclature and classification of disease, but it is the clinical

the one which, ever since medicine has existed, has been employed to investigate morbid states, to determine their characteristics, their causation, their correlations, and the modifications which they undergo by the influence of therapeutic agents. And facts of this kind, gentlemen, I beg you to observe, necessarily constitute the very foundation of every scientific construction in pathology, and without this basis the physiology of disease would be but a vain phrase.

If it is necessary, in the category of diseases of the nervous system, to show all the power of this method, it will suffice to recall a portion of the inimitable work of that great representative of French neuro-pathology, Duchenne (of Boulogne).[39] Without doubt his admirable study of muscular movements, made by the aid of localised electricity, could be, up to a certain point, claimed by the science of physiology. But it is not so with his grand discovery of those types of disease termed progressive muscular atrophy, infantile paralysis, pseudo-hypertrophic paralysis, glosso-laryngeal paralysis, and locomotor ataxy.[40] These results, undoubtedly the greatest achievements of his work, because they filled spaces hitherto empty, or occupied only by confused ideas, with animated living shapes, concrete realities, recognised by all; these results, I say, were accomplished entirely by the nosological method.

But this method need not necessarily be restricted to the observation of the outward manifestation of disease; it can, without changing its character, be appropriately applied in exploring the domain of morbid anatomy by following the patient into the post-mortem room.

It is often said that the progress of medicine and of pathological anatomy go side by side. This is specially true in diseases of the nervous system. One example will suffice to show that the discovery of a constant lesion in maladies of this kind is the result of such a co-operation.

The description given by Duchenne (of Boulogne) of locomotor ataxy, is most striking and vivid. It rightly takes rank as a masterpiece. However, there existed for a long time a hesitation in the minds of many about accepting the disease as a real entity until the spinal lesion … was known to be associated with this group of symptoms.

Some authors still continued to believe that the affection was functional in its origin. But all illusions of this kind vanished when it became realised that there existed, even in the earliest stages of the disease, an exact and easily recognised anatomical change, an anatomical lesion which could be detected even in the slight and aberrant forms of the disease.

…

In this case as in very many others, it is the intervention of pathological anatomy which gives the truly practical character. It furnishes to nosography more fixed, more material characters than appertain to the symptoms alone; and thus one does not fail to grasp the nature of the connections which unite the lesions to the outward signs.

---

method of investigation, in its widest sense, which is implied here; or that method of investigation which argues from effect to cause, commencing with a study of disease at the bedside.

[39]Guillaume-Benjamin-Amand Duchenne de Boulogne (1806–75) was a French physician who advanced electrophsiology and neurology through his experiments with clinical photography.

[40]These are all forms of a neurological lack of control of muscle movement.

Without detracting from the importance of the results obtained in this way, it is certain that the study of morbid lesions can be utilised in another way, and from a higher standpoint; more scientific if you like. It can, when the circumstances are favourable, furnish the basis of a physiological interpretation of normal or of morbid phenomena, and at the same time, as a natural consequence, give to diagnosis more penetration and exactitude.

American Nervousness: Its Causes and Consequences
George Miller Beard (1881)

The causes of American nervousness are complicated, but are not beyond analysis: first of all modern civilization. The phrase modern civilization is used with emphasis, for civilization alone does not cause nervousness. The Greeks were certainly civilized, but they were not nervous, and in the Greek language there is no word for that term. The ancient Romans were civilized, as judged by any standard. Civilization is therefore a relative term, and as such is employed throughout this treatise. The modern differ from the ancient civilizations mainly in these five elements – steam power, the periodical press, the telegraph, the sciences, and the mental activity of women. When civilization, plus these five factors, invades any nation, it must carry nervousness and nervous diseases along with it.

...

Edison's[41] electric light is now sufficiently advanced in an experimental direction to give us the best possible illustration of the effects of modern civilization on the nervous system. An electric machine of definite horse-power, situated at some central point, is to supply the electricity needed to run a certain number of lamps – say one thousand, more or less. If an extra number of lamps should be interposed in the circuit, then the power of the engine must be increased; else the light of the lamps would be decreased, or give out. This has been mathematically calculated, so that it is known, or believed to be known, by those in charge, just how much increase of horse-power is needed for each increase in the number of lamps. In all the calculations, however widely they may differ, it is assumed that the force supplied by any central machine is limited, and cannot be pushed beyond a certain point; and if the number of lamps interposed in the circuit be increased, there must be a corresponding increase in the force of the machine.

The nervous system of man is the centre of the nerve-force supplying all the organs of the body. Like the steam engine, its force is limited, although it cannot be mathematically measured – and, unlike the steam engine, varies in amount of force with the food, the state of health and external conditions, varies with age, nutrition, occupation, and numberless factors. The force in this nervous system can, therefore, be increased or diminished by good or evil influences, medical or hygienic, or by the natural evolutions – growth, disease and decline; but none the

---

[41]Thomas Alva Edison (1847–1931) was an American inventor and businessman who developed many devices that greatly influenced life around the globe, including the phonograph, the motion picture camera and the electric light bulb.

less it is limited; and when new functions are interposed in the circuit, as modern civilization is constantly requiring us to do, there comes a period, sooner or later, varying in different individuals, and at different times of life, when the amount of force is insufficient to keep all the lamps actively burning; those that are weakest go out entirely, or, as more frequently happens, burn faint and feebly – they do not expire, but give an insufficient and unstable light – this is the philosophy of modern nervousness. The invention of printing, the extension of steam power into manufacturing interests and into means of conveyance, the telegraph, the periodical press, the political machinery of free countries, the religious excitements that are the sequels of Protestantism – the activities of philanthropy, made necessary by the increase of civilization, and of poverty, and certain forms of disease – and, more than all, perhaps, the heightening and extending complexity of modern education in and out of schools and universities, the inevitable effect of the rise of modern science and the expansion of history in all its branches – all these are so many additional lamps interposed in the circuit, and are supplied at the expense of the nervous system, the dynamic power of which has not correspondingly increased.

Necessary Evils of Specialization: One evil, and hardly looked-for effect of the introduction of steam, together with the improved methods of manufacturing of recent times, has been the training in special departments or duties – so that artisans, instead of doing or preparing to do, all the varieties of the manipulations needed in the making of any article, are restricted to a few simple exiguous movements, to which they give their whole lives – in the making of a rifle, or a watch, each part is constructed by experts on that part. The effect of this exclusive concentration of mind and muscle to one mode of action, through months and years, is both negatively and positively pernicious, and notably so, when re-enforced, as it almost universally is, by the bad air of overheated and ill-ventilated establishments. Herein is one unanticipated cause of the increase of insanity and other diseases of the nervous system among the laboring and poorer classes. The steam engine, which would relieve work, as it was hoped, and allow us to be idle, has increased the amount of work done a thousand fold; and with that increase in quantity there has been a differentiation of quality and specialization of function which, so far forth, is depressing both to mind and body. In the professions – the constringing power of specialization is neutralized very successfully by general culture and observation, out of which specialties spring, and by which they are supported; but for the artisan there is no time, or chance, or hope, for such redeeming and antidotal influences.

Clocks and Watches – Necessity of Punctuality: The perfection of clocks and the invention of watches have something to do with modern nervousness, since they compel us to be on time, and excite the habit of looking to see the exact moment, so as not to be late for trains or appointments. Before the general use of these instruments of precision in time, there was a wider margin for all appointments; a longer period was required and prepared for, especially in travelling – coaches of the olden period were not expected to start like steamers or trains, on the instant – men judged of the time by probabilities, by looking at the sun, and needed not, as a rule, to be nervous about the loss of a moment, and had incomparably fewer experiences wherein a delay of a few moments might destroy the hopes of a lifetime. A nervous man cannot take out his watch and look at it when the time for an appointment or train is near, without affecting his pulse, and the effect on that pulse, if we could but measure and weigh it, would be found to be correlated to a loss to the nervous system.

Punctuality is a greater thief of nervous force than is procrastination of time. We are under constant strain, mostly unconscious, oftentimes in sleeping as well as in waking hours, to get somewhere or do something at some definite moment. Those who would relieve their nervousness may well study the manners of the Turks, who require two weeks to execute a promise that the Anglo-Saxon would fulfil in a moment. In Constantinople indolence is the ideal, as work is the ideal in London and New York; the follower of the Prophet is ashamed to be in haste, and would apologize for keeping a promise. There are those who prefer, or fancy they prefer, the sensations of movement and activity to the sensations of repose; but from the standpoint only of economy of nerve-force all our civilization is a mistake; every mile of advance into the domain of ideas, brings a conflict that knows no rest, and all conquests are to be paid for, before delivery often, in blood and nerve and life. We cannot have civilization and have anything else, the price at which nature disposes of this luxury being all the rest of her domain.

...

Rapid Development and Acceptance of New Ideas: The rapidity with which new truths are discovered, accepted and popularized in modern times is a proof and result of the extravagance of our civilization. Philosophies and discoveries as well as inventions which in the Middle Ages would have been passed by or dismissed with the murder of the author, are in our time – and notably in our country – taken up and adopted, in innumerable ways made practical – modified, developed, actively opposed, possibly overthrown and displaced within a few years, and all of necessity at a great expenditure of force.

The experiments, inventions, and discoveries of Edison alone have made and are now making constant and exhausting draughts on the nervous forces of America and Europe, and have multiplied in very many ways, and made more complex and extensive, the tasks and agonies not only of practical men, but of professors and teachers and students everywhere; the simple attempt to master the multitudinous directions and details of the labors of this one young man with all his thousands and thousands of experiments and hundreds of patents and with all the soluble and insoluble physical problems suggested by his discoveries would itself be a sufficient task for even a genius in science; and any high school or college in which his labors were not recognized and the results of his labors were not taught would be patronized only for those who prefer the eighteenth century to the twentieth.

On the mercantile or practical side the promised discoveries and inventions of this one man have kept millions of capital and thousands of capitalists in suspense and distress on both sides of the sea. In contrast with the gradualness of thought movement in the Middle Ages, consider the dazzling swiftness with which the theory of evolution and the agnostic philosophy have extended and solidified their conquests until the whole world of thought seems hopelessly subjected to their autocracy. I once met in society a young man just entering the silver decade, but whose hair was white enough for one of sixty, and he said that the color changed in a single day, as a sign and result of a mental conflict in giving up his religion for science. Many are they who have passed, or are yet to pass through such conflict, and at far greater damage to the nerve centres.

...

Repression of Emotion: One cause of the increase of nervous diseases is that the conventionalities of society require the emotions to be repressed, while the activity of our civilization gives an unprecedented freedom and opportunity for the expression of the intellect; the more we feel the more we must restrain our feelings. This expression of emotion and expression of reason, when carried to a high degree, as in the most active nations, tend to exhaustion, the one by excessive toil and friction, the other by restraining and shutting up within the mind those feelings which are best relieved by expression. Laughter and tears are safety-valves; the savage and the child laugh or cry when they feel like it – and it takes but little to make them feel like it; in all high civilization like the present, it is not polite either to laugh or to cry in public; the emotions which would lead us to do either the one or the other, thus turn in on the brain and expend themselves on its substance; the relief which should come from the movements of muscles in laughter and from the escape of tears in crying is denied us; nature will not, however, be robbed; her loss must be paid and the force which might be expended in muscular actions of the face in laughter and on the whole body in various movements reverberates on the brain and dies away in the cerebral cells.

Constant inhibition, restraining normal feelings, keeping back, covering, holding in check atomic forces, of the mind and body, is an exhausting process, and to this process all civilization is constantly subjected.

A modern philosopher of the most liberal school, states that he hates to hear one laugh aloud, regarding the habit, as he declares, a survival of barbarism.

Domestic and Financial Trouble: Family and financial sorrows, and secret griefs of various kinds, are very commonly indeed the exciting cause of neurasthenia. In very many cases where overwork is the assigned cause – and where it is brought prominently into notice, the true cause, philosophically, is to be found in family broils or disappointments, business failures or mishaps, or some grief that comes very near to one, and, rightly or wrongly, is felt to be very serious.

The savage has no property and cannot fail; he has so little to win of wealth or possessions, that he has no need to be anxious. If his wife does not suit he divorces or murders her; and if all things seem to go wrong he kills himself.

Mourning and Melancholia
Sigmund Freud (1917)

In mourning we found that the inhibition and loss of interest are fully accounted for by the work of mourning in which the ego is absorbed. In melancholia, the unknown loss will result in a similar internal work and will therefore be responsible for the melancholic inhibition. The difference is that the inhibition of the melancholic seems puzzling to us because we cannot see what it is that is absorbing him so entirely. The melancholic displays something else besides which is lacking in mourning – an extraordinary diminution in his self-regard, an impoverishment of his ego on a grand scale. In mourning it is the world which has become poor and empty; in melancholia it is the ego itself. The patient represents his ego to us as worthless, incapable of any achievement and morally despicable; he reproaches himself, vilifies himself and expects to be cast out and punished. He abases himself before everyone and commiserates with his own relatives for being connected with anyone so unworthy. He is not of the opinion that a change has taken place in him, but extends his self-criticism back over the past; he declares that he was never any better. This picture of a delusion of (mainly moral) inferiority is completed by sleeplessness and refusal to take nourishment, and – what is psychologically very remarkable – by an overcoming of the instinct which compels every living thing to cling to life.

It would be equally fruitless from a scientific and a therapeutic point of view to contradict a patient who brings these accusations against his ego. He must surely be right in some way and be describing something that is as it seems to him to be. Indeed, we must at once confirm some of his statements without reservation. He really is as lacking in interest and as incapable of love and achievement as he says.

But that, as we know, is secondary; it is the effect of the internal work which is consuming his ego – work which is unknown to us but which is comparable to the work of mourning. He also seems to us justified in certain other self-accusations; it is merely that he has a keener eye for the truth than other people who are not melancholic. When in his heightened self-criticism he describes himself as petty, egoistic, dishonest, lacking in independence, one whose sole aim has been to hide the weaknesses of his own nature, it may be, so far as we know, that he has come pretty near to understanding himself; we only wonder why a man has to be ill before he can be accessible to a truth of this kind. For there can be no doubt that if anyone holds and expresses to others an opinion of himself such as this (an opinion which Hamlet held both of himself and of everyone else), he is ill, whether he is speaking the truth or whether he is being more or less unfair to himself.

Nor is it difficult to see that there is no correspondence, so far as we can judge, between the degree of self-abasement and its real justification. A good, capable, conscientious woman will speak no better of herself after she develops melancholia than one who is in fact worthless; indeed, the former is perhaps more likely to fall ill of the disease than the latter, of whom we too should have nothing good to say. Finally, it must strike us that after all the melancholic does not behave in quite the same way as a person who is crushed by remorse and self-reproach in a normal fashion. Feelings of shame in front of other people, which would more than anything characterize this latter condition, are lacking in the melancholic, or at least they are not prominent in him. One might emphasize the presence in him of an almost opposite trait of insistent communicativeness which finds satisfaction in self-exposure.

The Repression of War Experience
W. H. Rivers (1917)

I do not attempt to deal in this paper with the whole problem of the part taken by repression in the production and maintenance of the war neuroses. Repression is so closely bound up with the pathology and treatment of these states that the full consideration of its role would amount to a complete study of neurosis in relation to the war.

The Process of Repression

It is necessary at the outset to consider an ambiguity in the term 'repression,' as it is now used by writers on the pathology of the mind and nervous system. The term is currently used in two senses which should be carefully distinguished from one another. It is used for the process whereby a person endeavours to thrust out of his memory some part of his mental content, and it is also used for the state which ensues when, either through this process or by some other means, part of the mental content has become inaccessible to manifest consciousness.

In the second sense the word is used for a state which corresponds closely with that known as dissociation, but it is useful to distinguish mere inaccessibility to memory from the special kind of separation from the rest of the mental content which is denoted by the term 'dissociation'.

The state of inaccessibility may therefore be called suppression in distinction from the process of repression. In this paper, I use repression for the active or voluntary process by which it is attempted to remove some part of the mental content out of the field of attention with the aim of making it inaccessible to memory and producing the state of suppression.

Using the word in this sense, repression is not in itself a pathological process, nor is it necessarily the cause of pathological states. On the contrary, it is a necessary element in education and in all social progress. It is not repression in itself which is harmful, but repression under conditions in which it fails to adapt the individual to his environment.

It is in times of special stress that these failures of adaptation are especially liable to occur, and it is not difficult to see why disorders due to this lack of adaptation should be so frequent at the present time. There are few, if any, aspects of life in which repression plays so prominent and so necessary a part as in the preparation for war.

The training of a soldier is designed to adapt him to act calmly and methodically in the presence of events naturally calculated to arouse disturbing emotions. His training should be such that the energy arising out of these emotions is partly damped by familiarity, partly diverted into other channels.

The most important feature of the present war in its relation to the production of neurosis is that the training in repression normally spread over years has had to be carried out in short spaces of time, while those thus incompletely trained have had to face strains such as have never previously been known in the history of mankind. Small wonder that the failures of adaptation should have been so numerous and so severe.

I do not now propose to consider this primary and fundamental problem of the part played by repression in the original production of the war neuroses. The process of repression does not cease when some shock or strain has removed the soldier from the scene of warfare, but it may take an active part in the maintenance of the neurosis.

New symptoms often arise in hospital or at home which are not the immediate and necessary consequence of the war experience, but are due to repression of painful memories and thoughts, or of unpleasant affective states arising out of reflection concerning this experience. It is with the repression of the hospital and of the home rather than with the repression of the trenches that I deal in this paper.

I propose to illustrate by a few sample cases some of the effects which may be produced by repression and the line of action by which these effects may be remedied.

I hope to show that many of the most trying and distressing symptoms from which the subjects of war neurosis suffer are not the necessary result of the strains and shocks to which they have been exposed in warfare, but are due to the attempt to banish from the mind distressing memories of warfare or painful affective states which have come into being as the result of their war experience.

The Attitude of Patients to War Memories:

Everyone who has had to treat cases of war neurosis, and especially that form of neurosis dependent on anxiety, must have been faced by the problem of what advice to give concerning the attitude the patient should adopt towards his war experience.

It is natural to thrust aside painful memories just as it is natural to avoid dangerous or horrible scenes in actuality, and this natural tendency to banish the distressing or the horrible is especially pronounced in those whose powers of resistance have been lowered by the long-continued strains of trench-life, the shock of shell-explosion, or other catastrophe of war.

Even if patients were left to themselves most would naturally strive to forget distressing memories and thoughts. They are, however, very far from being left to themselves, the natural tendency to repress being in my experience almost universally fostered by their relatives and friends, as well as by their medical advisors.

Even when patients have themselves realised the impossibility of forgetting their war experiences and have recognized the hopeless and enervating character of the treatment by repression, they are often induced to attempt the task in obedience to medical orders.

The advice which has usually been given to my patients in other hospitals is that they should endeavour to banish all thoughts of war from their minds. In some cases all conversation between patients or with visitors about the war is strictly forbidden, and the patients are instructed to lead their thoughts to other topics, to beautiful scenery and other pleasant aspects of experience.

To a certain extent this policy is perfectly sound. Nothing annoys a nervous patient more than the continual inquiries of his relatives and friends about his experiences of the front, not only because it awakens painful memories, but also because of the obvious futility of most of the questions and the hopelessness of bringing the realities home to his hearers.

Moreover, the assemblage together in a hospital of a number of men with little in common except their war experiences naturally leads their conversation far too frequently to this topic, and even among those whose memories are not especially distressing it tends to enhance the state for which the term 'fed up' seems to be the universal designation.

It is, however, one thing that those who are suffering from the shocks and strains of warfare should dwell continually on their war experience or be subjected to importunate inquiries; it is quite another to attempt to banish such experience from their minds altogether.

CHAPTER THREE

Consuming

from *Geneva*
Stephen Buck (1734)

> Bless'd be the Man! for ever bless'd his Name!
> Whose patriot Zeal excited him to move
> The *British* Senate to reverse the Law,
> So baneful, as its Force all Compound Drams,
> And *Gin*; the best, destroy'd: Now let us smile
> Since she revives; on her attendant wait
> *Clove, Cinamon*, and *Annis*, Cordial, all,
> But *Gin* more Cordial, most profusely good.
>
> O Sovereign Dram! How shall I speak thy Praise?
> Unequal to the Task, if not inspir'd
> By thy invigorating Drops, whose Heat
> Can in unlearned Minds raise Thoughts sublime.
>
> 'Tis Thou, that best dispel'st all human Woe,
> For meagre Want, with all her frightful Train
> Of Hunger, Thirst, Sickness, and Pain itself,
> From thee promiscuous fly, like heavy Mists
> Before the Morning Sun: The Winter's Cold,
> Bleak Winds, Frost, Snow, and Rain, lose all their Force
> In thy bless'd Presence; and the Body warm'd
> By thy puissant Drops, is more secure
> Than wrap'd in Wool, or Silks, or softest Furs.
> Inebriate by thee, the Captive Wretch
> Forgets Confinement, shudders not to hear
> Clashing of Chains, nor Clink of Fetters dire.
> The lash of Whips, Gibbets, and fiery Brands
> Oppos'd by thee, impending Terrors lose.
> Diffusive is thy Good to all Mankind
> As Air, or Water; for the lowest Rank
> Of Mortals can with Ease enjoy thy Charms,
> Nor Mendicants, nor Slaves are from thee barr'd.
>
> By thee the Passions that perplex the Mind
> Are soften'd, or subdu'd; Fear soon retires,

Hope centers but in thee, and Love alone
Reigns at the *Gin-Shop* with despotic Sway;
Not curb'd by Parents Rule or Av'rice vile,
For here both Nymphs and Swains with Hearts elate,
Quaff *Nectar* smiling, though in Rags they smile;
And laugh at Wretches that in gilded Cars
Triumphant ride, but with dejected Hearts.
Here no Ambition, nor distracting Cares
For fleeting Riches, ever dare approach,
But joyous all transmit the circling Glass.

from *The Art of Preserving Health: Diet*
John Armstrong (1744)

Prompted by instinct's never-erring power,
Each creature knows its proper aliment;
But man, the inhabitant of ev'ry clime,
With all the commoners of nature feeds.
Directed, bounded, by this power within,
Their cravings are well-aim'd: Voluptuous Man
Is by superior faculties misled;
Misled from pleasure even in quest of joy.
Sated with nature's boons, what thousands seek,
With dishes tortur'd from their native taste,
And mad variety, to spur beyond
Its wiser will the jaded appetite!
Is this for pleasure? Learn a juster taste;
And know that temperance is true luxury.
Or is it pride? Pursue some nobler aim.
Dismiss your parasites, who praise for hire;
And earn the fair esteem of honest men,
Whose praise is fame. Form'd of such clay as yours,
The sick, the needy, shiver at your gates.
Even modest want may bless your hand unseen,
Tho' hush'd in patient wretchedness at home.
Is there no virgin, grac'd with every charm
But that which binds the mercenary vow?
No youth of genius, whose neglected bloom
Unfoster'd sickens in the barren shade;
No worthy man, by fortune's random blows,
Or by a heart too generous and humane,
Constrain'd to leave his happy natal seat,
And sigh for wants more bitter than his own?
There are, while human miseries abound,
A thousand ways to waste superfluous wealth,

Without one fool or flatterer at your board,
Without one hour of sickness or disgust.
...
Gross riot treasures up a wealthy fund
Of plagues: but more immedicable ills
Attend the lean extreme. For physic[1] knows
How to disburden the too tumid veins,[2]
Even how to ripen the half-labour'd blood:
But to unlock the elemental tubes,
Collaps'd and shrunk with long inanity,
And with balsamic nutriment repair
The dried and worn-out habit, were to bid
Old age grow green, and wear a second spring;
Or the tall ash, long ravish'd from the soil,
Through wither'd veins imbibe the vernal dew.
When hunger calls, obey; nor often wait
Till hunger sharpen to corrosive pain:
For the keen appetite will feast beyond
What nature well can bear; and one extreme
Ne'er without danger meets its own reverse.
Too greedily th' exhausted veins absorb
The recent chyle, and load enfeebled powers
Oft to th' extinction of the vital flame.
To the pale cities, by the firm-set siege
And famine humbled, may this verse be borne;
And hear, ye hardiest sons that Albion breeds
Long toss'd and famish'd on the wintry main;
The war shook off, or hospitable shore
Attain'd, with temperance bear the shock of joy;
Nor crown with festive rites th' auspicious day:
Such feast might prove more fatal than the waves,
Than war or famine. While the vital fire
Burns feebly, heap not the green fuel on;
But prudently foment the wandering spark
With what the soonest feeds its kindred touch:
Be frugal ev'n of that: a little give
At first; that kindled, add a little more;
Till, by deliberate nourishing, the flame
Reviv'd, with all its wonted vigour glows.

---

[1]Physic: medical science.
[2]This and the next few lines refer to the widespread practice of bleeding (phlebotomy); the idea was that by opening and draining blood from the veins, noxious excesses would be released from the body, thereby re-establishing equilibrium.

But tho' the two (the full and the jejune)[3]
Extremes have each their vice; it much avails
Ever with gentle tide to ebb and flow
From this to that: So nature learns to bear
Whatever chance or headlong appetite
May bring. Besides, a meagre day subdues
The cruder clods by sloth or luxury
Collected, and unloads the wheels of life.
Sometimes a coy aversion to the feast
Comes on, while yet no blacker omen lours;
Then is a time to shun the tempting board.

The Smoking Doctor's Soliloquy over his Pipe
Francis Fawkes (1761)

Dulce tubo genitos haurire & reddere fumos.[4]

Emerging awful through a cloud of smoke,
The tall lean doctor snapt his box and spoke.
'Tho' scorn'd by fribbles all bedawb'd with snuff,
I value not their censures of a puff,
Who, if kind heav'n had furnish'd 'em with brains,
Would into pipes convert their taper canes,
Be sick that nauseous nostril-dust to see,
And substitute tobacco for rappee.[5]
I less regard the rage of female railings –
Some ladies have their waters, and their failings:
Tho' when gray prudence comes, and youth is past,
They'll learn to smoke (or I am deceiv'd) at last!
Peace to the beaux, and every scented belle,
Who cries, 'Tobacco has an odious smell:'
To men of sense I speak, and own with pleasure,
That smoking sooths my studies and my leisure;

It aids my eyes, inspires my mind to think,
And is a calm companion when I drink:
At home how sweetly does a pipe engage
My sense to relish Tully's moral page!
Or Homer's heav'n-aspiring muse divine,
And puffing measure each sonorous line![6]
But if to Tom's I stray to read the Daily,

---

[3]A jejune diet is deficient and lacking in nutrition.
[4]'Sweet tube allow the draw and make the smoke.'
[5]Rappee: snuff.
[6]Tully refers to the classical Roman orator and philosopher Marcus Tulius Cicero; Homer was the great epic poet of classical Greece.

Or at the tavern spend my evening gaily,
My pipe still adds, as the mild minutes pass,
Charms to the toast, and flavour to the glass.
Tho' by thy fumes the teeth are blacken'd o'er,
Thy ashes scour them whiter than before.

O with abundant riches amply blest!
He, who can buy one ounce of Freeman's best!
If in this fob my well-fill'd box I feel,
In that my short pipe, touchwood, flint, and steel,
Gold I regard not, I can live without;
I carry every requisite about.
Whether my stomach calls for drink or meat,
Whether the cold affects me, or the heat,
The weed of India answers the demand,
And is the pleasing remedy at hand.
O noblest proof of nature's genial power!
O weed more precious than the choicest flower!
Thy vapours bland through every state engage,
Charm us when young, and solace us in age;
Adorn when fortune showers her golden store,
And breathe kind comfort when she smiles no more:

Tranquil at home they lull with sweet content,
Abroad they give us no impediment;
But, mild associates, tend us night and day,
And if we travel cheer us on our way;
In town or country soft repose incite,
And puff us up with exquisite delight.'

On a Fit of the Gout: An Ode
Isaac Hawkins Browne (1768)

Wherefore was Man thus form'd with eye sublime,
With active joints to traverse hill or plain,
But to contemplate Nature in her prime,
Lord of this ample world, his fair domain?
Why on this various earth such beauty pour'd,
But for thy pleasure, Man, her sovereign lord?

Why does the mantling vine her juice afford
Nectareous, but to cheer with cordial taste?
Why are the earth and air and ocean stor'd
With beast, fish, fowl; if not for Man's repast?
Yet what avails to me, or taste, or sight,
Exil'd from every object of delight?

So much I feel of anguish, day and night
Tortur'd, benumb'd; in vain the fields to range
Me vernal breezes, and mild suns invite,
In vain the banquet smokes with kindly change
Of delicacies, while on every plate
Pain lurks in ambush, and alluring fate.

Fool, not to know the friendly powers create
These maladies in pity to mankind:
These abdicated Reason reinstate
When lawless Appetite usurps the mind;
Heaven's faithful centries at the door of bliss
Plac'd to deter, or to chastise excess.

Weak is the aid of wisdom to repress
Passion perverse; philosophy how vain!
'Gainst Circe's[7] cup, enchanting sorceress;
Or when the Syren[8] sings her warbling strain.
Whate'er or sages teach, or bards reveal,
Men still are men, and learn but when they feel.

As in some free and well-pois'd common-weal
Sedition warns the rulers how to steer,
As storms and thunders rattling with loud peal,
From noxious dregs the dull horizon clear;
So when the mind imbrutes in sloth supine,
Sharp pangs awake her energy Divine.

Cease then, oh cease, fond mortal, to repine
At laws, which Nature wisely did ordain;
Pleasure, what is it? rightly to define,
'Tis but a short-liv'd interval from pain:
Or rather, each, alternately renew'd,
Give to our lives a sweet vicissitude.

from *A Farewell to Tobacco*
Charles Lamb (1805)

Stinking'st of the stinking kind,
Filth of the mouth and fog of the mind,
Africa, that brags her foyson,[9]
Breeds no such prodigious poison,

---

[7] In Greek mythology, Circe was a goddess of magic, or sometimes a nymph, witch, enchantress or sorceress.
[8] Mythical sirens were beautiful creatures, who lured sailors with enchanting music and singing to shipwreck.
[9] Foyson: plenty.

Henbane, nightshade, both together,
Hemlock, aconite[10] –

– Nay, rather,
Plant divine, of rarest virtue;
Blisters on the tongue would hurt you.
'Twas but in a sort I blam'd thee;
None e'er prosper'd who defam'd thee;
Irony all, and feign'd abuse,
Such as perplexed lovers use,
At a need, when, in despair
To paint forth their fairest fair,
Or in part but to express
That exceeding comeliness
Which their fancies doth so strike,
They borrow language of dislike;
And, instead of Dearest Miss,
Jewel, Honey, Sweetheart, Bliss,
And those forms of old admiring,
Call her Cockatrice and Siren,
Basilisk, and all that's evil:
Witch, Hyena, Mermaid, Devil,
Ethiop, Wench, and Blackamoor,[11]
Monkey, Ape and twenty more;
Friendly Trait'ress, loving Foe –
Not that she is truly so,
But no other way they know
A contentment to express,
Borders so upon excess,
That they do not rightly wot[12]
Whether it be pain or not.

Or, as men, constrain'd to part
With what's nearest to their heart,
While their sorrow's at the height,
Lose discrimination quite,
And their hasty wrath let fall,
To appease their frantic gall,
On the darling thing whatever,
Whence they feel it death to sever,

---

[10]Henbane is a nightshade plant, source of the poison belladonna. Hemlock is the poison famous for having killed Socrates. Aconite is a sedative derived from the root of the herb monkhood.

[11]The cockatrice is a mythical two-legged dragon with a rooster's head; sirens lured sailors to their death with their enchanting music; the basilisk is a mythical reptile that could cause death with a single glance or breath; Blackamoor is a Moor.

[12]Wot: know.

Though it be, as they, perforce,
Guiltless of the sad divorce.

For I must (nor let it grieve thee,
Friendliest of plants, that I must) leave thee.
For thy sake, TOBACCO, I
Would do any thing but die,
And but seek to extend my days
Long enough to sing thy praise.
But, as she, who once hath been
A king's consort, is a queen
Ever after, nor will bate
Any title of her state,
Though a widow, or divorced,
So I, from thy converse forced,
The old name and style retain,
A right Katherine of Spain[13];
And a seat, too, 'mongst the joys
Of the blest Tobacco Boys;
Where, though I, by sour physician,
Am debarr'd the full fruition
Of thy favours, I may catch
Some collateral sweets, and snatch
Sidelong odours, that give life
Like glances from a neighbour's wife;
And still live in the by-places
And the suburbs of thy graces;
And in thy borders take delight,
An unconquer'd Canaanite.[14]

The Fat Man
John Greenleaf Whittier (1832)

Oh – wo for pursy[15] gentlemen –
The short and thick of frame;
With tun-like[16] bodies that would put
A Dutchman's vrou[17] to shame! –
Wo – for the round and bulky man –
The greasy and the fat –

---

[13]A reference to Catherine of Aragon, the divorced first wife of King Henry VIII.
[14]The Canaanites were an ancient polytheistic people.
[15]Pursy: fat.
[16]A tun was a large cask for holding beer.
[17]Vrou: wife.

The five feet high by four feet broad –
A walking tallow vat!
I have a handsome country-seat
And pleasant rooms in town,
I keep a noble pair of steeds,
For driving up and down –
My garb is of the costliest –
My steeds are dapple grey –
I've friends who sup with me by night,
And dine with me by day.

But I am one of those who bear
The curse of fat with them,
Enveloping their choicest gifts
Like earth around a gem.
And then I have an altitude
Too Pygmean[18] by far –
Out-measuring in circumference,
My perpendicular.

And with a spirit all alive,
And sensitive and proud,
I bear my massy frame about
Amidst the jesting crowd –
And some will smile and all will stare –
And some will roar with laughter;
And lanky skeletons will point
Their bony finger after.

The ladies, too, are dumb with fear,
Or struggling with a smile –
Whene'er I make my awkward bow,
And talk of love the while –
They turn them from my dashing greys,
And from my country seat –
And love each needy skeleton
That kneels before their feet.

Oh – tell me not that mirth and joy
To giant bodies fall –
Your over-grown and mammoth men
Are melancholy all!
Nay – rather than 'this hill of flesh' –
I'd be a Barber's post –

---

[18]Pygmies are small-statured people native to equatorial Africa. It refers disparagingly here to a small or dwarfish person; a person of small importance.

The mummy of an Esquimaux –
Or Calvin Edson's ghost.[19]

The Opium Eater
Mary Eliza Perine Tucker (1867)

Before taking a dose.

Life's pathway to me is dreary;
I am ill, and cold, and weary;
Would my lonely walk were done,
And my heavenly race begun!

Once all things to me were bright,
Things that now seem dark as night:
Is the darkness all within?
Dark without from inward sin?

The present dark; eyes dim with age
Can see no joy, save memory's page.
The present, future, ne'er can be
Bright as the past they once did see.

My hair is turning quite grey now;
I see some wrinkles on my brow;
My teeth – they must be failing too –
And corns are growing in my shoe.

I muffle up my aching face,
And pray from pangs a moment's grace.
Ah! now the misery seeks my head –
Would I were with the pangless dead!

There is a cure for pain and grief –
Come, Opium, come to my relief!
Soothed by thy influence, I shall find
A moment's rest, and peace of mind.

After taking a dose.

Ah! now I sit in bowers of bliss,
Soothed by an angel's balmy kiss!
Delicious languor o'er me stealing
Is now my only sense of feeling.

The breath of flowers perfumes the air;
The forms around are – oh, so fair!

---

[19]'The Human Skeleton', Calvin Edson (early 1800s), was a medical curiosity and circus 'freak' from Stafford, Connecticut.

The once cold air seems warm and bright,
And I, too, seem a being of light.

My hair is not so very grey –
Some dye will take that hue away;
A little powder shall, I vow,
Hide the small wrinkles on my brow.

My teeth are sound – I feel no pain –
Their slight ache was but sign of rain;
And then the twinging of my feet
Was nothing but a dream, a cheat.

To me, the night, though dark, seems day,
Colored by Hope's most beauteous ray:
No sorrow hence shall give me pain –
I know I'll never weep again!

The Opium Smoker
Arthur Symons (1889)

I am engulfed, and drown deliciously.
Soft music like a perfume, and sweet light
Golden with audible odours exquisite,
Swathe me with cerements for eternity.
Time is no more. I pause and yet I flee.
A million ages wrap me round with night.
I drain a million ages of delight.
I hold the future in my memory.

Also I have this garret which I rent,
This bed of straw, and this that was a chair,
This worn-out body like a tattered tent,
This crust, of which the rats have eaten part,
This pipe of opium; rage, remorse, despair;
This soul at pawn and this delirious heart.

I Had Been Hungry All The Years
Emily Dickinson (1891)

I had been hungry all the years;
My noon had come, to dine;
I, trembling, drew the table near,
And touched the curious wine.

'Twas this on tables I had seen,
When turning, hungry, lone,
I looked in windows, for the wealth
I could not hope to own.

I did not know the ample bread,
'Twas so unlike the crumb
The birds and I had often shared
In Nature's dining-room.

The plenty hurt me, 'twas so new,
Myself felt ill and odd,
As berry of a mountain bush
Transplanted to the road.

Nor was I hungry; so I found
That hunger was a way
Of persons outside windows,
The entering takes away.

The Absinthe Drinker
Arthur Symons (1892)

Gently I wave the visible world away.
Far off, I hear a roar, afar yet near,
Far off and strange, a voice is in my ear,
And is the voice my own? the words I say
Fall strangely, like a dream, across the day;
And the dim sunshine is a dream. How clear,
New as the world to lovers' eyes, appear
The men and women passing on their way!

The world is very fair. The hours are all
Linked in a dance of mere forgetfulness.
I am at peace with God and man. O glide,
Sands of the hour-glass that I count not, fall
Serenely: scarce I feel your soft caress.
Rocked on this dreamy and indifferent tide.

The Barley-Fever[20]
George Outram (1916)

Oh the Barley-fever!
The Barley-fever, the Barley-fever!
It sticks like a burr, or a plough in a fur,
An' it fells a man like a cleaver.
Yer beard turns lang, an' yer head turns bald,
An' yer face grows as white as the lipo' a scald;

---

[20]This poem is in a Scottish dialect. Barley-fever is a popular name for drunkenness.

Yer tae end is het, and the tither is cauld,
Like a rat wi' its tail in a siever.

Oh the Barley-fever!
The Barley-fever, the Barley-fever!
It gars the best soul grow as toom[21] as a bowl,
An'as flat as the doup[22] o'a weaver.
The Typhus tak's folk that are no very clean,
The Scarlet's content wi'a fat fozy wean[23];
But the Barley tak's rich, poor, clean, dirty, fat, lean,
The infidel and the believer.

Old Witherington
Dudley Randall (1943)

Old Witherington had drunk too much again.
The children changed their play and packed around him
To jeer his latest brawl. Their parents followed.

Prune black, with bloodshot eyes and one white tooth,
He tottered in the night with legs spread wide
Waving a hatchet. 'Come on, come on,' he piped,
'And I'll baptize these bricks with bloody kindling.
I may be old and drunk, but not afraid
To die. I've died before. A million times
I've died and gone to hell. I live in hell.
If I die now I die, and put an end
To all this loneliness. Nobody cares
Enough to even fight me now, except
This crazy bastard here.'

                              And with these words
He cursed the little children, cursed his neighbours,
Cursed his father, mother and his wife,
Himself, and God and all the rest of the world,
All but his grinning adversary, who, crouched,
Danced tenderly around him with a jag-toothed bottle,
As if the world compressed to one old man
Who was the sun, and he sole faithful planet.

---

[21]Toom: emptied or drained.
[22]Doup: buttocks.
[23]Scarlet refers to scarlet fever; a fat fozy wean is a fat, flabby baby.

My Papa's Waltz
Theodore Roethke (1948)

> The whiskey on your breath
> Could make a small boy dizzy;
> But I hung on like death:
> Such waltzing was not easy.
>
> We romped until the pans
> Slid from the kitchen shelf;
> My mother's countenance
> Could not unfrown itself.
>
> The hand that held my wrist
> Was battered on one knuckle;
> At every step you missed
> My right ear scraped a buckle.
>
> You beat time on my head
> With a palm caked hard by dirt,
> Then waltzed me off to bed
> Still clinging to your shirt.

Io Baccho!
William Carlos Williams (1950)

> God created alcohol
> and it wasn't privately for the Russians
> God created alcohol
> and it wasn't for Dr Goldsmith
>
> It was for Mrs Reiter
> who is bored with having children
> though she loves them.
> God created alcohol to release
> and engulf us. Shall I
> say it is the only evidence of God
> in this environment?
>
> Mrs R. doesn't drink
> but I drink and I told the angel,
> God created alcohol!
> – if it weren't for that I'd say
> there wasn't Any –
> thinking of Mrs R. who is
> one eighth American Indian
> and what with the pain in her guts

stands like an Indian
'If I had the strength'
Why should I bother to tell you?

God created alcohol
Shall I swoon like Mr Keats?
and not from looking
at a Grecian urn. God created alcohol
to allay us

Thalidomide[24]
Sylvia Plath (1962)

O half moon –

Half-brain, luminosity –
Negro, masked like a white,

Your dark
Amputations crawl and appal –

Spidery, unsafe.
What glove

What leatheriness
Has protected

Me from that shadow –
The indelible buds.

Knuckles at shoulder-blades, the
Faces that

Shove into being, dragging
The lopped

Blood-caul of absences.
All night I carpenter

A space for the thing I am given,
A love

Of two wet eyes and a screech.
White spit

---

[24]The drug Thalidomide was first marketed in 1957 in West Germany and primarily prescribed as a sedative to treat anxiety, insomnia, gastritis and tension. When it was later used to treat morning sickness in pregnancy, about 10,000 global cases were reported of infants born with malformed limbs (phocomelia), deformed eyes and hearts, deformed alimentary and urinary tracts, blindness and deafness, only half of whom survived.

Of indifference!
The dark fruits revolve and fall.

The glass cracks across,
The image

Flees and aborts like dropped mercury.

Confessions of an English Opium Smoker
D. J. Enright (1962)

In some sobriety
I offer to recall those images:
Damsel, dome and dulcimer,
Portentous pageants, alien altars,
Foul unimaginable imagined monster,
Façades of fanfares, Lord's Prayer
Tattooed backwards on a Manchu[25] fingernail,
Enigma, or a dread too well aware,
Swirling curtains, almond eyes or smell?

And I regain these images:
Rocked by the modern traffic of the town,
A grubby, badly lighted, stuffy shack –
A hollow in some nobody's family tree,
The undistinguished womb of anybody's
Average mother. And then me,
In all sobriety, slight pain in neck and back,
Expecting that and then a little more,
Right down to bedrock.
This was no coloured twopenny,
Just a common people's penny sheet –

To read with cool avidity.
And damsels, and such embarrassments?
Imagined beasts more foul than real monsters?
(No man at peace makes poetry.)
Thus I recall, despite myself, the images
That merely were. I offer my sedate respects
To those so sober entertainments,
Suited to our day and ages.

---

[25]In Manchurian high culture of the Qing dynasty (1644–1912), elite women sometimes wore long, elaborate, inlaid or carved gold or silver nail guards, to show they were above manual labour.

Anxiety
Frank O'Hara (1964)

I'm having a real day of it.

There was
something I had to do. But what?
There are no alternatives, just
the one something.

I have a drink,
it doesn't help – far from it!

I
feel worse. I can't remember how
I felt, so perhaps I feel better.
No, just a little darker.

If I could
get really dark, richly dark, like
being drunk, that's the best that's
open as a field. Not the best,

but the best except for the impossible
pure light, to be as if above a vast
prairie, rushing and pausing over
the tiny golden heads in deep grass.

The Addict
Anne Sexton (1966)

Sleepmonger,
deathmonger,
with capsules in my palms each night,
eight at a time from sweet pharmaceutical bottles
I make arrangements for a pint-sized journey.
I'm the queen of this condition.
I'm an expert on making the trip
and now they say I'm an addict.
Now they ask why.
WHY?

Don't they know
that I promised to die!
I'm keeping in practice.
I'm merely staying in shape.
The pills are a mother, but better,
every color and as good as sour balls.
I'm on a diet from death.

Yes, I admit
it has gotten to be a bit of a habit –
blows eight at a time, socked in the eye,
hauled away by the pink, the orange,
the green and the white goodnights.
I'm becoming something of a chemical
mixture.
that's it!

My supply
of tablets
has got to last for years and years.
I like them more than I like me.
Stubborn as hell, they won't let go.
It's a kind of marriage.
It's a kind of war
where I plant bombs inside
of myself.

Yes
I try
to kill myself in small amounts,
an innocuous occupation.
Actually I'm hung up on it.
But remember I don't make too much noise.
And frankly no one has to lug me out
and I don't stand there in my winding sheet.
I'm a little buttercup in my yellow nightie
eating my eight loaves in a row
and in a certain order as in
the laying on of hands
or the black sacrament.

It's a ceremony
but like any other sport
it's full of rules.
It's like a musical tennis match where
my mouth keeps catching the ball.
Then I lie on my altar
elevated by the eight chemical kisses.

What a lay me down this is
with two pink, two orange,
two green, two white goodnights.
Fee-fi-fo-fum –
Now I'm borrowed.
Now I'm numb.

Diabetes
James Dickey (1969)

SUGAR

One night I thirsted like a prince
Then like a king
Then like an empire   like a world
On fire. I rose and flowed away and fell
Once more to sleep. In an hour I was back
In the kingdom   staggering, my belly going round with self-
Made night-water, wondering what
The Hell. Months of having a tongue
Of flame convinced me: I had better not go
On this way. The doctor was young

And nice. He said, I must tell you,
My friend, that it is needless moderation
And exercise. You don't want to look forward
To gangrene and kidney

Failure   boils blindness infection skin trouble falling
Teeth coma and death.
O.K.
In sleep my mouth went dry
With my answer   and in it burned the sands
Of time with new fury. Sleep could give me no water
But my own. Gangrene in white
Was in my wife's hand at breakfast
Heaped like a mountain. Moderation, moderation,
My friend, and exercise. Each time the barbell
Rose   each time a foot fell
Jogging, it counted itself
One death   two death   three death and resurrection
For a little while. Not bad! I always knew it would have to be
somewhere around
The house: the real
Symbol of Time I could eat
And live with, coming true when I opened my mouth:
True in the coffee and the child's birthday
Cake   helping sickness be fire-
tongued, sleepless and water-
logged   but not bad, sweet sand
Of time, my friend, an everyday –
A livable death at last.

Gout[26]
Lewis Warsh (1971)

He changes into a bird, and that's
the only difference. Rain
on the improved sidewalk seems
inspired after so much heat.
Look at the objects
that have already wilted and died.
Someone is losing hair trying
to penetrate the meaning of death – rather
language which postpones dying
is inventing a drug to keep us alive.
Being similar never made this body more true. Bills
for electricity and answering
service are burning inside the hearth.
My dream, to have a hearth and
set an example for fading
youth. The conspicuous peacock
neither turns nor changes,
yet suddenly loses its feathers, buckles
in the dust and dies. The
meaning is as fantastic as any truth. Language
invents a painkilling drug for restoring youth – an
occasion inviting feelings which
jolt and never subside. I mean
he is dying again, slowly, as he gains time.

Pain-killers
Tony Harrison (1978)

My father haunts me in the old men that I find
holding the shop-queues up by being slow.
It's always a man like him that I'm behind
just when I thought the pain of him would go
reminding me perhaps it never goes,
with his pension book kept utterly pristine
in a plastic wrapper labelled *Pantihose*
as if they wouldn't pay if it weren't clean,

or learning to shop so late in his old age
and counting his money slowly from a purse
I'd say from its ornate clasp and shade of beige

---

[26]Caused by crystallized uric acid in the joints and tissues, gout is characterized by recurrent attacks of acute inflammatory arthritis and swollen joints. It is exacerbated by eating rich food and drinking alcohol.

was his dead wife's glasses' case. I curse,
but silently, secreting pain, at this delay,
the acid in my gut caused by dad's ghost –
I've got aerogrammes to buy. My love's away!
And the proofs of *Pain-Killers* to post!

Going for pills to ease the pain I get
from the Post Office on Thursdays, Pension Day,
the chemist's also gives me cause to fret
at more of my dad's ghosts, and more delay
as they queue for their prescriptions without hopes
and go looking for the old cures on the shelves,
stumbling into pyramids of scented soaps
they once called cissy when they felt 'themselves'.

There are more than in the Post Office in BOOTS[27]
and I try to pass the time behind such men
by working out the Latin and Greek roots
of cures, the *san-* that's in *Sanatogen*,[28]
compounds derived from *derm-* for teenage spots,
suntan creams and lotions prefixed *sol-*
while a double of my dad takes three wild shots
at pronouncing PARACETAMOL.

Anorexic
Eavan Boland (1980)

Flesh is heretic.
My body is a witch.
I am burning it.

Yes I am torching
her curves and paps and wiles.
They scorch in my self-denials.

How she meshed my head
in the half-truths
of her fevers till I renounced
milk and honey
and the taste of lunch.

I vomited
her hungers.
Now the bitch is burning.

---

[27]Boots is a British chain of chemists.
[28]Sanatogen is a 'brain tonic' invented by the Bauer Chemical Company in Germany 1898.

I am starved and curveless.
I am skin and bone.
She has learned her lesson.

Thin as a rib
I turn in sleep.
My dreams probe

a claustrophobia,
a sensuous enclosure.
How warm it was and wide

once by a warm drum,
once by the song of his breath
and in his sleeping side.

Only a little more,
only a few more days
sinless, foodless,

I will slip
back into him again
as if I had never been away.

Caged so
I will grow
angular and holy

past pain,
keeping his heart
such company

as will make me forget
in a small space
the fall

into forked dark,
into python needs
heaving to hips and breasts
and lips and heat
and sweat and fat and greed.

Medicine
Raymond Carver (1985)

All I know about medicine I picked up
from my doctor friend in El Paso
who drank and took drugs. We were buddies

until I moved East. I'm saying
I was never sick a day in my life.
But something has appeared
on my shoulder and continues to grow.
A wen, I think, and love the word
but not the thing itself, whatever
it is. Late at night my teeth ache
and the phone rings. I'm ill,
unhappy and alone. Lord!
Give me your unsteady knife,
doc. Give me your hand, friend.

De Quincey in Glasgow
Edwin Morgan (1990)

Twelve thousand drops of laudanum a day
kept him from shrieking. Wrapped in a duffle
buttoned to the neck, he made his shuffle,
door, table, window, table, door, bed, lay
on bed, sighed, groaned, jumped from bed, sat and wrote
till the table was white with pages, rang
for his landlady, ordered mutton, sang
to himself with pharmacies in his throat.
When afternoons grew late, he feared and longed
for dusk. In that high room in Rottenrow
he looks out east to the Necropolis.
Its crowded tombs rise jostling, living, thronged
with shadows, and the granite-bloodying glow
flares on the dripping bronze of a used kris.[29]

Obesity
Kathleen Peirce (1991)

Reception is a gesture of the will
opening, one peach rose widening the light, or
rain finally taking the abandoned room,
the walls newly alive with water, and the ceiling
raining. It must have been happening a long time;
the random, jewel-colored bottles on the floor
swallowing the intermittent drops to a point approaching fullness,
then over full, and every surface here is changed, bigger,
touched too much by something wonderful
and ruinous. She would hardly tell you how bakery cakes call to her,

---

[29]Kris: a Malay dagger.

but look; the tiniest prettiest woman, a decoration
for a cake, was saved inside the cupboard by the sink. One arm
is raised. The smallest spider imaginable has linked her as an object
to a world full of things, a strand at each hinge: shoulder,
elbow, wrist, and mouth, obedient to hunger, and the room falling in.

These Things Happen in the Lives of Women
Thomas Lynch (1994)

The first time he ever bought her lingerie
she was dead of gin and librium[30] and years
of trying to regain her innocence.
'These things happen in the lives of women ...'
is what the priest told him. 'They lose their way.'
And lost is what she looked like lying there
awash in her own puke and the disarray
of old snapshots and pill bottles,
bedclothes and letters and mementos of
the ones with whom she had been intimate.
She was cold already. Her lips were blue.
So he bought her a casket and red roses
and bought silk panties and a camisole
and garters and nylons and a dressing gown
with appliqués in the shape of flowers.
And after the burial he bought a stone
with her name and dates on it and wept aloud
and went home after that and kept weeping.

History of Medicine
Sharon Olds (1996)

Finally I fondly remember even Benylin,
Robitussin, Actifed,
Tedral, erythromycin,
penicillin, E. E. S., I can
see the tidy open mouth
and the spoon's regular journey toward it,
the bowl almost convex with its shuddering
load of blackish maroon.
Time slowed down as the spoon went in, I can
still feel the thrum, in the handle,
that little tug like nursing, and then
the pulling of the spoon out of the mouth,

---

[30]Librium is a drug for the treatment of severe anxiety and acute alcohol withdrawal syndrome.

ampicillin, ipecac, St
Joseph's, tetracycline, my body
turned to the four-hour intervals – we made
one being, the bottle and the child and I,
I remember it with longing. Even the ear-drops,
lice-shampoo, wart-glaze,
even the time when our son would not take
his Tedral, he was standing in his crib
and he spat it out and I gently jammed another
dose through his teeth and he spat it out
until the bars and cruising rail
were splattered with dots of heavy syrup and he
understood I cared about the matter
even more than he.
As I cleaned him up with a damp cloth
I told him the germs were strong, we had to
staunchly fight them – I can hear my voice,
calm and cheerful. I can see myself,
a young woman with an orderly array of
bottles behind her, she is struggling to be good, to be healed.

Lithium[31]
Robin Robertson (1997)

After the arc of ECT[32]
and the blunt concussion of pills,
they gave him lithium to cling to –
the psychiatrist's stone.
A metal that floats on water,
must be kept in kerosene,
can be drawn into wire.
(He who had jumped in the harbour,
burnt his hair off,
been caught hanging from the light.)
He'd heard it was once used
to make hydrogen bombs,
but now was a coolant for nuclear reactors,
so he broke out of hospital barefoot
and walked ten miles to meet me in the snow.

---

[31]Lithium is a drug for the treatment of bipolar and schizoaffective disorders, as well as other forms of mental illness associated with a chemical imbalance in the brain.
[32]ECT (electroconvulsive therapy or electroshock therapy) is a controversial psychiatric treatment.

from *The Wasting Game*
Philip Gross (1998)

'I'm fat, look, *fat ...*'

yes and the moon's made of cheese,
that chunk she won't touch in the fridge

dried, creviced, sweating in its cold
like someone with a killing fever.

Half a scrape-of-marmite sandwich,
last night's pushed-aside

potatoes greying like a tramp's teeth,
crusts, crumbs are a danger to her,

so much orbiting space junk
that's weightless for only so long.

Burn it up on re-entry, burn it,
burn it. So she trains

with weights, she jogs, she runs
as if the sky were falling.

Thin
Caitriona O'Reilly (2001)

It is chill and dark in my small room.
A wind blows through gaps in the roof,
piercing even the eiderdown. My skin
goose-pimples in front of the cloudy glass
though there was scalding tea for dinner
with an apple. I'm cold to the bone.

I don't sleep well either. My hip-bones
stick in the foam mattress, and the room's
so empty. My sister is having dinner
with a boy. Awake under the roof
I watch the stars bloom heavily through glass
and think, *how shatterproof is my skin?*

I doze till six, then drink semi-skim
milk for breakfast (the bare bones
of a meal) before nine o'clock class.
It's kind of hard to leave my room
for the walk to school. No roof
over me, and eight solid hours till dinner-

time. All day my dreams of dinner
are what really get under my skin,
not the boys. My tongue sticks to the roof
of my mouth again in class. I'm such a bone-
head! And my stomach's an empty room.
My face floats upwards in a glass

of Coke at lunchtime. One glass.
I make it last the whole day till dinner:
hot tea and an apple in my room.
My sister seems not to notice the skin
around my mouth or my ankle-bones.
If our parents knew they'd hit the roof

I suppose. My ribs rise like the roof
of a house that's fashioned from glass.
I might even ping delicately like bone-
china when flicked. No dinner
for six weeks has made this skin
more habitable, more like a room –

or a ceiling that shatters like glass
over those diners off gristle and bone.
This skin is a more distinguished room.

Fat Man
Kwame Dawes (2003)

How terrible the confession, *We are all dying.*
The way fat weighs us and the heart swells
from too long labouring to make us breathe, slouch
and snore with guttural dreadfulness (the terror
of it). I do not want to die. So absurd
this admission, this effort to confront
the unpredictable odds of our living. But fat
people die quickly – we know this – and I,
too, too solid with the mess of casualness
grow fat with age. So hard to come back.
I stare at my stranger self in hotel mirrors.
I am afraid to meet this stomach-glorious
creature, unable these days to find an angle
of satisfying grace. I am now a circle of errors,
the fat has taken over. Perhaps pride in this
plump existentialism will make it well,
but my child seems too, too small, helplessly
small in my clumsy cumbersome arms.

They, my children, will call me fat,
and I will resent their kindnesses
and compensations for my limp and waddle.
I dream of sweat, the familiar
hint of muscles beneath the inner flesh,
the rib, a round reminder of the body
so vulnerable beneath this cloak of flesh.
I dream of breathing easily when I bend
in two to touch my shoelaces. I dream
of better days when I will leap lightly,
a slender man gambolling in the mirror's face.

MEDICAL WRITING:

A Dissertation on the Gout[33]
William Cadogan (1771)

Now let us compare this simple idea of temperance with the common course of most men's lives, and observe their progress from health to sickness: for I fear we shall find but very few who have any pretensions to real temperance. In early youth we are insensibly led into intemperance by the indulgence and mistaken fondness of parents and friends wishing to make us happy by anticipation. Having thus exhausted the first degrees of luxury before we come to the dominion of ourselves, we should find no pleasure in our liberty did we not advance in new sensations, nor feel ourselves free but as we abuse it.

Thus we go on till some friendly pain or disease bids, or rather forces, us to stop. But in youth all the parts of our bodies are strong and flexible, and bear the first loads of excess with less hurt, and throw them off soon by their own natural vigor and action, or with very little assistance from artificial evacuations. As we grow older, either by nature in due time, or repeated excesses before our time, the body is less able to free itself, and wants more aid from art.

The man however goes on, taking daily more than he wants, or can possibly get rid of; he feels himself replete and oppressed, and, his appetite failing, his spirits sink for want of fresh supply. He has recourse to dainties, sauces, pickles, provocatives of all sorts. These soon lose their power; and though he washes down each mouthful with a glass of wine, he can relish nothing. What is to be done? Send for a physician. Doctor, I have lost my stomach; pray give me, says he, with great innocence and ignorance, something to give me an appetite; as if want of appetite was a disease to be cured by art. In vain would the physician, moved by particular friendship to the man, or that integrity he owes to all men, give him the best advice in two words, *quaere sudando*, seek it by labor. He would be thought a man void of all knowledge and skill in his profession, if he did not immediately, or after a few evacuations,

---

[33]In the eighteenth century, physicians debated whether gout – a painful arthritic condition – was hereditary or a 'disease of civilization' (i.e. caused by drinking alcohol, a rich diet and a lack of exercise).

prescribe stomachics, bitter spicy infusions in wine or brandy, vitriolic elixirs, bark, steel, etc. By the use of these things the stomach, roused to a little extraordinary action, frees itself, by discharging its crude, austere, coagulated contents into the bowels, to be thence forwarded into the blood. The man is freed for a time, finds he can eat again, and thinks all well.

But this is a short-liv'd delusion. If he is robust, the acrimony floating in the blood will be thrown out, and a fit of gout succeeds; if less so, rheumatism or colic, etc. as I have already said. But let us suppose it to be the gout, which if he bears patiently, and lives moderately, drinking no madeira or brandy to keep it out of his stomach, nature will relieve him in a certain time, and the gouty acrimony concocted and exhausted by the symptomatic fever that always attends, he will recover into health; if assisted by judicious, mild, and soft medicines, his pains might be greatly assuaged and mitigated, and he would recover sooner. But however he recovers, it is but for a short time; for he returns to his former habits, and quickly brings on the same round of complaints again and again, all aggravated by each return, and he less able to bear them; till he becomes a confirmed invalid and cripple for life, which, with a great deal of useless medication, and a few journies to Bath,[34] he drags on, till, in spite of all the doctors he has consulted, and the infallible quack medicines he has taken, lamenting that none have been lucky enough to hit his case, he sinks below opium and brandy, and dies long before his time.

...

If this be true of the common provocatives at every poor man's board, who is there that exceeds not nature's law? who is truly temperate? What shall we say of that studied, labored, refined extravagance at the tables of the rich, where the culinary arts are push'd to that excess, that luxury is become false to itself, and things are valued, not as they are good and agreeable to the natural and undebauch'd appetite; but high, inflammatory, rare, out of season, and costly; where, though variety is aimed at, every thing has the same taste, and nothing it's own. I am sorry and ashamed, that men professing luxury should understand it so little, as to think it lies in the dish or the sauce or multitude of either; or that urging beyond natural satiety can afford any real enjoyment.

But this they do by all the researches of culinary and medical art, introducing all the foreign aids to luxury, every stimulating provocative that can he found in acids, salts, fiery spices, and essences of all kinds, to rouse their nerves to a little feeling; not knowing the more they are chafed and irritated the more callous they still grow; and the same things must now be more frequently repeated, increased in quantity, and exalted in quality, till they know not where to stop, and every meal they make serves only to overload and oppress the stomach, to foul and inflame the blood, obstruct and choke all the capillary channels, bring on a hectic fever of irritation, that though it raise the spirits for the evening, leaves behind it all the horrid sensations of inanition and crapula[35] the next morning; and but that nature is

---

[34]In the eighteenth century, the spa town Bath became a popular destination for health tourists.
[35]Inanition is a lack of mental or spiritual vigour and enthusiasm. Crapula is sickness caused by excessive eating or drinking; a hangover.

so kind as to stop them in their career with a painful fit of gout or some other illness, in which she gets a little respite, they would soon be at the end of their course.

Men bring all these evils upon themselves, either not knowing or not attending to two things: the one, that pleasure is a coy coquet, and to be enjoy'd must not always be pursued; we must sometimes sit still, that she may come and court us in her turn: the other, that pleasure and happiness are as distinct things as riot and enjoyment: besides, pleasure is not infinite, and our sensations are limited: we can bear but a certain measure, and all urging beyond it, infallibly brings pain in its stead.

The Elements of Medicine
John Brown (1780; 1795 ed.)[36]

Since the general powers produce all the phenomena of life, and the only operation, by which they do so is stimulant; it follows, that the whole phenomena of life, every state and degree of health and disease, are also owing to stimulus, and to no other cause.

Excitement, the effect of the exciting powers, the true cause of life, is, within certain boundaries, proportional to the degree of stimulus. The degree of stimulus, when moderate, produces health; in a higher degree it gives occasion to diseases of excessive stimulus; in a lower degree, or excessively weak, it induces those that depend upon a deficiency of stimulus, or debility. And, as excitement is the cause both of diseases and perfect health, so that which restores the morbid to the healthy state is a diminution of excitement in diseases of excessive stimulus, and an increase of excitement in diseases of debility. These intentions are called Indications of Cure.

This mutual relation obtains betwixt excitability and excitement, that the more weakly the powers have acted, or the less the stimulus has been, the more abundant the excitability becomes; the more powerful the stimulus, the excitability becomes the more exhausted.

A mean stimulus, acting on a mean or half consumed excitability, produces the highest excitement. And the excitement becomes less and less, in proportion either as the stimulus is applied in a higher degree, or as the excitability is more accumulated. Hence the vigour of youth, and the weakness of childhood and old age. Hence, within a shorter period, a middle diet will produce vigour, and excess or abstemiousness, debility.

...

When the excitability is wasted by any one stimulus, there is still a reserve capable of being acted upon by any other. Thus a person, who has dined fully, or is either fatigued in body, or tired with intellectual exertion, and therefore has a disposition to sleep, will be refreshed by strong liquors; and when these have produced the same sleepiness, the more diffusible stimulus of opium will arouse him.

---

[36]Trans. from the Latin by Thomas Beddoes.

(A gentleman, engaged in a literary composition, which required an uninterrupted exertion of his mental faculties for more than forty hours, was enabled to go through it with alacrity, by supporting himself in this manner. After dining well and setting to business, he took a glass of wine every hour. Ten hours after he ate something nourishing, but sparing in quantity, and for some hours kept himself up with punch not too strong. And, when he found himself at last like to be overcome by an inclination to sleep, he changed all his stimuli for an opiate; and finished his business in forty hours. What he had wrote was now to be put to the press. He had next to watch and correct the proofs, which cost him between four or five hours further continuance of vigilance and activity. To effect this he took a glass with the master printer, while his men were going on with their part of the work. The succession of stimuli in this case was first food, next the stimulus of the intellectual function, then wine, then the food varied, then punch, then opium, then punch and conversation.)

Even after opium fails, and leaves him heavy and oppressed, a stimulus still higher and more diffusible, if there be any such, will have the same effect. A person fatigued with a journey will be roused by music to dance and skip; and he will be enabled to run after a flying beauty, if she fly so as to leave him hopes of overtaking her.

The exhaustion of excitability, by successive stimuli, is most difficultly repaired; because the more stimulant operation has been employed, that is, the more stimuli have been applied, there remains the less susceptibility to fresh stimuli, by which the failure of excitement might be removed.

The reason of the difficulty is that no means of reproducing the healthy state, or the proper degree of excitement are left; except those that occasioned the waste, that is, an excess of stimulant operation, rendering the body less and less susceptible of stimulus.

After this waste of excitement, there is danger of speedy death, unless proper measures be taken to preserve life by a powerful stimulus, but less than that which occasioned it, and then by one still less, till by means of the moderate stimulus, that is suitable to nature, or one somewhat greater, life may at last be secured. The difficult cure of drunkards and gluttons, affected with disease, sufficiently evinces, that this consideration applies to all the exciting powers that stimulate in excess. This proposition applies to the most difficult part of the practice of medicine.

...

The seat of excitability in the living body is the medullary nervous matter, and muscular solid; to which the appellation of *nervous system* may be given. In this the excitability is inherent, but is not different in different parts of its seat. This is evident, because the exciting powers will immediately rouse into exertion any of the functions that distinguish living animal systems; or, in other words, produce sense, motion, thought or passion.

Different exciting powers are applied to different parts of the nervous system, none to them all at once; but the mode of their action is such, that, wherever they are applied, every one immediately affects the whole excitability.

Every one of these powers always affects some one part more than any other, and different powers affect different parts in this unequal manner. The affected part is generally that to which the power is directly applied.

An Essay, Medical, Philosophical and Chemical on Drunkenness
Thomas Trotter (1804)

In medical language, I consider drunkenness, strictly speaking, to be a disease; produced by a remote cause, and giving birth to actions and movements in the living body, that disorder the functions of health. This being the case, besides the value of an accurate definition for the sake of system, it may be of some practical utility to point out the affinity which the paroxysm has with other affections. In assigning the character formerly, I was well aware of the difficulty of fixing on any symptom, or even concourse of symptoms, that are invariably present.

For this reason *delirium* seemed to be the most certain, as it is the most prominent and general. But objections may yet be made to this; for difference of age, and varieties of temperament and constitution, influence the accession and progress of wavering intellect during intoxication. Again, although the animal functions are evidently deranged, exhibited by all the shades and gradations of *delirium,* such as imbecility of mind or fatuity, erroneous judgment, imaginary perceptions, false relations, violent emotions called raving, etc. yet at the same time, the paroxysm is so generally attended with a partial or total abolition of the powers of sense and motion, that it assumes very much the nature of a *comatose* condition. Indeed the most frequent fatal termination of the drunken fit is *apoplexy*. It is certainly no uncommon occurrence to see an inebriate who can neither walk nor speak, exercise so considerable a degree of mental power, as to recollect every circumstance that passes; yet so conscious of his inability to move without staggering, that he cunningly watches the opportunity, when unperceived by his companions, to take his leave. The character of this disease therefore, partakes both of *delirium* and *coma*.

...

When inebriety has become so far habitual that some disease appears in consequence, the physician is for the first time called in, and a task the most ungrateful devolves upon him. If friends and relations had taken the alarm before to save the constitution of the patient, it will at once be found that their attempts proved unsuccessful. Whatever this disease may be, whether stomach complaints, with low spirits, premature gout, epilepsy, jaundice, or any other of the catalogue, it is in vain to prescribe for it till the evil genius of the habit has been subdued. On such an occasion it is difficult to lay down rules. The physician must be guided by his own discretion: he must scrutinize the character of his patient, his pursuits, his modes of living, his very passions and private affairs. He must consult his own experience of human nature, and what he has learned in the school of the world. The great point to be obtained is the confidence of the sick man, but this is not to be accomplished at a first visit. It is to be remembered that a bodily infirmity is not the only thing to be corrected. *The habit of drunkenness is a disease of the mind.* The soul itself has received impressions that are incompatible with its reasoning powers.

Confessions of an English Opium-Eater
Thomas De Quincey (1821)

And first, one word with respect to its bodily effects; for upon all that has been hitherto written on the subject of opium, whether by travellers in Turkey (who may plead their privilege of lying as an old immemorial right), or by professors of medicine, writing *ex cathedra*,[37] I have but one emphatic criticism to pronounce – Lies! lies! lies! ... I do by no means deny that some truths have been delivered to the world in regard to opium. Thus it has been repeatedly affirmed by the learned that opium is a dusky brown in colour; and this, take notice, I grant. Secondly, that it is rather dear, which also I grant, for in my time East Indian opium has been three guineas a pound, and Turkey eight. And thirdly, that if you eat a good deal of it, most probably you must – do what is particularly disagreeable to any man of regular habits, viz., die. These weighty propositions are, all and singular, true: I cannot gainsay them, and truth ever was, and will be, commendable. But in these three theorems I believe we have exhausted the stock of knowledge as yet accumulated by men on the subject of opium.

And therefore, worthy doctors, as there seems to be room for further discoveries, stand aside, and allow me to come forward and lecture on this matter. First, then, it is not so much affirmed as taken for granted, by all who ever mention opium, formally or incidentally, that it does or can produce intoxication. Now, reader, assure yourself, *meo periculo*,[38] that no quantity of opium ever did or could intoxicate. As to the tincture of opium (commonly called laudanum) *that* might certainly intoxicate if a man could bear to take enough of it; but why? Because it contains so much proof spirit, and not because it contains so much opium. But crude opium, I affirm peremptorily, is incapable of producing any state of body at all resembling that which is produced by alcohol, and not in *degree* only incapable, but even in *kind*: it is not in the quantity of its effects merely, but in the quality, that it differs altogether. The pleasure given by wine is always mounting and tending to a crisis, after which it declines; that from opium, when once generated, is stationary for eight or ten hours: the first, to borrow a technical distinction from medicine, is a case of acute – the second, the chronic pleasure; the one is a flame, the other a steady and equable glow. But the main distinction lies in this, that whereas wine disorders the mental faculties, opium, on the contrary (if taken in a proper manner), introduces amongst them the most exquisite order, legislation, and harmony. Wine robs a man of his self-possession; opium greatly invigorates it. Wine unsettles and clouds the judgement, and gives a preternatural brightness and a vivid exaltation to the contempts and the admirations, the loves and the hatreds of the drinker; opium, on the contrary, communicates serenity and equipoise to all the faculties, active or passive, and with respect to the temper and moral feelings in general it gives simply that sort of vital warmth which is approved by the judgment, and which would probably always accompany a bodily constitution of primeval or antediluvian health.

...

---

[37]*'with the full authority of the office'.*
[38]*'at my own risk'.*

This is the doctrine of the true church on the subject of opium: of which church I acknowledge myself to be the only member – the alpha and the omega: but then it is to be recollected that I speak from the ground of a large and profound personal experience: whereas most of the unscientific authors who have at all treated of opium, and even of those who have written expressly on the materia medica, make it evident, from the horror they express of it, that their experimental knowledge of its action is none at all. I will, however, candidly acknowledge that I have met with one person who bore evidence to its intoxicating power, such as staggered my own incredulity; for he was a surgeon, and had himself taken opium largely. I happened to say to him that his enemies (as I had heard) charged him with talking nonsense on politics, and that his friends apologized for him by suggesting that he was constantly in a state of intoxication from opium. Now the accusation, said I, is not *prima facie*[39] and of necessity an absurd one; but the defence *is*. To my surprise, however, he insisted that both his enemies and his friends were in the right. 'I will maintain,' said he, 'that I *do* talk nonsense; and secondly, I will maintain that I do not talk nonsense upon principle, or with any view to profit, but solely and simply, said he, solely and simply – solely and simply (repeating it three times over), because I am drunk with opium, and *that* daily.'

...

I confess, however, that the authority of a surgeon, and one who was reputed a good one, may seem a weighty one to my prejudice; but still I must plead my experience, which was greater than his greatest by 7,000 drops a-day; and though it was not possible to suppose a medical man unacquainted with the characteristic symptoms of vinous intoxication, it yet struck me that he might proceed on a logical error of using the word intoxication with too great latitude, and extending it generically to all modes of nervous excitement, instead of restricting it as the expression for a specific sort of excitement connected with certain diagnostics. Some people have maintained in my hearing that they had been drunk upon green tea; and a medical student in London, for whose knowledge in his profession I have reason to feel great respect, assured me the other day that a patient in recovering from an illness had got drunk on a beef-steak.

Having dwelt so much on this first and leading error in respect to opium, I shall notice very briefly a second and a third, which are, that the elevation of spirits produced by opium is necessarily followed by a proportionate depression, and that the natural and even immediate consequence of opium is torpor and stagnation, animal and mental. The first of these errors I shall content myself with simply denying; assuring my reader that for ten years, during which I took opium at intervals, the day succeeding to that on which I allowed myself this luxury was always a day of unusually good spirits.

With respect to the torpor supposed to follow, or rather (if we were to credit the numerous pictures of Turkish opium-eaters) to accompany the practice of opium-eating, I deny that also. Certainly opium is classed under the head of narcotics, and

---

[39]'*at first sight*', meaning evidently factual or true.

some such effect it may produce in the end; but the primary effects of opium are always, and in the highest degree, to excite and stimulate the system. This first stage of its action always lasted with me, during my noviciate, for upwards of eight hours; so that it must be the fault of the opium-eater himself if he does not so time his exhibition of the dose (to speak medically) as that the whole weight of its narcotic influence may descend upon his sleep.

'The Pains of Opium'

The opium-eater will find, in the end, as oppressive and tormenting as any other, from the sense of incapacity and feebleness, from the direct embarrassments incident to the neglect or procrastination of each day's appropriate duties, and from the remorse which must often exasperate the stings of these evils to a reflective and conscientious mind. The opium-eater loses none of his moral sensibilities or aspirations; he wishes and longs as earnestly as ever to realize what he believes possible, and feels to be exacted by duty; but his intellectual apprehension of what is possible infinitely outruns his power, not of execution only, but even of power to attempt. He lies under the weight of incubus[40] and night-mare; he lies in sight of all that he would fain perform, just as a man forcibly confined to his bed by the mortal languor of a relaxing disease, who is compelled to witness injury or outrage offered to some object of his tenderest love: he curses the spells which chain him down from motion; he would lay down his life if he might but get up and walk; but he is powerless as an infant, and cannot even attempt to rise.

I now pass to what is the main subject of these latter confessions, to the history and journal of what took place in my dreams; for these were the immediate and proximate cause of my acutest suffering. The first notice I had of any important change going on in this part of my physical economy, was from the reawaking of a state of eye generally incident to childhood, or exalted states of irritability. I know not whether my reader is aware that many children, perhaps most, have a power of painting, as it were, upon the darkness, all sorts of phantoms: in some that power is simply a mechanic affection of the eye; others have a voluntary or semi-voluntary power to dismiss or summon them; or, as a child once said to me, when I questioned him on this matter, 'I can tell them to go, and they go; but sometimes they come when I don't tell them to come.'

Corpulence: Or, Excess of Fat in the Human Body
Thomas King Chambers (1850)

It sometimes begins immediately after birth, and proceeds rapidly, as part of a general hypertrophic tendency affecting the whole body. The children come into the world very fat and strong, and grow very rapidly, so that at two or three years old they are as large as others at seven or eight, and are often at this stage made objects of curiosity at fairs and elsewhere.

...

---

[40]An incubus is a mythical demon that lies upon the sleeping victim.

One of these children was born in humble life, at Manchester, about three years ago. It was exhibited at six months old, at which time it weighed ninety pounds. What has since become of the poor infant I have been unable to learn. The only noticeable point about it was that the chest was small in proportion to the body. Another ... was also born at Manchester, in a higher station of life, being the seventh child of a medical man. It was, as you may see, born very large, and shortly before its death weighed eighty-seven pounds. At one year old he weighed forty pounds, and was thirty-one inches in height. The circumference of the head was twenty-one inches; of the thigh, seventeen and a half; of the ankle, eight inches. This child was introduced, through Sir James Clark, to Her Majesty, who was pleased to express her surprise at the ease with which it could walk. An interesting point about this case was, that, contrary to what is usually observed, the mental faculties were developed in an equal degree with the corporeal bulk, the understanding being very precocious. An early death, as is ordinarily the case, removed this child from further observation.

...

I think I have observed in families where there is a tendency to corpulency, that those members of them in whom the hereditary disease is likely to be developed, are distinguished by precocity of body [rapid development, including early menstruation], and that those in whom it is not found have a better chance of escaping the unfortunate entail. If further observation confirms this idea, it will afford a useful means of prognosis, and teach us when to be on our guard against future obesity, and when we may feel at ease on that point. It is not a mere matter of curiosity or overcautious prying into the future; for I firmly believe, that well-advised habits of living, and measures such as rational physiology will suggest, may in many cases prevent this bane of comfort and shortener of life, and in all much diminish its intensity. It may tend as caution also in our treatment of the acute diseases of young persons, lest in healing one disorder we give occasion to another, which will stick by them for life.

Habit
William James (1890)

The question of 'tapering-off' in abandoning such habits as drink and opium-indulgence, comes in here, and is a question about which experts differ within certain limits, and in regard to what may be best for an individual case. In the main, however, all expert opinion would agree that abrupt acquisition of the new habit is the best way, *if there be a real possibility of carrying it out*. We must be careful not to give the will so stiff a task as to insure its defeat at the very outset; but, *provided one can stand it*, a sharp period of suffering, and then a free time, is the best thing to aim at, whether in giving up a habit like that of opium, or in simply changing one's hours of rising or of work. It is surprising how soon a desire will die of inanition if it be *never* fed.

...

The physiological study of mental conditions is thus the most powerful ally of hortatory ethics.[41] The hell to be endured hereafter, of which theology tells, is no worse than the hell we make for ourselves in this world by habitually fashioning our characters in the wrong way. Could the young but realize how soon they will become mere walking bundles of habits, they would give more heed to their conduct while in the plastic state. We are spinning our own fates, good or evil, and never to be undone. Every smallest stroke of virtue or of vice leaves its never so little scar. The drunken Rip Van Winkle, in Jefferson's play,[42] excuses himself for every fresh dereliction by saying, 'I won't count this time!' Well! he may not count it, and a kind Heaven may not count it; but it is being counted none the less. Down among his nerve-cells and fibres the molecules are counting it, registering and storing it up to be used against him when the next temptation comes. Nothing we ever do is, in strict scientific literalness, wiped out. Of course, this has its good side as well as its bad one. As we become permanent drunkards by so many separate drinks, so we become saints in the moral, and authorities and experts in the practical and scientific spheres, by so many separate acts and hours of work.

Fasting Girls: Their Physiology and Pathology
William A. Hammond (1879)

Among the many remarkable manifestations by which hysteria exhibits itself, for the astonishment of the credulous and uneducated portion of the public, and – alas, that it should have to be said – for the delectation of an occasional weak-minded and ignorant physician, the assumption of the ability to live without food may be assigned a prominent place. I am not aware that this power has been claimed in its fullest development for the male of the human species. When he is deprived of food he dies in a few days, more or less, according to his physical condition as regards adipose tissue and strength of constitution; but if a weak emaciated girl asserts that she is able to exist for years without eating, there are at once certificates and letters from clergymen, professors, and even physicians, in support of the truth of her story. The element of impossibility goes for nothing against the bare word of such a woman, and her statements are accepted with a degree of confidence which is lamentable to witness in this era of the world's progress. The class of deceptions occasionally induced by hysteria and embracing these 'fasting girls,' has been known for many years, though it is only in comparatively recent times that the instances have been taken at their proper value.

...

About sixty-five years ago, a woman of Sudbury, in Staffordshire, England, named Ann Moore, declared that she did not eat, and a number of persons volunteered

---

[41]Hortatory: urging a course of action.
[42]Rip Van Winkle, a character in the story of the same name by American author Washington Irving (pub. 1819), is a Dutch-American colonist who enjoys solitude and shirks work, but is well-loved by his neighbours. Joseph Jefferson (or Joe Jefferson) (1829–1905) was one of the most celebrated nineteenth-century American comedians.

to watch her, in order to ascertain whether or not she was speaking the truth. The watch was continued for three weeks and then the watchers, as in other instances, reported that Ann Moore was a real case of abstinence from food of all kinds. The Bible was always kept open on Ann's bed. Her emaciation was so extreme that it was said her vertebral column could be felt through the abdominal walls. This sad condition was asserted to have been caused by her washing the linen of a person affected with ulcers. From that time she experienced a dislike for food, and even nausea at the sight or mention of it. As soon as the watchers reported in favor of the genuineness of Ann's pretensions her notoriety increased, and visitors came from all parts of the country, leaving donations to the extent of two hundred and fifty pounds in the course of two years. Doubts, however, again arose, and, bold from the immunity she had experienced from the first investigation, Ann in an evil moment, for the continuance of her fraud, consented to a second watching. This committee was composed of notable persons, among them being Sir Oswald Mosley, Bart., Reverend Legh Richmond, Dr Fox and his son, and many other gentlemen of the country. Two of them were always in her room night and day. At the suggestion of Mr Francis Fox, the bedstead, bedding, and the woman in it were placed on a weighing machine, and thus it was ascertained that she regularly lost weight daily. At the expiration of the ninth day of this strict watching, Dr Fox found her evidently sinking and told her she would soon die unless she took food. After a little prevarication, the woman signed a written confession that she was an impostor, and had 'occasionally taken sustenance for the last six years.' She also stated that during the first watch of three weeks her daughter had contrived, when washing her face, to feed her every morning, by using towels made very wet with gravy, milk, or strong arrowroot gruel, and had also conveyed food from mouth to mouth in kissing her, which it is presumed she did very often.

CHAPTER FOUR

Illness, Disease and Disability

from *Syphilis: Or, a Poetical History of the French Disease*
Nahum Tate (1686)[1]

In all productions of wise Nature's hand,
Whether Conceiv'd in Air on Sea, or Land;
No constant method does direct her way,
But various Beings various Laws obey;
Such things as from few Principles arise,
In every place and season meet our eyes;
But what are fram'd of Principles abstruse,
Such places only and such times produce.
Effects of yet a more stupendous Birth,
And such as Nature must with pangs bring forth,
Where violent and various Seeds unite,
Break slowly from the Bosom of the Night;
Long in the Womb of Fate the Embryo's worn,
Whole Ages pass before the Monster's born.

Diseases thus which various Seeds compound,
As various in their Birth and date are found.
Some always seen, some long in darkness hurl'd,
That break their chains at last to scourge the World.
To which black List this Plague must be assign'd,
Nights foulest Birth and Terror of Mankind.
Nor must we yet think this escape the first,
Since former Ages with the like were curst.
Long since he scatter'd his Infernal flame,
And always Being had, though not a Name,
At least what Name it bore is now unfound:
Both Names and things in time's Abyss lie drown'd.
How vainly then do we project to keep
Our Names remember'd when our Bodies sleep?
Since late Succession searching their descent,
Shall neither find our dust nor Monument.

---

[1]This is a translation from the Latin 1530 work of the Italian physician, poet and scholar Girolamo Fracastoro.

Yet where the Western Ocean finds its bound
(The World so lately by the *Spaniards* found)
Beneath this Pest the wretched Natives groan
In every Nation there and always known,
Such dire Effects depend upon a Clime,
On varying Skies and long Revolving time:
The temper of their Air this Plague brought forth,
The Soil itself dispos'd for such a Birth.
All things conspir'd to raise the Tyrant there,
But time alone could fix his Conquest here.
If therefore more distinctly we would know
Each Source from whence this deadly Bane did flow,
His Progress in the Earth we must survey
How many Cities groan beneath his sway.
And when his great Advancement we have trac'd,
We must allow his Principles as vast.
That Earth nor Sea th' Ingredients could prepare
And wholly must ascribe it to the Air,
The Tyrant's seat, his Magazine is there.
The Air that does both Earth and Sea surround,
As easily can Earth and Sea confound;
What Fence for Bodies when at every pore
The soft Invader has an open door?
What fence, where poison's drawn with vital Breath,
And Father Air the Authour proves of Death?
Of subtle substance that with ease receives
Infection, which as easily it gives.
Now by what means this dire Contagion first,
Was form'd aloft, by what Ingredients nurs'd,
Our Song shall tell; and in this wondrous Course,
Revolving times and varying Planets force.

First then the Sun with all his train of Stars,
Amongst our Elements raise endless Wars;
And when the Planets from their Stations Range,
Our Orb is influenc'd, and feels the Change.
The chiefest instance is the Sun's retreat,
No sooner he withdraws his vital heat,
But fruitless Fields with Snow are cover'd o'er,
The pretty Fountains run and talk no more.
Yet when his Chariot to the *Crab* returns,
The Air, the Earth, the very Ocean burns.
The Queen of Night can boast no less a sway,
At least all humid things her power obey.
Malignant *Saturn's* Star as much can claim,

With friendly *Jove's*, bright *Mars*, and *Venus* flame,
And all the host of Lights without a Name.

Plague
Daniel Defoe (1722)

A dreadful plague in London was
In the year sixty-five,
Which swept an hundred thousand souls
Away; yet I alive!

Saturday: The Small-Pox
Lady Mary Wortley Montagu (1747)

The wretched FLAVIA[2] on her couch reclin'd,
Thus breath'd the anguish of a wounded mind;
A glass revers'd in her right hand she bore,
For now she shun'd the face she sought before.

'How am I chang'd! alas! how am I grown
A frightful spectre, to myself unknown!
Where's my complexion? where my radiant bloom,
That promis'd happiness for years to come?
Then with what pleasure I this face survey'd!
To look once more, my visits oft delay'd!
Charm'd with the view, a fresher red would rise,
And a new life shot sparkling from my eyes!

Ah! faithless glass, my wonted bloom restore;
Alas! I rave, that bloom is now no more.
The greatest good the gods on men bestow,
Ev'n youth itself to me is useless now.
There was a time (oh! that I cou'd forget!)
When opera-tickets pour'd before my feet;
And at the ring,[3] where brightest beauties shine,
The earliest cherries of the spring were mine.
Witness, O *Lilly*; and thou, *Motteux*,[4] tell,
How much japan these eyes have made ye sell.
With what contempt ye saw me oft despise
The humble offer of the raffled prize;
For at the raffle still each prize I bore,

---

[2]Flavia, from the Latin meaning 'blonde'; a beauty.
[3]The ring refers to the fashionable West Carriage Drive, dividing Hyde Park and Kensington Gardens.
[4]Charles Lillie was a celebrated perfumer, and Peter Anthony Motteux was first an author, then seller of Indian and Chinese goods. 'Japan' in the next line refers to Japanese porcelain, silk and other coveted goods.

With scorn rejected, or with triumph wore.
Now beauty's fled, and presents are no more!

For me the Patriot has the house⁵ forsook,
And left debates to catch a passing look:
For me the Soldier has soft verses writ:
For me the Beau has aim'd to be a wit.
For me the Wit to nonsense was betray'd;
The Gamester has for me his dun⁶ delay'd,
And overseen the card he would have play'd.
The bold and haughty by success made vain,
Aw'd by my eyes, have trembled to complain:
The bashful 'Squire touch'd by a wish unknown,
Has dar'd to speak with spirit not his own:
Fir'd by one wish, all did alike adore;
Now beauty's fled, and lovers are no more!

As round the room I turn my weeping eyes,
New unaffected scenes of sorrow rise.
Far from my sight that killing picture bear,
The face disfigure, and the canvas tear:
That picture, which with pride I us'd to show,
The lost resemblance but upbraids me now.
And thou, my toilette, where I oft have sate,
While hours unheeded pass'd in deep debate,
How curls should fall, or where a patch to place;
If blue or scarlet best became my face;
Now on some happier nymph your aid bestow;
On fairer heads, ye useless jewels, glow;
No borrow'd lustre can my charms restore;
Beauty is fled, and dress is now no more.

Ye meaner beauties, I permit ye shine;
Go, triumph in the hearts that once were mine;
But, 'midst your triumphs with confusion know,
'Tis to my ruin all your arms ye owe.
Wou'd pitying Heav'n restore my wonted mien,
Ye still might move unthought of and unseen:
But oh, how vain, how wretched is the boast
Of beauty faded, and of empire lost!
What now is left but weeping, to deplore
My beauty fled, and empire now no more?

Ye cruel Chymists, what with-held your aid!
Could no pomatums save a trembling maid?

---

⁵House: Parliament.
⁶Dun: demand for payment.

How false and trifling is that art ye boast!
No art can give me back my beauty lost.
In tears, surrounded by my friends I lay,
Mask'd o'er, and trembled at the sight of day;
MIRMILLIO[7] came my fortune to deplore,
(A golden-headed cane well carv'd he bore)
Cordials, he cry'd, my spirits must restore!
Beauty is fled, and spirit is no more!

GALEN,[8] the grave; officious Squirt was there,
With fruitless grief and unavailing care:
MACHAON too, the great MACHAON,[9] known
By his red cloak and his superior frown;
And why, he cry'd, this grief and this despair,
You shall again be well, again be fair;
Believe my oath; (with that an oath he swore)
False was his oath; my beauty is no more!
Cease, hapless maid, no more thy tale pursue,
Forsake mankind, and bid the world adieu!
Monarchs and beauties rule with equal sway;
All strive to serve, and glory to obey:
Alike unpitied when depos'd they grow –
Men mock the idol of their former vow.
Adieu! ye parks! – in some obscure recess,
Where gentle streams will weep at my distress,
Where no false friend will in my grief take part,
And mourn my ruin with a joyful heart;
There let me live in some deserted place,
There hide in shades this lost inglorious face,
Plays, operas, circles, I no more must view!
My toilette, patches, all the world adieu!'

After the Small Pox
Mary Jones (1750)

When skillful traders first set up,
To draw the people to their shop,
They strait hang out some gaudy sign,

---

[7]Mermillio refers to Sir Hans Sloane, a famous physician.
[8]Galen of Pergamon (129–c.216 AD) was a prominent Greek physician, surgeon and philosopher. But, here refers to the playwright John Gay's nickname for the physician Dr. John Woodward, who condemned popular treatments of smallpox.
[9]In Greek mythology, Machaon was a son of Asclepius and a highly skilled surgeon and medic, but here refers to Lady Mary's own doctor.

Expressive of the goods within.
The Vintner has his boy and grapes,
The Haberdasher thread and tapes,
The Shoemaker exposes boots,
And Monmouth Street old tatter'd suits.

So fares it with the nymph divine;
For what is Beauty but a Sign?
A face hung out, through which is seen
The nature of the goods within.
Thus the coquet her beau ensnares
With study'd smiles, and forward airs:
The graver prude hangs out a frown
To strike th' audacious gazer down;
But she alone, whose temp'rate wit
Each nicer medium can hit,
Is still adorn'd with ev'ry grace,
And wears a sample in her face.

What tho' some envious folks have said,
That *Stella* now must hide her head,
That all her stock of beauty's gone,
And ev'n the very sign took down:
Yet grieve not at the fatal blow;
For if you break a while, we know,
'Tis bankrupt like, more rich to grow.
A fairer sign you'll soon hang up,
And with fresh credit open shop:
For nature's pencil soon shall trace,
And once more finish off your face,
Which all your neighbours shall out-shine,
And of your Mind remain the Sign.

To Disease
John Scott (1782)

Disease! Man's dread, relentless foe,
Fell source of fear, and pain, and woe!
O say, on what ill-fated coast
They mourn thy tyrant reign the most?
On Java's bogs, or Gambia's sand,
Or Persia's sultry southern strand;
Or Egypt's annual-flooded plain,
Or Rome's neglected, waste domain;
Or where her walls Byzantium rears,
And mosques and turrets crescent-crown'd,

And from his high serail the sultan hears
The wide Propontis'[10] beating waves resound.

I'll ask no more – Our clime, tho' fair,
Enough thy tyrant reign must share;
And lovers there, and friends, complain,
By Thee their friends and lovers slain:
And yet our Avarice and our Pride
Combine to spread thy mischiefs wide;
While that the captive wretch confines,
To hunger, cold, and filth resigns –
And this the funeral pomp attends
To vaults, where mouldering corpses lie –
Amid foul air thy form unseen ascends,
And like a vulture hovers in the sky.

On the Education of the Blind
Huard (1786)[11]

Typographies, by which imprest,
The learned's thoughts embodied shine,
Their immortality attest:
Treasures, O France, which now are thine.
Eyeless, thank heav'n's supreme decree,
We can to late posterity,
Transmit the light of every sage;
Though blind, we can in open day,
Truth's venerable form display,
And show the glories of our age.

Greece, fruitful source of arts resin'd,
To mortals raptur'd and surpriz'd,
Gave perfect masters of each kind,
At once beheld and idoliz'd.
Yet though their times we justly praise,
Illum'd by such effulgent rays,
Did then the dumb articulate?
Or had the hopeless blind been taught,
From tactile signs to construe thought,
To read, to write, and calculate?

---

[10]The Propontis, or Sea of Marmara, is the inland sea in Turkey, connecting the Black Sea to the Aegean Sea.
[11]Huard, about whom little is known, was a blind pensioner at Haüy's Royal Institute for Blind Youth in Paris, where Louis Braille would attend some years later. This is an English translation of the poem, in the collected works of the blind Scottish poet Thomas Blacklock.

Though Nature from our darken'd eyes,
For ever veils her charms sublime,
The form of earth, and ev'n of skies,
By Fancy's aid, we figuring climb;
We trace the rivers to their source,
Of stars we calculate the course;
From Europe to th' Atlantic shore,
Successive journies we pursue,
Thanks to the hand, whose prudence due,
Guides us in Geographic lore.

Mildew
Charlotte Dacre (1805)

Behold, within that cavern drear and dank,
Whose walls in rainbow tints so dimly shine,
A wretch, with swollen eyes and tresses lank,
Does on a heap of mould'ring leaves recline.

Unwholsome dews for ever him surround,
From his damp couch he scarcely ever hies,
Save when blue vapours, issuing from the ground,
Lure him abroad, to catch them as they rise.

Or else at eve the dripping rock he loves,
Or the moist edge of new-dug grave, full well;
To get the sea spray too at night he roves,
And, gem'd with trickling drops, then seeks his cell.

Such his delights, his green and purple cheek,
His bloated form, his chill, discolour'd hand
He would not change; and if he guests would seek,
He steals among the church-yard's grisly hand.

Cholera Cured Before-Hand
Samuel Taylor Coleridge (1832)

Pains ventral, subventral,
In stomach or entrail,
Think no longer mere prefaces
For grins, groans, and wry faces;
But off to the doctor, fast as ye can crawl!
Yet far better 'twould be not to have them at all.

Now to 'scape inward aches,
Eat no plums nor plum-cakes;
Cry avaunt! new potato –

And don't drink, like old Cato.[12]
Ah! beware of Dispipsy,[13]
And don't ye get tipsy!
For tho' gin and whiskey
May make you feel frisky,

They're but crimps to Dispipsy;
And nose to tail, with this gipsy
Comes, black as a porpus,
The diabolus ipse,
Call'd Cholery Morpus[14];
Who with horns, hoofs, and tail, croaks for carrion to feed him,
Tho' being a Devil, no one never has seed him!

Ah! then my dear honies,
There's no cure for you
For loves nor for monies –
You'll find it too true.
Och! the hallabaloo!
Och! och! how you'll wail,
When the offal-fed vagrant
Shall turn you as blue
As the gas-light unfragrant,
That gushes in jets from beneath his own tail; –
'Till swift as the mail,
He at last brings the cramps on,
That will twist you like Samson.[15]
So without further blethring,
Dear mudlarks! my brethren!
Of all scents and degrees,
(Yourselves and your shes)
Forswear all cabal, lads,
Wakes, unions, and rows,
Hot dreams and cold salads,
And don't pig in styes that would suffocate sows!
Quit Cobbett's, O'Connell's and Beelzebub's[16] banners,
And whitewash at once bowels, rooms, hands, and manners!

---

[12]The Roman Cato the Elder wrote about wine.
[13]Dispepsia: indigestion.
[14]Cholera morbus was what would now be called acute gastroenteritis.
[15]According to the Biblical narrative, Samson died when he grasped two pillars of the Temple of Dagon, and 'bowed himself with all his might' (Judges 16:30), causing the temple to buckle and collapse.
[16]William Cobbett (1763–1835) was an English pamphleteer, farmer and journalist, who agitated for the reform of Parliament. Daniel O'Connell (1775–1847) was an Irish political leader, referred to as The Liberator or The Emancipator, who campaigned for Catholic emancipation – including the right for Catholics to sit in the Westminster Parliament, denied for over 100 years – and repeal of the Act of Union which combined Great Britain and Ireland. Beelzebub: the devil.

The Mowers: An Anticipation of Cholera[17]
Charles Mackay (1848)

Dense on the stream the vapours lay,
Thick as wool on the cold highway;
Spongy and dim, each lonely lamp
Shone o'er the streets so dull and damp;
The moonbeam could not pierce the cloud
That swathed the city like a shroud.
There stood three Shapes on the bridge alone,
Three figures by the coping-stone;
Gaunt, and tall, and undefined,
Spectres built of mist and wind;
Changing ever in form and height,
But black and palpable to sight.

'This is a city fair to see,'
Whisper'd one of the fearful three;
'A mighty tribute it pays to me.
Into its river, winding slow,
Thick and foul from shore to shore,
The vessels come, the vessels go,
And teeming lands their riches pour.
It spreads beneath the murky sky
A wilderness of masonry;
Huge, unshapely, overgrown,
Dingy brick and blacken'd stone.
Mammon is its chief and lord,
Monarch slavishly adored;
Mammon sitting side by side
With Pomp, and Luxury, and Pride;
Who calls his large dominion theirs,
Nor dream a portion is Despair's.

'Countless thousands bend to me
In rags and purple, in hovel and hall,
And pay the tax of Misery
With tears, and blood, and spoken gall.
Whenever they cry
For aid to die,
I give them courage to dare the worst,
And leave their ban on a world accursed.
I show them the river so black and deep,

---

[17]Cholera is an often deadly infection of the small intestine caused by the bacterium *Vibrio cholerae*. There were three major cholera pandemics in the nineteenth century.

They take the plunge, they sink to sleep;
I show them poison, I show them rope,
They rush to death without a hope.
Poison, and rope, and pistol-ball,
Welcome either, welcome all!
I am the lord of the teeming town –
I mow them down, I mow them down!'

'Aye, thou art great, but greater I,'
The second spectre made reply;
'Thou rulest with a frown austere,
Thy name is synonym of Fear.
But I, despotic and hard as thou,
Have a laughing lip, an open brow.
I build a temple in every lane,
I have a palace in every street;
And the victims throng to the doors amain,
And wallow like swine beneath my feet.
To me the strong man gives his health,
The wise man reason, the rich man wealth;
Maids their virtue, youth its charms,
And mothers the children in their arms.
Thou art a slayer of mortal men –
Thou of the unit, I of the ten;
Great thou art, but greater I,
To decimate humanity.
'Tis I am the lord of the teeming town –
I mow them down, I mow them down!'

'Vain boasters to exult at death,'
The third replied, 'so feebly done;
I ope my jaws, and with a breath
Slay thousands while you think of one.
All the blood that Cæsar[18] spill'd,
All that Alexander[19] drew,
All the hosts by 'glory' kill'd,
From Agincourt to Waterloo,[20]

---

[18]Julius Caesar (100–44 BC) was Roman general, statesman and when emperor, was assassinated by Marcus Junius Brutus and his associated senators in 44 BC.
[19]Alexander the Great (356–323 BC) was one of history's most celebrated military commanders, who remained undefeated in battle.
[20]The Battle of Agincourt, Friday 25 October 1415, near modern-day Azincourt, in northern France, was a major English victory in the Hundred Years' War. At the Battle of Waterloo, Sunday 18 June 1815, in present-day Belgium, the French, commanded by Napoleon, were defeated by the Duke of Wellington.

Compared with those whom I have slain,
Are but a river to the main.
'I brew disease in stagnant pools,
And wandering here, disporting there,
Favour'd much by knaves and fools,
I poison streams, I taint the air;
I shake from my locks the spreading Pest,
I keep the Typhus[21] at my behest;
In filth and slime
I crawl, I climb –
I find the workman at his trade,
I blow on his lips, and down he lies;
I look in the face of the ruddiest maid,
And straight the fire forsakes her eyes –
She droops, she sickens, and she dies;
I stint the growth of babes new-born,
Or shear them off like standing corn;
I rob the sunshine of its glow,
I poison all the winds that blow;
Whenever they pass, they suck my breath,
And freight their wings with certain death.
'Tis *I* am the lord of the crowded town –
I mow them down, I mow them down!

'But great as we are, there cometh one
Greater than you – greater than I,
To aid the deeds that shall be done,
To end the work that we've begun,
And thin this thick humanity.
I see his footmarks east and west,
I hear his tread in the silence fall.
He shall not sleep, he shall not rest –
He comes to aid us one and all!

Were men as wise as men might be,
They would not work for you, for me,
For him that cometh over the sea;
But they will not heed the warning voice.
The Cholera comes, rejoice! rejoice!
He shall be lord of the swarming town,
And mow them down, and mow them down!'

---

[21]Typhus, not to be confused with typhoid fever, refers to any of several similar diseases caused by *Rickettsia* bacteria. The name comes from the Greek *typhos*, meaning 'smokey' or 'hazy', describing the state of mind of those affected.

The Plague
Christina Rossetti (1848)

'Listen, the last stroke of death's noon has struck –
The plague is come,' a gnashing Madman said,
And laid him down straightway upon his bed.
His writhèd hands did at the linen pluck;
Then all is over. With a careless chuck
Among his fellows he is cast. How sped
His spirit matters little: many dead
Make men hard-hearted. 'Place him on the truck.
Go forth into the burial-ground and find
Room at so much a pitful for so many.
One thing is to be done; one thing is clear:
Keep thou back from the hot unwholesome wind,
That it infect not thee.' Say, is there any
Who mourneth for the multitude dead here?

The Water That John Drinks
Anonymous (1849)

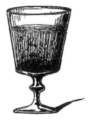

This is the water that JOHN drinks.

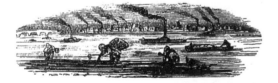

This is the Thames with its cento of stink,
That supplies the water that JOHN drinks.

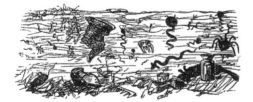

These are the fish that float in the ink-
y stream of the Thames with its cento of stink,
That supplies the water that JOHN drinks.

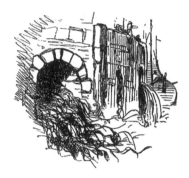

This is the sewer from cesspool and sink,
That feeds the fish that float in the ink-
y stream of the Thames with its cento of stink,
That supplies the water that JOHN drinks.

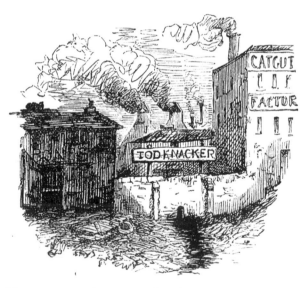

These are vested int'rests, that fill to the brink,
The network of sewer from cesspool and sink,
That feed the fish that float in the ink-
y stream of the Thames with its cento of stink,
That supplies the water that JOHN drinks.

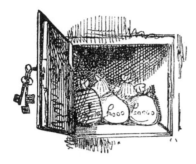

This is the price that we pay to wink,
At the vested int'rests, that fill to the brink,
The network of sewer from cesspool and sink,
That feed the fish that float in the ink-
y stream of the Thames with its cento of stink,
That supplies the water that JOHN drinks.

The Hunchback
W. J. Linton (1865)

God lays his burden on each back:
But who
What is within the pack
May know?

All pointed at the Hunchback. He, they said,
Was hideous; and their scorn
Doubled the anguish which bow'd down his head –
So friendlessly forlorn.

Low bow'd his head, even lower than was need,
For all his Atlas[22] weight;
Bow'd with men's scorn, and with his own sad heed
Of what might be the freight

'Neath which so painfully his being creep'd;
'Was it a heritage,
Growth of his father's sins on him upheap'd?
Or his own sinful wage?'

Ask'd he of lawgiver and sage and priest,
Of all the esteem'd and wise;

---

[22]In Greek mythology, Atlas was the primordial Titan who held up the heavens on his shoulders.

And gat no answer. Nay! not even the least
From worshipp'd Beauty's eyes.

Not that they spake not. Some said – It was nought,
There was no hump at all;
And some that – It was nothing which he sought –
The why such did befall;

Some laugh'd; and some long visages did pull;
Some knew not what he meant;
But the Belovéd was so pitiful
He cursed her as he went.

Some bade him quit vain inquest, and delight
Each sense with pleasant things;
And some swore 'twas the sign that Heaven would blight
His highest imagings;

And some – An operation would remove
The mere excrescent flesh;
While others – Pruning it would only prove
How fast 'twould grow afresh.

And some, who cited law and gospel, laid
New heaviness on his neck:
Let him that hath have ever more, they said,
And let the wreck'd bear wreck!

Yet after every check, repulse, and scoff,
He ask'd again, again –
What is this burthen? Can none take it off?
Is there no end of pain?

Flung back on his own soul, what he inquired
Was hardly, sadly taught;
With desperate travail he at length acquired
Something of what he sought.

He found there was a meaning: that was much:
He trusted God was Good:
These thoughts made patience earnest, out of such
He earn'd some spirit-food.

And grew: for all the evil hump remain'd,
Like Sindbad's Man o' the Sea.[23]
Only he had no hope to be unchain'd:
How from himself get free?

---

[23]Sinbad the Sailor was a fictional Middle Eastern hero known for his adventures on the high seas; according to legend, the Old Man of the Sea rides, maddeningly, on Sinbad's shoulders.

At last came Time, who from the chrysalis
Brings forth the rainbow'd fly;
Of Time he ask'd – What was this weight of his?
And Time gave full reply.

Time mask'd as Death, yet smiling, did unpack
The worn man's crushing load:
Two wings sprang forth; high o'er the cloudy wrack
The Angel, whom men call'd *That Poor Hunchback*,
Through farthest heavens rode.

So, looking westward yestereve, I knew
A figure of warm cloud:
A very humpback till his load he threw,
As Lazarus[24] left his shroud.

Dust and Disease[25]
Lord Charles Neaves (1875)

Of the wonderful things that lie round us concealed,
How much have the true Sons of Science revealed!
Good Faraday[26] long was the foremost of these,
And now Tyndall[27] has told us of Dust and Disease.

If a long beam of light crosses through a dark room,
It seems peopled with motes that shine bright in the gloom:
But the gay dancing things, that the gazer thus sees,
Are in fact nothing better than Dust and Disease.

Around us, above us, on all sides they float:
They light on our skin, and they slide down our throat:
Though we don't feel or see them, yet go where we please,
The atmosphere's laden with Dust and Disease.

All the varying ills to which flesh is an heir,
All the foes of both body and mind may be there.
Lusts and Fevers that burn, Fears and Agues that freeze,
May be mixed in these atoms of Dust and Disease.

---

[24]In the Bible, Jesus miraculously restored Lazarus of Bethany to life, four days after his death.
[25]In the last half of the nineteenth century, the germ theory of disease supplanted earlier models of disease, such as 'miasma theory', which held that diseases such as plague and cholera were caused by a noxious form of 'bad air'.
[26]Michael Faraday (1791–1867) was an English scientist who contributed to the fields of electromagnetism and electrochemistry.
[27]John Tyndall (1820–93) was a prominent nineteenth-century physicist, who discovered an effective way to eradicate bacterial spores, affirming 'germ theory' against its critics.

All places alike these intruders infest,
And 'tis thought that St Stephen's is none of the best:
Where Faction and Folly are busy as bees,
There will always be plenty of Dust and Disease.

In Westminster Hall, where the Lawyers convene,
These pestilent particles ever are seen:
Where wrangling and wrath can be hired with big fees,
You are sure of a market for Dust and Disease.

The Church should be free; but some heretics say
That at present the Vatican's in a bad way:
And some other Assemblies of learned D. D.'s[28]
Are perhaps not exempted from Dust and Disease.

The Dissenters[29] are thought a peculiar people,
More pious than those that sit under a Steeple:
But some one-sided views and intolerant pleas
Seem to savour a little of Dust and Disease.

But what of the Doctors? are *they* without flaw?
Is Medicine more pure than Religion or Law?
I suspect that some even with Doctors' degrees
Love to kick up a Dust and shake hands with Disease.

Diplomacy dresses her visage in smiles,
To conceal all the better her treacherous wiles:
But behind her false front a keen critic may seize
On strong proofs of her traffic with Dust and Disease.

Where Fashion and Luxury glitter like gold,
But where Beauty is bartered and Honour is sold,
Though the surface show little to shock or displease,
Yet beneath – all is Misery, Dust, and Disease.

Some attacks on the lungs, that of woe would be full,
Are repelled by a filter of loose Cotton Wool:
But a barrier of brass, or a *chevaux-de-frise*,[30]
Won't exclude some descriptions of Dust and Disease.

How long will these poison-germs stifle the day?
When will Truth's blessed light shed a purified ray?

---

[28]D. D.: Doctor of Divinity.
[29]Protestants who refused to recognize the supremacy of the Established Anglican Church were known as Dissenters.
[30]A *chevaux-de-frise* was a medieval anti-cavalry defence consisting of a portable frame and many projecting long iron or wooden spikes.

When will Phoebus[31] send heat, or Favonius a breeze,
To destroy or disperse all this Dust and Disease?

Behold the Plague-wind, from some Orient Fen
Evelyn Douglas (John Evelyn Barlas) (1887)

Behold the plague-wind. From some orient fen
It rises spreading out its foggy wings
And wreathing in long curls its smoke-like rings –
A great wise serpent, darting far its ken,
Eager to see the cities of strange men,
To quench the thirst of knowledge at pure springs,
To spread itself over the face of things,
River and sea, mountain and flowery glen.
Sinuous it glides, and lengthens from the hills,
Gathering up its train of shortening folds.
With earnest love the monster onward sweeps.
A blue steam rises mantling o'er the rills,
And o'er the cities and the spreading wolds,
And the dead lie about the plains in heaps.

Indian Fevers
Sir Ronald Ross (1890–93)

In this, O Nature, yield I pray to me.
I pace and pace, and think and think, and take
The fever'd hands, and note down all I see,
That some dim distant light may haply break.

The painful faces ask, can we not cure?
We answer, No, not yet; we seek the laws.
O God, reveal through all this thing obscure
The unseen, small, but million-murdering cause.

Bangalore, 1890–93

The Scourge of God
Frederick William Orde Ward (F. Harald Williams) (1894)

We come from the fiery East,
From the land of the yellow face –
We come to the funeral feast,
To our own appointed place;

---

[31]In mythology, Phoebus Appollo was the god of sun and light; Favonius was the Roman god of the western wind.

From the dismal swamps that breed
Fever and woe and pain,
With the slimy toad and reed
And the belt of scorching plain;
On the back of the stormwind's breath,
In the right of the judgment rod,
With our mission of doom and death
We come as the Scourge of God.

We are sent by an awful Power
And its sentences we wreak,
And we laugh at the radiant flower
That glows on the maiden's cheek;
We regard not the snows of age
Nor the fulness of the years,
And the bud in its opening stage
Folds up at our blasting fears;
As we march on our silent path,
The thrones of the highest nod
And the bravest flee our wrath,
For we are the Scourge of God.

We mock at the wisest plan
As we hurry on to slay,
All the barriers built by man
Cannot bind our course a day;
For his false and foolish lore
Tricked out in the learnèd names,
And the medicines in his store,
Are but fuel to our flames;
He may baffle the shot and shell
And triumph as others trod,
Against us there is no spell,
For we are the Scourge of God.

We follow the wake of sin
As the shadow falls with night,
When our armies enter in
The angels have taken flight;
For we must perform our task,
While we purge the temple floor
And the guilty land unmask,
As we knock at every door;
And the hidden vice starts up
Though in pearls and purple shod,
Though it grasps the golden cup,
For we are the Scourge of God.

Malaria
Sir Ronald Ross (1897)[32]

This day relenting God
Hath placed within my hand
A wondrous thing; and God
Be praised. At His command,

Seeking His secret deeds
With tears and toiling breath,
I find thy cunning seeds,
O million-murdering Death.

I know this little thing
A myriad men will save.
O Death, where is thy sting?
Thy victory, O Grave?

Yellow Jack of '97[33]
Samuel Alfred Beadle (1899)

With a shudder still I remember
The alarm of Yellow Jack:
Sent out in the daily number,
Of the 'Times-Democrat.'[34]

Also the 'Daily Picayune'[35]
Made the dreaded tidings known;
The paper venders caught the tune
And heralded it around the town.

'Here's your Daily Picayune,'
And 'Here's your Times-Democrat!'
'Paper, sir, Daily Picayune,
All about the Yellow Jack!'

'At Ocean Springs and Scranton, sir,
Biloxi[36] and ev'rywhere
Along the coast – Picayune, sir?
All about the fever hit there!

---

[32]From the longer poem 'Exile'; Ronald Ross was awarded the Nobel Prize in 1902 for the discovery that mosquitoes transmit malaria (1897–98). Malaria is a mosquito-borne infectious disease caused by parasitic microorganisms.
[33]Yellow Jack, or yellow fever, is an acute viral disease whose symptoms include fever, chills, loss of appetite, nausea and back pain.
[34]*The Times Democrat*: New Orleans newspaper, 1881–1914.
[35]*The Times-Picayune* (originally *The Picayune*): New Orleans newspaper, since the 1830s.
[36]Ocean Springs, Scranton and Biloxi are coastal towns on the Gulf of Mexico, Mississippi.

'There 'tis, sir! a catastrophe,
Strikes our business interest square,
And leaves us a wreck in mid sea,
With fever and despair.'

'If it's fever, it's dengue,[37]
Or malaria from lack
Of cleanliness, in a few
Coast towns. It's not Yellow Jack,'

Said all the doctors, looking wise.
But the restless feeling grew,
And all the people, with glaring eyes,
And ashen lips, said 'It's true!'

From the start business stopped, congealed,
And strong men gathered the crowd
About the public streets, to feel
The business pulse, sigh aloud;

And then to troop it out of town:
For their fancy paints so well,
Until it kinder brings them down,
To unwholesome views of – Well –

You understand; roasting scenes in that
Sultry country where the swell
Epidemic fiend, grim Yellow Jack,
The conductor acts so well.

You talk of being panic struck,
Routed friend and all of that;
You should see the bulletin stuck
To the alarm of Yellow Jack.

For yellow fever 'larms from press
And newsboys, can clear the earth
With inflated yells of distress
In twenty minutes without death.

And then the faithful few, who stand
At duty's post; because
They cannot escape, understand,
Prohibitory laws.

---

[37]Dengue fever (also known as breakbone fever) is a mosquito-borne tropical disease; symptoms include fever, headache, muscle and joint pains, and a characteristic skin rash similar to measles.

They quarantine the empty void
With a mailed guard so well,
That 'twould terrorize the alloid
Visage of the host of Hell.

Then gnaws the formidable thought,
Quarantined away from home:
This experience so dearly bought,
So vividly paints our own:

Till we see the ghost of all our hopes
Floating down the yellow stream;
Our empty homes along the copse
And grim Yellow Jack between.

And hear the stroke of the sturdy oar,
The surge of the awful wave;
As Yellow Jack trips our loved ones o'er –
The druggist into the grave.

Song of the Dwarf
Rainer Maria Rilke (1906)[38]

My soul may be straight and good;
but my heart, my bent blood,
all that hurts me inside;
it can't hold upright.
It has no garden, it has no bed,
it clings to my sharp skeleton
with horrified beating of wings.

Nor will anything ever come of my hands.
Look at how stunted they are:
sluggishly they hop, damp and heavy,
like little toads after the rain.
And the rest of me is
worn out and old and dreary;
why does God hesitate to throw
all this on the heap.

Could it be that he hates me for my face
with its grumpy jowls?
So often it was ready with all its heart

---

[38]Trans. Edward Snow.

to be friendly and appealing;
but nothing ever came up close
the way the big dogs do.
And the dogs couldn't care less.

With Cholera Morbus[39]
John Banister Tabb (1907)

I am so sick I'd like to be
A clock, to have them open me
And regulate the jerks,
When on the pendulum a Pain
Is riding forth and back again,
And pulling at my works.

Going Blind
Rainer Maria Rilke (1908)[40]

She sat just like the others at the table.
But on second glance, she seemed to hold her cup
a little differently as she picked it up.
She smiled once. It was almost painful.

And when they finished and it was time to stand
and slowly, as chance selected them, they left
and moved through many rooms (they talked and laughed),
I saw her. She was moving far behind

the others, absorbed, like someone who will soon
have to sing before a large assembly;
upon her eyes, which were radiant with joy,
light played as on the surface of a pool.

She followed slowly, taking a long time,
as though there were some obstacle in the way;
and yet: as though, once it was overcome,
she would be beyond all walking, and would fly.

Malade
D. H. Lawrence (1916)

The sick grapes on the chair by the bed lie prone; at the window
The tassel of the blind swings gently, tapping the pane,

---

[39]Cholera morbus is now known as acute gastroenteritis.
[40]Trans. Stephen Mitchell.

As a little wind comes in.
The room is the hollow rind of a fruit, a gourd
Scooped out and dry, where a spider,
Folded in its legs as in a bed,
Lies on the dust, watching where is nothing to see but twilight and walls.

And if the day outside were mine! What is the day
But a grey cave, with great grey spider-cloths hanging
Low from the roof, and the wet dust falling softly from them
Over the wet dark rocks, the houses, and over
The spiders with white faces, that scuttle on the floor of the cave!
I am choking with creeping, grey confinedness.

But somewhere birds, beside a lake of light, spread wings
Larger than the largest fans, and rise in a stream upwards
And upwards on the sunlight that rains invisible,
So that the birds are like one wafted feather,
Small and ecstatic suspended over a vast spread country.

Disabled
Wilfred Owen (1916)

He sat in a wheeled chair, waiting for dark,
And shivered in his ghastly suit of grey,
Legless, sewn short at elbow. Through the park
Voices of boys rang saddening like a hymn,
Voices of play and pleasure after day,
Till gathering sleep had mothered them from him.

About this time Town used to swing so gay
When glow-lamps budded in the light blue trees,
And girls glanced lovelier as the air grew dim –
In the old times, before he threw away his knees.
Now he will never feel again how slim
Girls' waists are, or how warm their subtle hands.
All of them touch him like some queer disease.

There was an artist silly for his face,
For it was younger than his youth, last year.
Now, he is old; his back will never brace;
He's lost his colour very far from here,
Poured it down shell-holes till the veins ran dry,
And half his lifetime lapsed in the hot race
And leap of purple spurted from his thigh.

One time he liked a blood-smear down his leg,
After the matches, carried shoulder-high.

It was after football, when he'd drunk a peg,
He thought he'd better join. He wonders why.
Someone had said he'd look a god in kilts,
That's why; and maybe, too, to please his Meg,
Aye, that was it, to please the giddy jilts
He asked to join. He didn't have to beg;
Smiling they wrote his lie: aged nineteen years.

Germans he scarcely thought of; all their guilt,
And Austria's, did not move him. And no fears
Of Fear came yet. He thought of jewelled hills
For daggers in plaid socks; of smart salutes;
And care of arms; and leave; and pay arrears;
Esprit de corps; and hints for young recruits.
And soon, he was drafted out with drums and cheers.

Some cheered him home, but not as crowds cheer Goal.
Only a solemn man who brought him fruits
Thanked him; and then enquired about his soul.

Now, he will spend a few sick years in institutes,
And do what things the rules consider wise,
And take whatever pity they may dole.
Tonight he noticed how the women's eyes
Passed from him to the strong men that were whole.
How cold and late it is! Why don't they come
And put him into bed? Why don't they come?

The Germ
Ogden Nash (1925)

A mighty creature is the germ,
Though smaller than the pachyderm.
His customary dwelling place
Is deep within the human race.
His childish pride he often pleases
By giving people strange diseases.
Do you, my popet, feel infirm?
You probably contain a germ.

Fever 103°
Sylvia Plath (1962)

Pure? What does it mean?
The tongues of hell
Are dull, dull as the triple

Tongues of dull, fat Cerberus[41]
Who wheezes at the gate. Incapable
Of licking clean

The aguey tendon, the sin, the sin.
The tinder cries.
The indelible smell

Of a snuffed candle!
Love, love, the low smokes roll
From me like Isadora's scarves, I'm in a fright

One scarf will catch and anchor in the wheel.[42]
Such yellow sullen smokes
Make their own element. They will not rise,

But trundle round the globe
Choking the aged and the meek,
The weak

Hothouse baby in its crib,
The ghastly orchid
Hanging its hanging garden in the air,

Devilish leopard!
Radiation turned it white
And killed it in an hour.

Greasing the bodies of adulterers
Like Hiroshima[43] ash and eating in.
The sin. The sin.

Darling, all night
I have been flickering, off, on, off, on.
The sheets grow heavy as a lecher's kiss.

Three days. Three nights.
Lemon water, chicken
Water, water make me retch.

---

[41]In Greek and Roman mythology, Cerberus was a multi-headed dog, with a serpent's tail, a mane of snakes, and a lion's claws. He guarded the entrance of the underworld to prevent the dead from escaping, and the living from entering.
[42]Refers to the American dancer Isadora Duncan (1877–1927), who died in an automobile accident in Nice, France, when her silk scarf became entangled in the car's wheel, breaking her neck.
[43]Hiroshima, Japan, was the first city in history to be targeted by a nuclear weapon when the US Army Air Forces (USAAF) dropped an atomic bomb at 8:15 am on 6 August 1945.

I am too pure for you or anyone.
Your body
Hurts me as the world hurts God. I am a lantern –

My head a moon
Of Japanese paper, my gold beaten skin
Infinitely delicate and infinitely expensive.

Does not my heat astound you. And my light.
All by myself I am a huge camellia
Glowing and coming and going, flush on flush.

I think I am going up,
I think I may rise –
The beads of hot metal fly, and I, love, I

Am a pure acetylene
Virgin
Attended by roses,

By kisses, by cherubim,
By whatever these pink things mean.
Not you, nor him.

Not him, nor him
(My selves dissolving, old whore petticoats) –
To Paradise.

Suffering
Miroslav Holub (1963)[44]

Ugly creatures, ugly grunting creatures,
Completely concealed under the point of the needle,
    behind the curve of the Research Task Graph,
Disgusting creatures with foam at the mouth,
    with bristles on their bottoms,
One after the other
They close their pink mouths
They open their pink mouths
They grow pale

---

[44]Trans. George Theiner.

Flutter their legs
   as if they were running a very
   long distance,

They close ugly blue eyes,
They open ugly blue eyes
   and
   they're
   dead.

But I ask no questions,
no one asks any questions.

And after their death we let the ugly creatures
   run in pieces along the white expanse
   of the paper electrophore.

We let them graze in the greenish-blue pool
   of the chromatogram
And in pieces we drive them for a dip
   in alcohol
   and xylol
And the immense eye of the ugly animal god
   watches their every move
   through the tube of the microscope
And the bits of animals are satisfied
like flowers in a flower-pot
   like kittens at the bottom of a pond
   like cells before conception.
But I ask no questions,
   no one asks any questions,
Naturally no one asks
Whether these creatures wouldn't have preferred
   to live all in one piece,
   their disgusting life
   in bogs
   and canals,
Whether they wouldn't have preferred to eat
   one another alive,
Whether they wouldn't have preferred to make love
   in between horror and hunger,
Whether they wouldn't have preferred to use
   all their eyes and pores to perceive
   their muddy stinking little world

Incredibly terrified,
Incredibly happy
In the way of matter which can do no more.

But I ask no questions,
    no one asks any questions,
Because it's all quite useless,
Experiments succeed and experiments fail,
Like everything else in this world,
    in which the truth advances
    like some splendid silver bulldozer
    in the tumbling darkness,

Like everything else in this world,
    in which I met a lonely girl
    inside a shop selling bridal veils,
In which I met a general covered
        with oak leaves,
In which I met ambulance men who could find no
        wounded,
In which I met a man who had lost
        his name,
In which I met a glorious and famous, bronze,
        incredibly terrified rat,
In which I met people who wanted to lay down
        their lives and people who wanted to lay down
        their heads in sorrow,
In which, come to think of it, I keep meeting my
        own self at every step.

A New Year Greeting[45]
W. H. Auden (1969)
(After an article by Mary J. Marples in *Scientific American*, January, 1969)

On this day tradition allots
to taking stock of our lives,
my greetings to all of you, Yeasts,
Bacteria, Viruses,
Aerobics and Anaerobics:

---

[45]W. H. Auden had Touraine–Solente–Golé syndrome, a rare genetic skin disorder also known as pachydermoperiostosis, which affects both bones and skin and is mainly characterized by pachydermia (thickening of the skin), accounting for Auden's recognizable facial wrinkles.

A Very Happy New Year
to all for whom my ectoderm
is as Middle-Earth to me.

For creatures your size I offer
a free choice of habitat,
so settle yourselves in the zone
that suits you best, in the pools
of my pores, in the tropical
forests of arm-pit and crotch,
in the deserts of my fore-arms,
or the cool woods of my scalp.

Build colonies: I will supply
adequate warmth and moisture,
the sebum and lipids[46] you need,
on condition you never
do me annoy with your presence,
but behave as good guests should,
not rioting into acne
or athlete's-foot or a boil.

Does my inner weather affect
the surfaces where you live?
Do unpredictable changes
record my rocketing plunge
from fairs when the mind is in tift
and relevant thoughts occur,
to fouls when nothing will happen
and no one calls and it rains.

I should like to think that I make
a not impossible world,
but an Eden it cannot be:
my games, my purposive acts,
may turn to catastrophes there.
If you were religious folk,
how would your dramas justify
unmerited suffering?

---

[46]Sebum is an odourless, waxy secretion, but when broken down by bacteria, produces strong odors. Lipids are body fats.

By what myths would your priests account
for the hurricanes that come
twice every twenty-four hours,
each time I dress or undress,
when, clinging to keratin rafts,
whole cities are swept away
to perish in space, or the Flood
that scalds to death when I bathe?

Then, sooner or later, will dawn
a Day of Apocalypse,
when my mantle suddenly turns
too cold, too rancid, for you,
appetising to predators
of a fiercer sort, and I
am stripped of excuse and nimbus,
a Past, subject to Judgement.

The Patient
Peter Meinke (1977)

disease has expanded my horizons
and pain
spread the good word

since I've been sick
I feel close to the blighted things of nature
(I myself am a blighted thing of nature)
burnt oaks
gutted houses
(for surely houses are as natural as beehives)
broken foxes lying by the highway

bugs crawl along the rims of my glasses
my body pocked with spiraled holes
like those punched in butter
in each hole something moving

hooked on disease (it gives
meaning to my life) I wriggle wormlike
around the pain and God
is the large-mouthed bass circling
below me

Two Years
Muriel Rukeyser (1978)

Two years of my sister's bitter illness;
the wind whips the river of her last spring.
I have burned the beans again.

Typhus
Louis Aston Marantz Simpson (1979)

'The whole earth was covered with snow,
and the Snow Queen's sleigh came gliding.
I heard the bells behind me,
and ran, and ran, till I was out of breath.'

During the typhus epidemic
she almost died, and would have
but for the woman who lived next door
who cooked for her and watched by the bed.

When she came back to life
and saw herself in a mirror
they had cut off all her hair.
Also, they had burned her clothing,
and her doll, the only one she ever had,
made out of rags and a stick.

Afterwards, they sent her away
to Odessa,[47] to stay with relatives.
The day she was leaving for home
she bought some plums, as a gift
to take back to the family.
They had never seen such plums!
They were in a window, in a basket.
To buy them she spent her last few kopecks.[48]

The journey took three days by train.
It was hot, and the plums were beginning to spoil.
So she ate them ...

---

[47]Odessa is the third largest city in Ukraine, located on the north-western shore of the Black Sea.
[48]The Russian ruble is divided into 100 kopecks.

until, finally, all were gone.
The people on the train were astonished.
A child who would eat a plum
and cry … then eat another!

…

Her sister, Lisa, died of typhus.
The corpse was laid on the floor.

They carried it to the cemetery
in a box, and brought back the box.
'We were poor – a box was worth something.'

from C
Peter Reading (1984)

Disseminated spinal carcinoma.[49]
I have lost all control and movement of
the abdomen, legs, feet and back. The growth
(particularly painful) on the spine
prevents my lying on my back. Bedsores
daily increase in size, restrict still more
manipulation of me on the bed –
nurses change my position every hour.
the open bedsores suppurate and stink …
I am abusive to a social worker.

We, trained Caregivers, can identify
symptoms like this – he is withdrawn and craves
attentive sympathy. Each afternoon
I persist – my ability to bear
his poor responses helps him to contain
his desperation. So there is much comfort.

…

My fistulae ooze blood and stink,
I vomit puce spawn in the sink,
diarrhoea is exuded.
Do not be deluded:
mortality's worse than you think.

---

[49]A spreading cancer of the spine.

Pneumoconiosis[50]
Duncan Bush (1985)

This is The Dust:

black diamond dust.

I had thirty years in it, boy,
a laughing red mouth
coming up to spit smuts black
into a handkerchief.

But it's had forty years
in me now:
so fine
you could inhale it
through a gag.
I'll die with it now.
It's in me,
like my blued scars.

But I try not to think about it.

I take things pretty easy, these days;
one step at a time.
Especially the stairs.
I try not to think about it.

I saw my own brother: rising,
dying in panic, gasping
worse than a hooked
carp drowning in air.
Every breath was his last.

I try not to think about it.

                But
know me by my slow step,
       the occasional little cough, involuntary
and delicate as a consumptive's,

and my lungs full of budgerigars.

---

[50]Pneumoconiosis is an occupational lung disease caused by the inhalation of dust.

Fever
Eavan Boland (1986)

is what remained or what they thought
remained after the ague and the sweats
were over and the shock of wild flowers
at the bedside had been taken away;

is what they tried to shake out of
the crush and dimple of cotton,
the shy dust of a bridal skirt;
is what they beat, lashed, hurt like

flesh as if it were a lack of virtue
in a young girl sobbing her heart out
in a small town for having been seen
kissing by the river; is what they burned

alive in their own back gardens
as if it were a witch and not the full-
length winter gabardine and breathed again
when the fires went out in charred dew.

When grandmother died in her fever ward,
younger than I am and far from
the sweet chills of a Louth spring –
its sprigged light and its wild flowers –

with five orphan daughters to her name.
Names, shadows, visitations, hints
and a half-sense of half-lives remain.
And nothing else, nothing more unless

I re-construct the soaked-through midnights;
vigils; the histories I never learned
to predict the lyric of; and re-construct
risk; as if silence could become rage,

as if what we lost is a contagion
that breaks out in what cannot be
shaken out from words or beaten out
from meaning and survives to weaken

what is given, what is certain
and burns away everything but this
exact moment of delirium when
someone cries out someone's name.

Cancer and Nova
Hyam Plutzik (1987)

The star exploding in the body;
The creeping thing, growing in the brain or the bone;
The hectic cannibal, the obscene mouth.

The mouths along the meridian sought him,
Soft as moths, many a moon and sun,
Until one
In a pale fleeing dream caught him.

Waking, he did not know himself undone,
Nor walking, smiling, reading that the news was good,
The star exploding in his blood.

Pestilence [Epidemic]
Charles Reznikoff (1919; 1989)[51]

Streamers of crepe idling before doors.
Now the huge moon
at the end of the street like a house afire.

Thinking about Bill, Dead of AIDS
Miller Williams (1990)

We did not know the first thing about
how blood surrenders to even the smallest threat
when old allergies turn inside out,

the body rescinding all its normal orders
to all defenders of flesh, betraying the head,
pulling its guards back from all its borders.

Thinking of friends afraid to shake your hand,
we think of your hand shaking, your mouth set,
your eyes drained of any reprimand.

Loving, we kissed you, partly to persuade
both you and us, seeing what eyes had said,
that we were loving and were not afraid.

If we had had more, we would have given more.
As it was we stood next to your bed,
stopping, though, to set our smiles at the door.

---

[51]This is the 1919 version; in 1989, only the first line of the poem was published as 'Epidemic'.

Not because we were less sure at the last.
Only because, not knowing anything yet,
we didn't know what look would hurt you least.

The Weakness
Bernard O'Donoghue (1991)

It was the frosty early hours when finally
The cow's despairing groans rolled him from bed
And into his boots, hardly awake yet.
He called 'Dan! come on, Dan!
She's calving,' and stumbled without his coat
Down the icy path to the haggard.

Castor and Pollux[52] were fixed in line
Over his head but he didn't see them,
This night any more than another.
He crossed to the stall, past the corner
Of the fairy-fort[53] he'd levelled last May.
But this that stopped him, like the mind's step

Backward: what was that, more insistent
Than the calf's birth-pangs? 'Hold on, Dan.
I think I'm having a weakness.
I never had a weakness, Dan, before.'
And down he slid, groping for the lapels
Of the shocked boy's twenty-year-old jacket.

The Man with Night Sweats
Thom Gunn (1992)

I wake up cold, I who
Prospered through dreams of heat
Wake to their residue,
Sweat, and a clinging sheet.

My flesh was its own shield:
Where it was gashed, it healed.

I grew as I explored
The body I could trust

---

[52]In Greek and Roman mythology, Castor and Pollux (or Polydeuces) were twin brothers, known as the Dioskouri. When Castor was killed, Pollux asked Zeus to let him share his immortality with his twin, and they were transformed into the constellation Gemini.
[53]Fairy forts, also known as *raths* from the Irish, are the earthen mounds marking the remains of ring forts, hill forts and other circular dwellings in Ireland. Thought to be the abode of fairies and 'little people'.

Even while I adored
The risk that made robust,

A world of wonders in
Each challenge to the skin.

I cannot but be sorry
The given shield was cracked,
My mind reduced to hurry,
My flesh reduced and wrecked.

I have to change the bed,
But catch myself instead

Stopped upright where I am
Hugging my body to me
As if to shield it from
The pains that will go through me,

As if hands were enough
To hold an avalanche off.

Ankylosing Spondylitis[54]
Simon Armitage (1993)

Ankylosing meaning bond or join
and spondylitis meaning of the bone or spine.
That half explains the cracks and clicks,
the clockwork of my joints and discs,
the ratchet of my hips. I'm fossilising –
every time I rest
I let the gristle knit, weave, mesh.

My dear, my skeleton will set like biscuit overnight,
like glass, like ice, and you can choose
to snap me back to life before first light,
or let me laze until
the shape I take becomes the shape I keep.

Don't leave me be. Don't let me sleep.

---

[54]Ankylosing spondylitis, is a chronic inflammatory disease of the skeleton, which mainly affects joints in the spine and the sacro-iliac joint in the pelvis. In severe cases, it can eventually cause complete fusion and rigidity of the spine.

Fog
Mark Doty (1993)

> The crested iris by the front gate waves
> its blue flags three days, exactly,
>
> then they vanish. The peony buds'
> tight wrappings are edged crimson;
>
> when they open, a little blood-color
> will ruffle at the heart of the flounced,
>
> unbelievable white. Three weeks after the test,
> the vial filled from the crook
>
> of my elbow, I'm seeing blood everywhere:
> a casual nick from the garden shears,
>
> a shaving cut and I feel the physical rush
> of the welling up, the wine-fountain
>
> dark as Siberian iris. The thin green porcelain
> teacup, our homemade Ouija's planchette,
>
> rocks and wobbles every night, spins
> and spells. It seems a cloud of spirits
>
> numerous as lilac panicles vie for occupancy –
> children grabbing for the telephone,
>
> happy to talk to someone who isn't dead yet?
> Everyone wants to speak at once, or at least
>
> these random words appear, incongruous
> and exactly spelled: *energy, immunity, kiss.*
>
> Then: *M. has immunity. W. has.*
> And that was all. One character, Frank,
>
> distinguishes himself: a boy who lived
> in our house in the thirties, loved dogs
>
> and gangster movies, longs for a body,
> says he can watch us through the television,
>
> asks us to stand before the screen
> and kiss. *God in garden*, he says.
>
> Sitting out on the back porch at twilight,
> I'm almost convinced. In this geometry
>
> of paths and raised beds, the green shadows
> of delphinium, there's an unseen rustling:

some secret amplitude
seems to open in this orderly space.

Maybe because it contains so much dying,
all these tulip petals thinning

at the base until any wind takes them.
I doubt anyone else would see that, looking in,

and then I realize my garden has no outside, only *is*
subjectively. As blood is utterly without

an outside, can't be seen except out of context,
the wrong color in alien air, no longer itself.

Though it submits to test, two,
to be exact, each done three times,

though not for me, since at their first entry
into my disembodied blood

there was nothing at home there.
For you they entered the blood garden over

and over, like knocking at a door
because you know someone's home. Three times

the Elisa Test,[55] three the Western Blot,[56]
and then the incoherent message. We're

the public health care worker's
nine o'clock appointment,

she is a phantom hand who forms
the letters of your name, and the word

that begins with P. I'd lie out
and wait for the god if it weren't

so cold, the blue moon huge
and disruptive above the flowering crab's

foaming collapse. The spirits say *Fog*
when they can't speak clearly

and the letters collide; sometimes
for them there's nothing outside the mist

---

[55]The ELISA test uses components of the immune system and chemicals to detect immune responses in the body (for instance, to infectious microbes).
[56]The western blot, sometimes called the protein immunoblot detects specific antibodies and proteins in a tissue sample, in this case for HIV.

of their dying. Planchette,
peony, I would think of anything

not to say the word. Maybe the blood
in the flower is a god's. Kiss me,

in front of the screen, please,
the dead are watching.

They haven't had enough yet.
Every new bloom is falling apart.

I would say anything else
in the world, any other word.

The Plague of Painlessness
Eve Merriam (1995)

A pin shall prick thy finger and thou shalt feel it not

Thy tooth shall be extracted and thou shalt be anaesthetized

Thou shalt be bitten by a mad dog and injected with serum
and the mad dog be shot and neither of you feel any pain

Thou shalt pass every day a bundle of rags
and lo the bundle of rags shall arise
and cry Woe Woe Give unto me
a quarter a dime a nickel help oh help me for I am homeless
and thou shalt be anaesthetized and pass on

Thou shalt be in the antechamber of the hospital awaiting
birth or death
and thou shalt peruse the news of the world
and the pages shall offer up unto thine eyes
FAMINE IN CENTRAL AFRICA
LATEST FASHION BIKINI LEAVES NO
STRAPMARKS
DIOXIN
DIET COOKBOOK
FILM STAR OF THE YEAR
ASSASSINATION OF THE YEAR

and no one thing shall be worse
and none better
and thou shalt ingest them all
the painless smiling same

have a nice have a nice have a not nice
have a nice nice not nice not nice.

Fragments: Mrs Reuben Chandler writes to her Husband During a Cholera Epidemic[57]
Anne Stevenson (1996)

En route from New York to New Orleans aboard the 'General Wayne',
August 1849

Two weeks aboard the 'General Wayne'
is little more than a floating hospital
vomiting spells. I attribute them to
is truly ill. For two days he has
in his bunk.
Belle seems to recover. At least
fretful which indicates improvement.
struck by a nervous disorder.
I sleep very little and take no solid food.
    (page torn)

(Second page)
Yesterday evening poor little Cookie died.
She was seized suddenly with spasms, poor thing,
and died in an hour. You will accuse me of
but it was truly frightful.
I have not slept for weeping.
only a dog!
    (page torn)

(Third page)
arrived safely in New Orleans but
embark. We are all in quarantine
might be better, but Belle is
all day by her bedside. Doctor
plague and gives me no hope
pray for survival.
    (page torn)

(Fourth page)
have not been able to put pen to
all over. Our dear little girl
among the blessed, my beautiful

---

[57]Author's note: Most of this journal, written on shipboard, seems to have been destroyed, probably by fire. What remains suggests that Mrs Chandler journeyed to New Orleans without her husband's permission, thus in her mind becoming an indirect cause of her baby's death.

authorities let no one near.
darkies. I am full of
one who was without fault and so
lies shrouded in my sister's
blame God and myself, dear
why you have left me without support?
    (*page torn*)

Psoriasis[58]
Sarah Maguire (1997)

After all this time on my knees
I am starting to bleed –

the cushion, the dark sheets
are foxed with my dead skin

worn from love
from the way you move me,

the cream dust like meal,
spoor in the tracks.

Again you kneel back
to look at me like this

opened before you, patient
your hand encircling my ankle.

It has rained all afternoon,
the light fretting of water on glass

seeps into my breathing,
your musk on my lips.

I lay my cheek on the pillow
to take you in.

I could be a child again
suckling my own thumb.

---

[58]Psoriasis is a chronic disease characterized by red, scaly, itchy patches and papules on the skin.

Lymphoma[59]
Julia Kasdorf (1998)

Perhaps I should call your disease by its name
and admit that pain has no meaning, nothing to redeem it,

but I was gripped by beauty again this morning,
peeling the shell off a hard-boiled egg;

outside, the hydrangeas were heaps of light
on the lawn, harsh and brilliant. (Your skin

is now that pale.) And in the meadow
cabbage butterflies lifted like flakes

of lead white paint above white crests
of Queen Anne's lace in light so pure,

I ached. The lit stove: that vital blue exists
in the intricate veins of your wrist

and the map I now see on your scalp.
Clearly as a child, you sketch death –

the back of a rabbi walking fluorescent wards,
his long, black coat and *pais* blowing out –

and the delivery from death – yourself the Pietà[60]
in a blue hospital gown. Claiming no formal faith,

you draw out these meanings as I cling to words,
binding whatever I know to what I do not,

calling it all other names: your lymph nodes,
for instance, are new potatoes lodged against

a loaf of lung. Anything to comfort,
to tame. How can I think we have not found

meaning in this – or faith in the way we clutch
each other, each time I arrive or leave?

Metaphor as Illness
Ronald Wallace (1998)

He wakes up seasick, sleep's calm given way
to ocean swells, the roll of a distant storm.
He's damp and chilled, as if by the salt spray

---

[59]Lymphomas are a group of cancers affecting the lymph system.
[60]The Pietà is a common subject in Christian art depicting the Virgin Mary cradling the dead body of Jesus

slapping the sails, and when the tardy alarm
sounds, he's too far gone to heed it. The body
mutinies – it's every man for himself.
Who'll handle the bilge pumps? Claim the booty?
Steer the helpless ship through the terrible rough

night? Metaphor is too easy. Illness
demands the literal; none of this 'under the weather,'
none of this 'touch of the flu,' none of this
evasion and euphemism. Whole ships are lost,
all hands gone, the cargo and the treasure
lost to tropes – and those with health and leisure.

Prognoses
Carole Satyamurti (1998)

'She'll walk something like this ...'
Springing from his chair
he waddles, knees crumpled,
on the outer edges of his feet
– a hunchback, jester, ape,
a wind-up toy
assembled by a saboteur.
I turn away, concentrate
on the caesarean sting.

I wander corridors.

Far off, approaching,
a couple, hand in hand,
the girl, lurching
against the window's light.
I hear them laugh, pick up
the drift – a private joke,
the film they saw last night.
Long after they are gone, I hear
the jaunty click-creak of her callipers.

Salvador
Simon Armitage (2002)

He has come this far for the English to see,
arrived by bubble through a twelve-hour dream
of altitude sickness and relative speed, of leg room
and feet, headphone headache, reclining sleep.

Jet-lag slung from the eyes like hammocks at full stretch,
Meflaquin[61] pellets riding shotgun in a blister-pack.
This far south for the English to see, as they say.
The hotel drives towards him up the street,
he turns the keyhole anti-clockwise with the key,
the water spins the plug-hole backwards as it drains.
He counts the track-marks in his upper arm
and those in the buttocks and those in the calves,
the pins and needles of shots and jabs, strains and strands,
spores going wild in the tunnels and tubes of veins,
mushrooming into the brain. A polio[62] spider
abseils the drop from the sink to the bath.
Larium[63] country – this far south to broaden the mind.
Look, learn, rise to the day, throw back the blind:
the blue-green flowers of the meningitis[64] tree,
the two-note singing of the hepatitis[65] bird,
the two-stroke buzz of the tetanus[66] bee.
In a puff of chalk a yellow-fever[67] moth
collides and detonates against the window frame.
Malaria witters and whines in the radio waves.
A warm, diphtherial[68] breeze unsettles the pool.
Three hours behind and two days' growth –
hey you in the mirror, shaving in soap,
brushing your teeth in duty-free rum and mini-bar coke,
you with the look, you with the face – it's me, wake up.

Too Heavy
Julia Darling (2003)

Dear Doctor,
I am writing to complain about these words
you have given me, that I carry in my bag
lymphatic, nodal, progressive, metastatic

---

[61]Meflaquin (Mefloquine) is an anti-malarial drug.
[62]Poliomyelitis is an infectious disease, the symptoms of which incllude neck stiffness, pains in the arms and legs, and the wasting of the limbs.
[63]Lariam (Mefloquine) is an anti-malarial drug.
[64]Meningitis is the acute inflammation of the protective membranes covering the brain and spinal cord.
[65]Hepatitis is a medical condition defined by the inflammation of the liver, which often leads to yellow discoloration of the skin, poor appetite and malaise.
[66]Tetanus, also known as lockjaw, is an infection characterized by muscle spasms.
[67]Yellow fever, yellow jack or yellow plague is an acute viral disease. In most cases, symptoms include fever, chills, nausea and muscle pains particularly in the back.
[68]Diphtheria is an upper respiratory tract illness caused by bacteria and characterized by sore throat, low fever and blocked airway.

They must be made of lead. I haul them everywhere.
I've cricked my neck, I'm bent
with the weight of them
palliative, metabolic, recurrent

And when I get them out and put them on the table
they tick like bombs and overpower my own
sweet tasting words
orange, bus, coffee, June

I've been leaving them
crumpled up in pedal bins
where they fester and complain.
diamorphine, biopsy, inflammatory

And then you say
Where are your words Mrs Patient?
What have you done with your words?

Or worse, you give me that dewy look
Poor Mrs Patient has lost all her words, but shush,
don't upset her. I've got spares in the files.
Thank god for files.

So I was wondering,
Dear Doctor, if I could have
a locker,
my own locker
with a key.
I could collect them
one at a time,
and lay them on a plate
morphine-based, diagnostically,

with a garnish of
lollypop, monkey, lip.

The Ingliss Touriste Patient
Kelvin Corcoran (2004)

What do you mean too late? Is he in danger?

And I was afraid and thought I would die,
lifting off the table, only the ceiling above me
and the vertiginous air for your voice Melanie,
– Yesterday you should bring him, you must
be like sleep now, you must go to the hospital.

Next to Yorta, unconscious – ella Yorta, ella ella,
wake up wake up my daughter, my child;
Yorta – Aorta – Iota not caring one jot,
there's something wrong with a letter,
a letter is unconscious, a letter is Maria's daughter
next to Aorta, mine, something is wrong with the invisible.

Stand up.
Close your eyes.
Stand feet together.
You have the hurt problem.

I was there and not there,
under the great weight of the water
with the silver jackals and companions of the sea
suspended by a taste for the shape they once had;
diamonds of light dance over them,
they sit in a shining circle and grin,
– look at me, look at these anchors, look at these roots,
– down here the mind is overcome.

And I was there and not there,
wheeled off to brain scan land.
Where is my wife? Will I come back here? Where is she please?
Πού είναι η γυναίκα μου; Θα έρθει πίσω εδώ; Πού είναι παρακαλώ;
She's with the gypsies from the big camp
sliding along the corridors, riding hips,
I was back in the cardboard town by the airport,
– where do they come from?
– from here, they come from here.
Sliding along the dark corridors,
her hand holding up the baby's head to light the world.

Gracious Maria found us cold water;
she sat by her daughter all night,
drowsy Yorta recovering, Yorta the beautiful,
and Melanie thanked her for her help,
– oh but we are all people, yes.

I was there and not there:
Pound[69] in the olive grove raging,
a ghost white man waving a broken branch
in the perfect climate for the human nervous system;
the olive tree blown green and white and

---

[69]Ezra Pound (1885–1972) was an expatriate American poet and critic and a major figure of the early modernist movement.

the air like a lens for the Earth given a fair chance;
Pound went down to the ship, Europa, the wreckage,
raging, raging at the innocent ants of my harbour,
its arms open to the various world.

I was there and not there with my wife and my mother;
we stared at a small television at our feet, the size of a dark footlight;
it was the emergency services concert,
– firemen, bare-chested, singing Bohemian Rhapsody,
which was not to my taste;
we stood around the dark hole at our feet,
companionable and variously entertained.

My head was away and singing:
an' war'ly cares an' war'ly men / May a' gae tapsalteerie, O
my girls wait by the sea, longing for the waves,
green grow the rashes, O standing up so straight,

My head was away and singing:
all night I saw with my eyes closed
squares of blue-black landscape,
villages and tracks, cisterns, temples, bus lanes and hospitals;
a series of design features made for civilisation
before it was named; and talking of watercourses,
a mythology rising at every turn, local, particular and useful.
At last with my eyes open on the first day,
surprised not to see the landscapes imprinted on the world,
looking again and again, I was ready.

From Cambos, the air heavy with eucalyptus rolled over the car,
sweet pine and burnt dust off Taygetos drenched the road
and through Kardhamyli jasmine in waves fell upon us;
so you kept driving and I lay down and the full moon
made its path across the water and I was there.

A Great Stink
Paul Farley (2006)

> ... but in fifty years the Commons will complain
> they can't sit in this river's smell and soak
> their curtains in chloride of lime to take
> the edge off what they'll liken to a drain.
> 'King Cholera' will rise from *Punch* and walk[70]

---

[70]Known as 'King Cholera' for the way in which it controlled the fate of whole populations, cholera was personified as 'King' in a *Punch* cartoon in 1858 at the height of 'The Great Stink', when hot weather exacerbated the smell of untreated human waste in the Thames.

abroad with a peg on his nose. No poetry
will get written, save those olfactory
pieces papers commission: *This smell's a baulk*
to anything the eye can register
and crossing here is hazardous to health
at dawn, when all the night soil of Westminster
meets with a flood tide. Citizens of wealth,
flee for the summer while the city festers
and strike out for the coast like merde *yourselves.*

MEDICAL WRITING:

A Journal of the Plague Year
Daniel Defoe (1722)

They ran to conjurers and witches, and all sorts of deceivers, to know what should
become of them; who fed their fears, and kept them always alarmed and awake
on purpose to delude them and pick their pockets, so they were as mad upon their
running after quacks and mountebanks,[71] and every practising old woman, for
medicines and remedies; storing themselves with such multitudes of pills, potions,
and preservatives, as they were called, that they not only spent their money but
even poisoned themselves beforehand for fear of the poison of the infection;
and prepared their bodies for the plague, instead of preserving them against it.
On the other hand, it is incredible and scarce to be imagined, how the posts of
houses and corners of streets were plastered over with doctors' bills and papers
of ignorant fellows, quacking and tampering in physic, and inviting the people to
come to them for remedies, which was generally set off with such flourishes as
these, viz.: 'Infallible preventive pills against the plague.' 'Never failing preservatives
against the infection.' 'Sovereign cordials against the corruption of the air.' 'Exact
regulations for the conduct of the body, in case of an infection.' 'Anti-pestilential
pills.' 'Incomparable drink against the plague, never found out before.' 'An universal
remedy for the plague.' 'The only true plague water.' 'The royal antidote against
all kinds of infection' – and such a number more that I cannot reckon up; and if I
could, would fill a book of themselves to set them down.

Others set up bills to summon people to their lodgings for directions and advice
in the case of infection. These had specious titles also, such as these:

'An eminent High Dutch physician, newly come over from Holland, where he
resided during all the time of the great plague last year in Amsterdam, and cured
multitudes of people that actually had the plague upon them.'

'An Italian gentlewoman just arrived from Naples, having a choice secret to
prevent infection, which she found out by her great experience, and did wonderful
cures with it in the late plague there, wherein there died 20,000 in one day.'

---

[71]A mountebank is a swindler, particularly one who sells quack medicines.

'An ancient gentlewoman, having practised with great success in the late plague in this city, anno 1636, gives her advice only to the female sex. To be spoken with,' etc.

'An experienced physician, who has long studied the doctrine of antidotes against all sorts of poison and infection, has, after forty years' practice, arrived to such skill as may, with God's blessing, direct persons how to prevent their being touched by any contagious distemper[72] whatsoever. He directs the poor gratis.'

I take notice of these by way of specimen. I could give you two or three dozen of the like and yet have abundance left behind. 'Tis sufficient from these to apprise any one of the humour of those times, and how a set of thieves and pickpockets not only robbed and cheated the poor people of their money, but poisoned their bodies with odious and fatal preparations; some with mercury, and some with other things as bad, perfectly remote from the thing pretended to, and rather hurtful than serviceable to the body in case an infection followed.

...

It is scarce credible what dreadful cases happened in particular families every day. People in the rage of the distemper, or in the torment of their swellings, which was indeed intolerable, running out of their own government, raving and distracted, and oftentimes laying violent hands upon themselves, throwing themselves out at their windows, shooting themselves, etc.; mothers murdering their own children in their lunacy, some dying of mere grief as a passion, some of mere fright and surprise without any infection at all, others frighted into idiotism and foolish distractions, some into despair and lunacy, others into melancholy madness.

The pain of the swelling was in particular very violent, and to some intolerable; the physicians and surgeons may be said to have tortured many poor creatures even to death. The swellings in some grew hard, and they applied violent drawing-plaisters or poultices[73] to break them, and if these did not do they cut and scarified them in a terrible manner. In some, those swellings were made hard partly by the force of the distemper and partly by their being too violently drawn, and were so hard that no instrument could cut them, and then they burnt them with caustics, so that many died raving mad with the torment, and some in the very operation. In these distresses, some, for want of help to hold them down in their beds, or to look to them, laid hands upon themselves as above. Some broke out into the streets, perhaps naked, and would run directly down to the river if they were not stopped by the watchman or other officers, and plunge themselves into the water wherever they found it.

It often pierced my very soul to hear the groans and cries of those who were thus tormented, but of the two this was counted the most promising particular in the whole infection, for if these swellings could be brought to a head, and to break and run, or, as the surgeons call it, to digest, the patient generally recovered;

---

[72]Distemper is a viral disease (particularly of animals, especially dogs) causing fever, coughing and catarrh in humans. Here, Defoe conjures its political meaning, as the spread of disordered sentiment, a theme which is continued in subsequent paragraphs.

[73]A poultice is a soft, moist mass of natural herbs applied to the body to relieve soreness and inflammation and kept in place with a cloth.

whereas those who, like the gentlewoman's daughter, were struck with death at the beginning, and had the tokens come out upon them, often went about indifferent easy till a little before they died, and some till the moment they dropped down, as in apoplexies and epilepsies[74] is often the case. Such would be taken suddenly very sick, and would run to a bench or bulk, or any convenient place that offered itself, or to their own houses if possible, as I mentioned before, and there sit down, grow faint, and die. This kind of dying was much the same as it was with those who die of common mortifications, who die swooning, and, as it were, go away in a dream. Such as died thus had very little notice of their being infected at all till the gangrene was spread through their whole body; nor could physicians themselves know certainly how it was with them till they opened their breasts or other parts of their body and saw the tokens.

We had at this time a great many frightful stories told us of nurses and watchmen who looked after the dying people; that is to say, hired nurses who attended infected people, using them barbarously, starving them, smothering them, or by other wicked means hastening their end, that is to say, murdering of them; and watchmen, being set to guard houses that were shut up when there has been but one person left, and perhaps that one lying sick, that they have broke in and murdered that body, and immediately thrown them out into the dead-cart! And so they have gone scarce cold to the grave.

...

It is true that, as several physicians told my Lord Mayor, the fury of the contagion was such at some particular times, and people sickened so fast and died so soon, that it was impossible, and indeed to no purpose, to go about to inquire who was sick and who was well, or to shut them up with such exactness as the thing required, almost every house in a whole street being infected, and in many places every person in some of the houses; and that which was still worse, by the time that the houses were known to be infected, most of the persons infected would be stone dead, and the rest run away for fear of being shut up; so that it was to very small purpose to call them infected houses and shut them up, the infection having ravaged and taken its leave of the house before it was really known that the family was any way touched.

This might be sufficient to convince any reasonable person that as it was not in the power of the magistrates or of any human methods of policy, to prevent the spreading the infection, so that this way of shutting up of houses was perfectly insufficient for that end. Indeed it seemed to have no manner of public good in it, equal or proportionable to the grievous burden that it was to the particular families that were so shut up; and, as far as I was employed by the public in directing that severity, I frequently found occasion to see that it was incapable of answering the end.

---

[74]Apoplexy is an unconsciousness or incapacity resulting from a cerebral haemorrhage or stroke. Also meaning 'extreme anger'. Epilepsy is a neurological disorder marked by sudden recurrent episodes of sensory disturbance, loss of consciousness or convulsions, associated with abnormal electrical activity in the brain.

Letters on the Blind
Denis Diderot (1749)

I believe that we who see never imagine any shape without colouring it, and that if we are given little balls in the dark, whose substance and colour are unknown to us, we shall immediately think of them as black or white, or some other colour; and that if we did not, we, like the blind man, should have the remembrance only of little sensations excited at our fingers' ends, and such as little round bodies may occasion. This remembrance be very fleeting with us, if we have very little idea how one born blind fixes, recalls and combines the sensations of touch, it is owing to the custom we derive from our eyes of realising everything in our imagination by means of colours.

It has happened, however, that during the agitations of a violent passion I felt a thrill run through my whole hand, and I felt the impression of the bodies I had touched some time ago revived as vividly as if they had been still present to my touch, and I realised very distinctly that the limits of sensation exactly coincided with those of these absent bodies.

Although sensation by itself is indivisible, it occupies, if one may use the word, an extension in space to which the blind man is able to add and subtract mentally by enlarging or diminishing the parts affected. By this means he compares points, surfaces, and solids; and he could imagine a solid as large as this terrestrial globe, if he were to imagine his fingers' ends as large as this globe, and occupied by sensation in its length, breadth, and depth. I know of nothing which is a better proof of the reality of this internal sense than this faculty, weak in us, but strong in those born blind, of feeling or recalling the sensation of bodies when they are absent and no longer acting on us.

We cannot make a blind man understand how imagination represents absent objects as present to us, but we can easily recognise in ourselves the faculty that the blind possess of feeling at one's fingers' ends an absent body. To do this, press the forefinger and thumb together, shut your eyes; separate your fingers, and immediately after this separation examine yourself and tell me if the sensation does not linger after the pressure has ceased; if, while the pressure lasted, your mind appears to be in your head rather than at the ends of your fingers, and if this pressure does not convey the nature of a surface by the space which the sensation occupies? We only distinguish the presence of external things from their picture in our imagination by the strength or weakness of the impression; and similarly, the blind only distinguish the sensation from the actual presence of an object at their fingers' ends, by the strength or weakness of that sensation.

If ever a philosopher, blind and deaf from his birth, were to construct a man after the fashion of Descartes,[75] I can assure you, madam, that he would put the seat of the soul at the fingers' ends, for thence the greater part of the sensations and

---

[75]René Descartes (1596–1650) was a major figure in Western philosophy, perhaps best known for the philosophical statement 'Cogito ergo sum' (I think, therefore I am). Descartes surmised that the seat of the soul, the place where thoughts are formed, may be the pineal gland, which is located in the centre of the brain.

all his knowledge are derived. Who is to inform him that his head is the seat of his thoughts? If the labours of the imagination tire our brain, this is because the effort we make to imagine is somewhat similar to that to perceive very near or very small objects.

...

Our senses bring us back to symbols more suited to our comprehension and the conformation of our organs. We have arranged that these signs should be common property and serve, as it were, for the staple in the exchange of our ideas. We have made them for our eyes in the alphabet, and for our ears in articulate sounds; but we have none for the sense of touch, although there is a way of speaking to this sense and of obtaining its responses.

For lack of this language, there is no communication between us and those born deaf, blind, and mute. They grow, but they remain in a condition of mental imbecility. Perhaps they would have ideas, if we were to communicate with them in a definite and uniform manner from their infancy; for instance, if we were to trace on their hands the same letters we trace on paper, and associated always the same meaning with them.

Is not this language, madam,[76] as good as another? Is it not ready to hand, and would you dare to say that you have never been communicated with by this method? Nothing remains but to fix it, and make its grammar and dictionaries, if it is found that the expression by the common characters of writing is too slow for the sense of touch. Knowledge has three entrances by which it reaches our mind, and we keep one barricaded for want of signs. If the two others had been neglected we should now be little better than beasts. Just as a pressure is the only sign we have to the touch, so a cry would have been the only sign to the hearing. We have to lose one sense before we realise the advantage of symbols given to the remainder, and people who have the misfortune to be born deaf, blind, and mute, or who have lost these three senses by some accident, would be delighted if there existed a clear and precise language of touch.

'Cases'

Everyone has heard of the famous surgeon Daviel.[77] I was often present during his operations. He removed a cataract from the eyes of a blacksmith who had contracted this disease from exposure to the fire of his forge; and during twenty-five years of blindness he had grown so accustomed to the guidance of touch that he had to be forced to use the sense which had been restored to him. Daviel would beat him and say, 'Use your eyes, you wretch!' He walked and moved, and did all that we do with our eyes open, with his eyes shut.

We are drawn to the conclusion that the eye is not so necessary nor so essential to our happiness as we are inclined to believe. If the spectacle of nature had no charms for the blind smith Daviel operated on, what object is there to the loss of which we should be otherwise than indifferent, after long deprivation of sight

---

[76]Diderot addresses his intimate friend, the feminist writer Madeleine de Puisieux (1720-98).
[77]Jacques Daviel (1696–62) was a surgeon who was renowned for his skillful eye surgeries.

accompanied by no pain? The sight of a beloved woman? I don't believe it. ... We imagine that if one had passed a long time without seeing, one would never be weary of looking; but that is not the case. What a contrast between momentary and constant blindness!

An Essay on the Nature and Origin of the Contagion of Fevers
John Alderson (1788)

In the earliest ages of the world, when men had not yet formed themselves into large communities, and when they led a wandering Life, removing from place to place, determined in their choice of settlement alone by the convenience of pasturage, the operations of nature underwent no constraint, and the means intended by the all-wise Creator, produced their full effect. For no sooner was the *Liquidum Vitale* absorbed, and human effluvia[78] evolved, than the pure vapour from the running stream, or fertile plain, supplied the waste, and decomposed the noxious matter.

But when the human race, relinquishing the comforts of independence, began to place their happiness in large communities, and individuals formed themselves into societies for the improvement of those arts which could alone be brought to perfection by the conjunction and assistance of many, they crowded in to cities, and breathed their own destruction, crimes increased, and confinement became necessary. Taste and luxury devote myriads to destruction for their gratification, by the accumulation of sedentary arts, or of machines to shorten labour; nor is it the least of the horrors of war (the necessary consequence of an increase of wealth and power) that it shortens the period of our existence, by other methods than the sword. An invested camp, or a garrisoned town, have proved an inglorious grave to many a brave man, who had long resisted the sword of the enemy; and even in the projects of humanity to abate these miseries how often are we compelled to lament, that its generosity is defeated by an ill-constructed hospital, or the negligence of those who are appointed to superintend it?

Family Letters on the Yellow Fever
Benjamin Rush (1792)

Philadelphia, 25 August 1793.
MY DEAR JULIA,

Since my letter to you of Friday, the fever has assumed a most alarming appearance. It not only mocks in most instances the power of medicine, but it has spread through several parts of the city remote from the spot where it originated. Water Street

---

[78]*Liquidium vitale* signifies here 'life-giving' waters and human effluvia refers to excrement. Alderson praises the natural recycling of the less populated communities of the rural past.

between Arch and Race Streets is nearly desolated by it. This morning I witnessed a scene there, which reminded me of the histories I had read of the plague. In one house I lost two patients last night, a respectable young merchant and his only child. His wife is frantic this evening with grief. Five other persons died in the neighbourhood yesterday afternoon and four more last night at Kensington. The College of Physicians met this afternoon to consult upon the means of checking the progress of this dreadful disease. They appointed a Committee to draw up directions for that purpose. The Committee imposed this business upon me, and I have just finished them. They will be handed to the Mayor when adopted by the College and published by him in a day or two. I hope, and believe that they will be useful. After this detail of the state of the fever, I need hardly request you to remain for a while with all the children where you are. Many people are flying from the city, and some by my advice. Continue to commit me by your prayers to the protection of that Being who has so often manifested his goodness to our family by the preservation of my life, and I hope I shall do well. I endeavour to have no will of my own. I enjoy good health and uncommon tranquillity of mind. While I depend upon divine protection, and feel that at present I live, move, and have my being in a more especial manner in God alone, I do not neglect to use every precaution that experience has discovered, to prevent taking the infection. I even strive to subdue my sympathy for my patients, otherwise I should sink under the accumulated loads of misery I am obliged to contemplate. You can recollect how much the loss of a single patient once in a month used to affect me. Judge then how I must feel, in hearing every morning of the death of three or four! I shall confine John and Richard to the house, and oblige them to use precautions against the disorder. My mother and sister are so kind and attentive as to prevent all our wants and wishes. My love to your uncle and aunt and all the children. I am afraid you will burden our good relations, No this cannot be. They love you, and they love to do offices of kindness and humanity. Adieu; from your sincere and affectionate BENJ N RUSH.

Philadelphia, 28 October 1793
MY DEAR JULIA,

A new clamor has been excited against me in which many citizens take a part. I have asserted that the yellow fever was generated in our city. This assertion they say will destroy the character of Philad [elphia] for healthiness, and drive Congress from it. Truth in science as in morals never did any harm. If I prove my assertion, which I can most easily do, I shall at the same time point out the means of preventing its ever being generated among us again. I am urged to bring forward my proofs immediately. To this I have objected, until I am able to call upon a number of persons for the privilege of using their names. To a gentleman who pressed the matter upon me this day, I said that the good opinion of the citizens of Philad [elphia] was now of little consequence to me, for that I thought it probable from present appearances, that I should begin to seek a retreat and subsistence in some other part of the United States.

On the Mode of Communication of Cholera[79]
John Snow (1855)

'Evidence Of This Mode Of Communication In The Crowded Habitations Of The Poor'

Deficiency of light is a great obstacle to cleanliness, as it prevents dirt from being seen, and it must aid very much the contamination of the food with the cholera evacuations. Now the want of light, in some of the dwellings of the poor, in large towns, is one of the circumstances that has often been commented on as increasing the prevalence of cholera.

The involuntary passage of the evacuations in most bad cases of cholera, must also aid in spreading the disease. Mr Baker, of Staines, who attended two hundred and sixty cases of cholera and diarrhea in 1849, chiefly among the poor, informed me, in a letter with which he favored me in December of that year, that 'when the patients passed their stools involuntarily the disease evidently spread.' It is amongst the poor, where a whole family live, sleep, cook, eat, and wash in a single room, that cholera has been found to spread when once introduced, and still more in those places termed common lodging-houses, in which several families were crowded into a single room. It was amongst the vagrant class, who lived in this crowded state, that cholera was most fatal in 1832; but the Act of Parliament for the regulation of common lodging houses, has caused the disease to be much less fatal amongst these people in the late epidemics. When, on the other hand, cholera is introduced into the better kind of houses, as it often is, by means that will be afterwards pointed out, it hardly ever spreads from one member of the family to another. The constant use of the hand-basin and towel, and the fact of the apartments for cooking and eating being distinct from the sick room, are the cause of this.

The great prevalence of cholera in institutions for pauper children and pauper lunatics, whenever it has gained access to these buildings, meets with a satisfactory explanation according to the principles here laid down. In the asylum for pauper children at Tooting, one hundred and forty deaths from cholera occurred amongst a thousand inmates, and the disease did not cease till the remaining children had been removed. The children were placed two or three in a bed, and vomited over each other when they had the cholera. Under these circumstances, and when it is remembered that children get their hands into everything, and are constantly putting their fingers in their mouths, it is not surprising that the malady spread in this manner, although I believe as much attention was paid to cleanliness as is possible in a building crowded with children. Pauper lunatics are generally a good deal crowded together, especially in their sleeping wards, and as the greater number of them are in a state of imbecility, they are no more careful than children in the use of their hands. It is with the greatest difficulty that they can be kept even moderately clean. As might be expected, according to the views here explained, the lunatic

---

[79]Cholera is a severe infection of the intestine by the bacterium *Vibrio cholerae*, which is ingested through faecally contaminated water. Symptoms include severe diarrhoea, vomiting, muscle cramping, dehydration, resulting in sunken eyes, cold blue skin and very often, quick death.

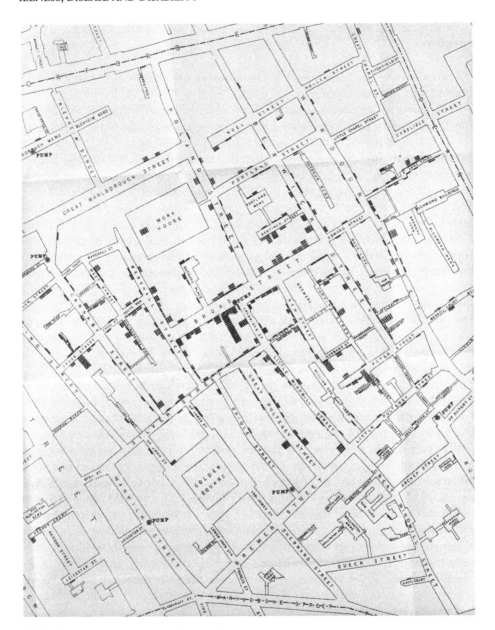

FIGURE 2: John Snow, *Street Map of Soho*, showing the situation of cholera deaths in and around Broad Street, Golden Square, from 19th August to 30th September 1854. A black bar indicates the house of the deceased. The Broad Street Pump is also indicated, as well as that of all the surrounding public pumps. Courtesy Wellcome Library, London.

patients generally suffered in a much greater proportion than the keepers and other attendants.

'Explanation Of The Map Showing The Situation Of The Deaths In And Around Broad Street, Golden Square'

The deaths which occurred during this fatal outbreak of cholera are indicated in the accompanying map [see Figure 2 above], as far as I could ascertain them.

...

The dotted line on the map surrounds the sub-districts of Golden Square, St. James's, and Berwick Street, St. James's, together with the adjoining portion of the sub-district of St. Anne, Soho, extending from Wardour Street to Dean Street, and a small part of the sub-district of St. James's Square enclosed by Marylebone Street, Titchfield Street, Great Windmill Street, and Brewer Street. All the deaths from cholera which were registered in the six weeks from 19th August to 30th September within this locality, as well as those of persons removed into Middlesex Hospital, are shown in the map by a black line in the situation of the house in which it occurred, or in which the fatal attack was contracted. In addition to these the deaths of persons removed to University College Hospital, to Charing Cross Hospital, and to various parts of London, are indicated in the map, where the exact address was given in the 'Weekly Return of Deaths,' or, when I could learn it by private inquiry. The pump in Broad Street is indicated on the map, as well as all the surrounding pumps to which the public had access at the time.

It requires to be stated that the water of the pump in Marlborough Street, at the end of Carnaby Street, was so impure that many people avoided using it. And I found that the persons who died near this pump in the beginning of September, had water from the Broad Street pump. With regard to the pump in Rupert Street, it will be noticed that some streets which are near to it on the map, are in fact a good way removed, on account of the circuitous road to it. These circumstances being taken into account, it will be observed that the deaths either very much diminished, or ceased altogether, at every point where it becomes decidedly nearer to send to another pump than to the one in Broad Street. It may also be noticed that the deaths are most numerous near to the pump where the water could be more readily obtained. The wide open street in which the pump is situated suffered most, and next the streets branching from it, and especially those parts of them which are nearest to Broad Street. If there have been fewer deaths in the south half of Poland Street than in some other streets leading from Broad Street, it is no doubt because this street is less densely inhabited.

In some of the instances, where the deaths are scattered a little further from the rest on the map, the malady was probably contracted at a nearer point to the pump. A cabinet-maker, who was removed from Philip's Court, Noel Street, to Middlesex Hospital, worked in Broad Street. A boy also who died in Noel Street, went to the National school at the end of Broad Street, and having to pass the pump, probably drank of the water. A tailor, who died at 6, Heddon Court, Regent Street, spent most of his time in Broad Street. A woman, removed to the hospital from 10, Heddon Court, had been nursing a person who died of cholera in Marshall Street. A little girl, who died in Ham Yard, and another who died in Angel Court, Great Windmill Street, went to the school in Dufour's Place, Broad Street, and were in the habit of drinking the pump-water, as were also a child from Naylor's Yard, and several others, who went to this and other schools near the pump in Broad Street. A woman who died at 2, Great Chapel Street, Oxford Street, had been occupied for two days preceding her illness at the public washhouses near the pump, and used to drink a good deal of water whilst at her work; the water drank there being sometimes from the pump and sometimes from the cistern.

The limited district in which this outbreak of cholera occurred, contains a great variety in the quality of the streets and houses; Poland Street and Great Pulteney Street consisting in a great measure of private houses occupied by one family, whilst Husband Street and Peter Street are occupied chiefly by the poor Irish. The remaining streets are intermediate in point of respectability. The mortality appears to have fallen pretty equally amongst all classes, in proportion to their numbers.

Dr Koch on the Cholera[80]
The Lancet (1884)

Dr Koch commenced by remarking that what was required for the prevention of cholera was a scientific basis. Many and diverse views as to its mode of diffusion and infection prevailed, but they furnished no safe ground for prophylaxis.[81] On the one hand, it was held that cholera is a specific disease originating in India; on the other, that it may arise spontaneously in any country, and own no specific cause. One view regards the infection to be conveyed only by the patient and his surroundings; and the other that it is spread by merchandise, by healthy individuals, and by atmospheric currents. There is a like discrepancy in the views on the possibility of its diffusion by drinking water, on the influence of conditions of soil, on the question whether the dejecta contain the poison or not, and on the duration of the incubation period. No progress was possible in combating the disease until these root questions of the etiology of cholera are decided.

Hitherto the advances in knowledge upon the etiology of other infective diseases have done little toward the etiology of cholera. These advances have been made within the last ten years, during which time no opportunity – at least not in Europe – has occurred to pursue researches; and in India, where there is abundant material for such research, no one has undertaken the task. The opportunity given by the outbreak of cholera in Egypt last year to study the disease before it reached European soil was taken advantage of by various governments, who sent expeditions for the purpose. He [Koch] had the honor to take part in one of these, and in accepting it he well knew the difficulties of the task before him, for hardly anything was known

---

[80]This is a report, in the medical journal *The Lancet*, of the important work of the German microbiologist Robert Koch (1843-1910). Koch made groundbreaking discoveries in bacteriology, including the causes of tuberculosis, cholera, anthrax and other infectious diseases.

[81]Prophylaxis refers to the prevention of disease, which, Koch argues, is dependent on understanding the etiology (the causes) of disease.

about the cholera poison, or where it should be sought; whether it was to be found only in the intestinal canal, or in the blood, or elsewhere. Nor was it known whether it was of bacterial nature, or fungoid, or an animal parasite – e.g., an amoeba. But other difficulties appeared in an unexpected direction.

...

Microscopical examination of the intestine and its contents revealed, especially in the cases where the margins of Peyer's patches[82] were reddened, a considerable invasion of bacteria, occurring partly within the tubular glands, partly between the epithelium and basement membrane,[83] and in some parts deeper still. Then he found cases in which, besides bacteria of one definite and constant form, there were others also accumulated within and around the tubular glands, of various size, some short and thick, others very fine; and he soon concluded that he had to do here with a primary invasion of pathogenic bacilli,[84] which, as it were, prepared the tissues for the entrance of the non-pathogenic forms, just as he had observed, in the necrotic, diphtheritic changes in the intestinal mucosa and in typhoid ulcers.[85]

Passing to speak of the microscopical character of the contents of the bowel, Dr Koch said that owing to the sanguinolent and putrescent character of these in the cases first examined, no conclusion was arrived at for some time. Thus he found multitudes of bacteria of various kinds, rendering it impossible to distinguish any special forms, and it was not until he had examined two acute and uncomplicated cases, before hæmorrhage had occurred, and where the evacuation had not decomposed, that he found more abundantly the kind of organism which had been seen so richly in the intestinal mucosa. He then proceeded to describe the characters of this bacterium. It is smaller than the tubercle bacillus, being only about half or at most two-thirds the size of the latter, but much more plump, thicker, and slightly curved. As a rule, the curve is no more than that of a comma (,) but sometimes it assumes a semicircular shape, and he has seen it forming a double curve like an S.

...

The diffusion of cholera in India depends on human intercourse, especially on pilgrimages, which are carried on to an inconceivable extent – e.g., hundreds of thousands flock yearly to Hurdivar and Puri, remain there many weeks herded together, bathing in the tanks that supply them also with drinking-water. Over the borders of India the cholera is carried to Persia, and in the old caravan days thence to the south of Europe; but the route now is by the Red Sea and Suez Canal. Every year the danger to Europe by this route increases, for Bombay, which is seldom free from cholera, is but eleven days distant from Egypt, sixteen from Italy, and eighteen or twenty from France. It is also clear that the greatest danger lies in ships carrying large numbers of people, as troops, pilgrims, coolies, and emigrants, and not the

---

[82]Peyer's patches, named after the seventeenth-century Swiss anatomist Johann Conrad Peyer, are usually found in the lowest portion of the small intestine, the ileum.
[83]These are layers of tissue.
[84]Pathogenic bacteria are disease causing.
[85]Necrotic refers to the localized death of cells; here, as caused by diphtheria and typhus.

merchant vessels with small crews, for in the former the outbreak of an epidemic would be likely to last till Europe was reached.

...

In conclusion, Dr Koch adverted to the subject of treatment, and reminded those who say that such discoveries do not enable us to cure the disease better than formerly, that a rational treatment of most diseases, and especially of infectious diseases, cannot be adopted until their cause and nature are known. But even yet the discovery of the cholera bacillus is important, as furnishing an aid in diagnosis which would facilitate the detection of the first case occurring in a district, and the adoption of measures to prevent its spread. Knowing also the nature and properties of the bacillus, and especially the readiness with which it is killed by drying, the right direction of prophylaxis is assured and the lavish expenditure of disinfectants checked, so that there will not be a repetition of what happened in the last epidemic, when millions of gallons were poured into the gutters and sewers without the slightest need.

Spanish Influenza – Three-Day Fever – The Flu
United States Public Health Service (1918)

What is Spanish Influenza? Is it something new? Does it come from Spain?

The disease now occurring in this country and called 'Spanish Influenza' resembles a very contagious kind of 'cold' accompanied by fever, pains in the head, eyes, ears, back or other parts of the body, and a feeling of severe sickness. In most of the cases the symptoms disappear after three or four days, the patient then rapidly recovering; some of the patients, however, develop pneumonia, or inflammation of the ear, or meningitis, and many of these complicated cases die. Whether this so-called 'Spanish' influenza is identical with the epidemics of influenza of earlier years is not yet known.

Epidemics of influenza have visited this country since 1647. It is interesting to know that this first epidemic was brought here from Valencia, Spain. Since that time there have been numerous epidemics of the disease. In 1889 and 1890 an epidemic of influenza, starting somewhere in the Orient, spread first to Russia, and thence over practically the entire civilized world. Three years later there was another flare-up of the disease. Both times the epidemic spread widely over the United States.

Although the present epidemic is called 'Spanish influenza,' there is no reason to believe that it originated in Spain. Some writers who have studied the question believe that the epidemic came from the Orient and they call attention to the fact that the Germans mention the disease as occurring along the eastern front in the summer and fall of 1917.

How can 'Spanish influenza' be recognized?

There is as yet no certain way in which a single case of 'Spanish influenza' can be recognized; on the other hand, recognition is easy where there is a group of cases. In contrast to the outbreaks of ordinary coughs and colds, which usually occur in the cold months, epidemics of influenza may occur at any season of the year, thus the present epidemic raged most intensely in Europe in May, June, and July. Moreover, in the case of ordinary colds, the general symptoms (fever, pain, depression) are by no means as severe or as sudden in their onset as they are in influenza. Finally, ordinary colds do not spread through the community so rapidly or so extensively as does influenza.

In most cases a person taken sick with influenza feels sick rather suddenly. He feels weak, has pains in the eyes, ears, head or back, and may be sore all over. Many patients feel dizzy, some vomit. Most of the patients complain of feeling chilly, and with this comes a fever in which the temperature rises to 100 to 104. In most cases the pulse remains relatively slow.

In appearance one is struck by the fact that the patient looks sick. His eyes and the inner side of his eyelids may be slightly 'blood-shot', or 'congested', as the doctors say. There may be running from the nose, or there may be some cough. These signs of a cold may not be marked; nevertheless the patient looks and feels very sick.

In addition to the appearance and the symptoms as already described, examination of the patient's blood may aid the physician in recognizing 'Spanish influenza', for it has been found that in this disease the number of white corpuscles shows little or no increase above the normal. It is possible that the laboratory investigations now being made through the National Research Council and the United States Hygienic Laboratory will furnish a more certain way in which individual cases of this disease can be recognized.

What causes the disease and how is it spread?

Bacteriologists who have studied influenza epidemics in the past have found in many of the cases a very small rod-shaped germ called, after its discoverer, Pfeiffer's bacillus.[86] In other cases of apparently the same kind of disease there were found pneumococci, the germs of lobar pneumonia. Still others have been caused by streptococci, and by other germs with long names.

No matter what particular kind of germ causes the epidemic, it is now believed that influenza is always spread from person to person, the germs being carried with the air along with the very small droplets of mucus, expelled by coughing or sneezing, forceful talking, and the like by one who already has the germs of the disease. They may also be carried about in the air in the form of dust coming from dried mucus, from coughing and sneezing, or from careless people who spit on the floor and on the sidewalk. As in most other catching diseases, a person who has only a mild attack of the disease himself may give a very severe attack to others.

What should be done by those who catch the disease?

It is very important that every person who becomes sick with influenza should go home at once and go to bed. This will help keep away dangerous complications and will, at the same time, keep the patient from scattering the disease far and wide. It is highly desirable that no one be allowed to sleep in the same room with the patient. In fact, no one but the nurse should be allowed in the room.

---

[86]Richard Friedrich Johannes Pfeiffer (1858–1945) was a German physician and bacteriologist, who first described Pfeiffer's bacillus, or *Bacillus influenza*, in 1892.

If there is cough and sputum or running of the eyes and nose, care should be taken that all such discharges are collected on bits of gauze or rag or paper napkins and burned. If the patient complains of fever and headache, he should be given water to drink, a cold compress to the forehead, and a light sponge. Only such medicine should be given as is prescribed by the doctor. It is foolish to ask the druggist to prescribe and may be dangerous to take the so-called 'safe, sure, and harmless' remedies advertised by patent-medicine manufacturers.

If the patient is so situated that he can be attended only by someone who must also look after others in the family, it is advisable that such attendant wear a wrapper, apron, or gown over the ordinary house clothes while in the sick room, and slip this off when leaving to look after the others.

Nurses and attendants will do well to guard against breathing in dangerous disease germs by wearing a simple fold of gauze or mask while near the patient.

How can one guard against influenza?

In guarding against disease of all kinds, it is important that the body be kept strong and able to fight off disease germs. This can be done by having a proper proportion of work, play, and rest, by keeping the body well clothed, and by eating sufficient, wholesome, and properly selected food. In connection with diet, it is well to remember that milk is one of the best all-around foods obtainable for adults as well as children. So far as a disease like influenza is concerned health authorities everywhere recognize the very close relation between its spread and overcrowded homes. While it is not always possible, especially in times like the present, to avoid such overcrowding, people should consider the health danger and make every effort to reduce the home overcrowding to a minimum. The value of fresh air through open windows cannot be over emphasized.

Where crowding is unavoidable, as in street cars, care should be taken to keep the face so turned as not to inhale directly the air breathed out by another person. It is especially important to beware of the person who coughs or sneezes without covering his mouth and nose. It also follows that one should keep out of crowds and stuffy places as much as possible, keep homes, offices, and workshops well aired, spend some time out of doors each day, walk to work if at all practicable – in short make every possible effort to breathe as much, pure air as possible.

'Cover up each cough and sneeze,
If you don't you'll spread disease.'

CHAPTER FIVE

Treatment

from *The Poetical History of Finnesbury Mad-house*
James Carkesse (1679)

The Dr—of *Finnesbury-House*
Knows, how to dissect an *Oyster*;
Whether *Man*, no more than a Mouse,
Be fit for *Bedlam*, or *Cloyster*.
I'll tell you his way of Proceeding,
All you, that here shall enter;
Purges, *Vomits*, and *Bleeding*,
Are his method of Cure, at a Venture.
By the way you must know, this *Else*
Both Bedlams does haunt, like the *Louse*;
And sways, as *Chair-man* himself,
Both upper and lower House.
Let him therefore be trusted by none,
But *Fools*, that are Fortunes *Minions*;
For, to Rule both these Houses alone,
Is to halt between two *Opinions*.
...
The *Doctor* his *Argument* urges;
This *Parson* must needs be *Mad*,
For on him, neither *Vomits* nor *Purges*,
Any Influence have had.
Fond *Doctor*, you beg the *Question*,
And you might have spar'd your pains;
For my *Blood's* from a good digestion,
And your *Physick* is lost in my *Veins*.
Nay, I prescrib'd Chains of *Iron*,
To take him off of his Mettle;
But *Brass* did him environ,
He had rub'd his Face with a *Kettle*.
My *Fetters* they were but *Straw*,
To the Sinews of his Armes;
And he burst Bars and Doors, as I saw,

By I know not what mighty Charmes.
Moreover I him in the *Hole*,
As under a Bushel, confin'd;
Lest God's Word, the Light of the Soul,
In my Mad-house should have Shin'd:
Ne're the less into the *Dungeon*,
He let in the Rayes of the *Sun*,
And i'th'Pit, where him I did plunge in,
Made Night and Day meet in one.
In a place I did him stow,
Where *Rats* and *Mice* do swarm;
These by Instinct the Madmen know,
And therefore do them no harm.
Now as *Weasel*, *Squirrel*, and *Ermine*
Are, then *Rats* of a higher strain
Rats and *Mice*, the nobler *Vermine*,
Might awe the *Worm* in his *Brain*.
Yet he fear'd, lest the *Rats* and *Mice*,
Of his Senses should bereave him;
Therefore I taking good advice,
Sent *Catmore* in to Relieve him.
I laid him in *Straw* for a Bed,
Lest *Feathers* should make him *light-headed*;
That there his wild Oats he might shed,
And again to his Wits be wedded.
Without either Shirt, or Cloaths,
I lodg'd my merry Mad Youth;
For of Kin we may well suppose,
The *Sober* to *Naked-Truth*.
His *Diet* was most of it *Milk*,
To reduce him again to a *Child*;
And *Butter* as soft as *Silk*,
To smooth the *Fierce* and the *Wild*.
My *Potions* he turn'd into *Drenches*,
For he freely would take ne're a jot;
But by *Thomas* and the *Wenches*,
They were forced down his Throat.
To feel his *Pulse*, I never thought;
I a Month I see him but once:
And how my Mad *Physick* has wrought,
If I know in the least I'm a *Dunce*.
For, in Truth and sober sadness,
This *Parson* I found so smart,
That I fear'd his *Wit*, more than his *madness*,
The *March-Hare* I never dare start.

My chirurgeon[1] he fiercely withstood,
And he led him such a Dance;
That to let this same Gown-man *Blood*,
A *Sword* was more fit than a *Lance*.
I order'd his *Keeper*, at Large,
On occasion to ply him with Blows,
That what *Jugular* did not discharge,
The mad *Blood* might come out at his *Nose*.
Enough: *Doc* has done his Endeavour,
It must be confest, though a weak one;
His Wits gather Wool for a *Beaver*,
But he's no *Fool* to speak on.
However, I'll *Sue* out his *Pardon*,
The man's not so much to be blam'd;
For to make a *Swan* white is unheard on,
And *Sobriety* never was tam'd.
Then pray all, the *mad-Devil* ne're touch you,
Nor yet the Cholick or Tissick[2];
Pray, MUFTI and MAMAMOUCHI,[3]
Mr Parson and Doctor of Physick.

from *A Description of Bath*[4]
Mary Chandler (1733)

Safe from the Ruin of a thousand Years.
These salutary Streams alone can boast
Their Virtues not in thrice five Ages lost.
The floating Waters, from their hidden Source,
Thro' the same *Strata* keep unerring Course;
The flowing *Sulphur* meets dissolving *Steel*,
And heat in *Combat*, till the Waters boil:
United then, enrich the healing Stream,
HEALTH to the *Sick* they give, and to the *Waters*, FAME.

Thus oft contending *Parties* rage and hate,
Malignant both, and push each other's Fate;
At last, their Fury spent, and cloy'd with Blood,
They *join* in *Friendship* for the *Publick* Good.

---

[1]Chirurgeon is the archaic term for surgeon.
[2]Cholick (or colic) refers to sudden pain caused by muscle contractions; tissick is the archaic term for pulmonary tuberculosis or asthma.
[3]A mufti is an interpreter of Islamic law. Mamamouchi is a mock-Turkish term for a pompous, self-important figure, coined by Molière in his play *Le Bourgeois Gentilhomme*.
[4]In the eighteenth century, the English town of Bath Spa, with its natural mineral springs, became a fashionable destination for health tourists, who came to take the waters.

Hither foul SCURVY, odious to the Sight:
And VAPOURS, which, in *ev'ry Form*, affright;
Sharp COLIC, groaning with a *Jaundice* Face;
White LEPROSY, of old *Egyptian* Race;
The shaking PALSY, RHEUMATISM lame[5];
And meager INDIGESTION pining came;
With many dreadful *Ails*, without a Name.

Fatal Effects of LUXURY and EASE!
We *drink* our POISON, and we *eat* DISEASE;
Indulge our SENSES at our REASON's Cost,
Till *Sense* is Pain and *Reason's hurt,* or *lost.*

Not so, O TEMP'RANCE bland! when rul'd by thee,
The *Brute's* obedient, and the *Man* is free:
Soft are his *Slumbers,* balmy is his *Rest,*
His *Veins* not boiling from the *Midnight Feast;*
Touch'd by AURORA's[6] rosy Hand, he wakes,
Peaceful and calm; and with the World partakes
The joyful Dawnings of returning Day,
For which their grateful Thanks the whole Creation pay!
All but the *human Brute;* 'Tis he alone
Whose Deeds of Darkness fly the rising Sun.

'Tis to thy Rules, O TEMPERANCE! we owe
All Pleasures which from *Health* and *Strength* can show;
Vigour of *Body, Purity* of *Mind,*
Unclouded *Reason, Sentiments* refin'd,
Unmix'd, untainted Joys, without *Remorse,*
Th' intemp'rate Sinner's never-failing Curse.

Our *Waters* with those num'rous Ills away,
And grant the *trembling Wretch* a *longer Day.*
O may returning Health more *Wisdom* give!
Let *Death's* Approaches teach us how to *live.*

---

[5]Scurvy is a disease resulting from a deficiency of vitamin C. Symptoms include malaise depression, fever, loss of teeth and partial immobility. Vapours refers to what we would not call depression. Colic: painful muscle contractions. Jaundice is a yellowish pigmentation of the skin, the conjunctival membranes over the whites of the eyes and other mucous membranes. Leprosy is a contagious disease that results in mottled, discoloured skin and disfigurement; it is associated with poverty. Palsy refers to various types of paralysis, often accompanied by loss of feeling and uncontrolled body movements such as shaking. Rheumatism is a non-specific term for medical problems affecting the joints and/or connective tissues.
[6]In mythology, Aurora was the goddess of dawn.

If but *one* Leper cur'd, makes Jordan's Stream,[7]
In Sacred Writ, a venerable Theme,
What Honour's to thy sov'reign Waters due,
Where Sick, by Thousands do their Health renew!

The Min'ral Streams which from the Baths arise,
From noxious Vapours clear the neighb'ring Skies:
When Fevers bore an epidemic Sway,
Unpeopled Towns, swept Villages away;
While Death abroad dealt Terror, and Despair,
The Plague but gently touch'd within their Sphere.

Blest Source of Health, seated on rising Ground,
With friendly Hills by Nature guarded round;
From Eastern Blasts, and sultry South secure;
The Air's balsamic, and the Soil is pure.

from *Relief from Accidental Death*
Alexander Johnson (1789)

'Recovery of Life, from Apparent Death, by Drowning'

In every instance of departed life,
Nature, still struggling, holds a doubtful strife.
In cases the most common that we meet,
Ere death the last decisive stroke complete,
Some time elapses – yet uncertainty
Attends that space – it long or short may be:
Therefore employ that interval to try
If yet some sparks of life may dormant lie,
And either a recov'ry safe procure,
Or from that worst of horrors thus ensure
Of quick interment. For experience shows,
That many women, from child-bearing throes,
And new-born infants, breathless long remain
In swooning 'strances, yet revive again
By means here recommended. Then beware
None perish through your want of thought or care;
But try those means which every willing hand,
At any time and place, may well command.

At first discov'ry of apparent death,
Lose not a moment; for the fleeting breath
Ay yet be stay'd – while life's last spark remains,
Patient attend, nor spare or time or pains.

---

[7]The River Jordan has significance in Judaism, Christianity and Islam as the site where the Israelites crossed
into the Promised Land and where Jesus was baptized by John the Baptist.

Avoid the dangerous practice now decry'd,
By ignorance and prejudice oft try'd,
Rolling with violence, nor shaking try,
Nor yet suspending – who those means apply
To force discharge of water, to the grave
Consign the wretch whom gentler means might save.
First, from wet cloaths the body free, with care
Wrap it in flannels soft and warm; beware
You no sharp salt, nor yet corrosive ply;
Nor rub with wetted cloths, but keep all dry.

These early steps when taken with the drown'd,
(On whom success first ascertain'd was found)
What follows equally relates to all
Those who into a death-like swooning fall,
Or seeming choak'd – like treatment will demand,
Cheering and rubbing with a gentle hand.

The purple stream of life alike beware
Not to diminish; and, with anxious care,
Avoid emetics, which may ills diffuse
Through all the frame, deem'd fatal by the muse.
Shun all those cruel methods that impair
The skin, nor, by your ill-directed care,
Congeal those humours, which to keep alive,
In fluid state, you anxiously should strive.
Attempt not, by excruciating pain,
Some knowledge of the patient's state to gain;
For know, those trials are a vain pretence,
While all sensation lies in dead suspense.
With patience wait, lest, by such cruel haste,
Life's feeble lamp you ignorantly waste:
From care and caution better comfort flows,
And jaws, tho' lock'd, will of themselves unclose.

With cordial drops endeavour to revive
The fleeting spirits, and life's current drive
Back to its native channels. Try to heal,
With opiate draughts, the irritated feel,
Caus'd by reviving sensation. Next attend,
With needful help, and frequent turn or bend,
Provoking motion in the languid breast,
Nor leave the body in lethargic rest.

Inject warm vapour, and blow in fresh air;
And let it likewise by your constant care
To chase the temples, palms, on every part
Most sensible, exert that needful art.

Take a clean feather, with it, tickle, teaze
The throat, and up the nose, to force a sneeze.

In suffocations caused by noxious air,
Or bodies frost bitten, be it your care
With water icy cold, or even snow,
Repeatedly apply'd to raise a glow:
Despising all absurd exploded ways,
With shock electrical the dead to raise,
Or reeking sheep's-blood pour'd in human veins;
True judgment all those vain attempts disdains.

Convulsions, swoonings, wear the face of death,
Still is the pulse, suspended is the breath;
Here spirits volatile and hartshorn use,
With gentle friction – ne'er inactive muse
O'er the extended patient; but apply
Means unremitted, every method try;
Raise, turn, and chase the temples, give not o'er,
Watch 'till returning breath your friend restore.
In this, and ev'ry case, quick help and care,
With gentle friction, change of posture, air,
With patience infinite, with watchful eye,
And frequent touch, each symptom to descry
Of faint pulsation, warmth, or rising glow,
Are the best helps attendants can bestow.

These symptoms a return to life portend,
And with assiduous care these signs attend;
Contractions of the muscles, face and eyes,
A spreading blush o'er cheek and lips arise,
Then spasms and sufferings strong exertions cause,
Break out in sad complaints, deep groaning draws;
Vomitings, head-ache, fail not to succeed,
The patient then your quickest help will need;
Pain-stilling drops, and saline draughts apply,
With camphor julep,[8] cooling mixtures try,
Ease and some kind refreshing sleep to gain,
Which, in few hours, may happiest ends obtain.

Yet stop not at the first faint glimpse of life;
While struggling nature holds a doubtful strife,
Continue still the means, nor spare your pain,
Lest in lethargic sleep they sink again.

---

[8]Camphor is a strong aromatic which, like spirits volatile (alcoholic solution) and hartshorn (smelling salts), is a stimulant.

Epitaph on a Patient Killed by a Cancer Quack
Lemuel Hopkins (1793)

Here lies a fool flat on his back,
The victim of a Cancer Quack;
Who lost his money and his life,
By plaster, caustic, and by knife.
The case was this – a pimple rose,
South-east a little of his nose;
Which daily redden'd and grew bigger,
As too much drinking gave it vigour:
A score of gossips soon ensure
Full three score diff'rent modes of cure;
But yet the full-fed pimple still
Defied all petticoated skill;
When fortune led him to peruse
A hand-bill in the weekly news;
Sign'd by six fools of diff'rent sorts,
All cur'd of cancers made of warts;
Who recommend, with due submission,
This cancer-monger as magician;
Fear wing'd his flight to find the quack,
And prove his cancer-curing knack;
But on his way he found another,
A second advertising brother:
But as much like him as an owl
Is unlike every handsome fowl;
Whose fame had rais'd as broad a fog,
And of the two the greater hog:
Who us'd a still more magic plaister,
That sweat forsooth, and cur'd the faster.
This doctor view'd, with moony eyes
And scowl'd up face, the pimple's size;
Then christen'd it in solemn answer,
And cried, 'This pimple's name is CANCER.
But courage, friend, I see you're pale,
My sweating plaisters never fail;
I've sweated hundreds out with ease,
With roots as long as maple trees;
And never fail'd in all my trials –
Behold these samples here in vials!
Preserv'd to show my wond'rous merits,
Just as my liver is – in spirits.
For twenty joes the cure is done – '
The bargain struck, the plaister on,
Which gnaw'd the cancer at its leisure,

And pain'd his face above all measure.
But still the pimple spread the faster,
And swell'd, like toad that meets disaster.
Thus foil'd, the doctor gravely swore,
It was a right rose-cancer sore;
Then stuck his probe beneath the beard,
And show'd them where the leaves appear'd;
And rais'd the patient's drooping spirits,
By praising up the plaister's merits.
Quoth he, 'The roots now scarcely stick –
I'll fetch her out like crab or tick;
And make it rendezvous, next trial,
With six more plagues, in my old vial.'
Then purg'd him pale with jalap[9] drastic,
And next applies th'infernal caustic.
But yet, this semblance bright of hell
Serv'd but to make the patient yell;
And, gnawing on with fiery pace,
Devour'd one broadside of his face –
'Courage, 'tis done,' the doctor cried,
And quick th'incision knife applied:
That with three cuts made such a hole,
Out flew the patient's tortur'd soul!

Go, readers, gentle, eke and simple,
If you have wart, or corn, or pimple;
To quack infallible apply;
Here's room enough for you to lie.
His skill triumphant still prevails,
For Death's a cure that never fails.

Cleanliness
Charles Lamb (1809)

Come my little Robert near –
Fie! what filthy hands are here!
Who that e'er could understand
The rare structure of a hand,
With its branching fingers fine,
Work itself of hands divine,
Strong, yet delicately knit,
For ten thousand uses fit,
Overlaid with so clear skin
You may see the blood within,

---

[9]Jalap is a cathartic drug, which purges the bowels, preparing him for the caustic, or corrosive substance that will destroy his tissues in the next lines.

And the curious palm, disposed
In such lines, some have supposed
You may read the fortunes there
By the figures that appear –
Who this hand would chuse to cover
With a crust of dirt all over,
Till it look'd in hue and shape
Like the fore-foot of an Ape?
Man or boy that works or plays
In the fields or the highways
May, without offence or hurt,
From the soil contract a dirt,
Which the next clear spring or river
Washes out and out for ever –
But to cherish stains impure,
Soil deliberate to endure,
On the skin to fix a stain
Till it works into the grain,
Argues a degenerate mind,
Sordid, slothful, ill inclin'd,
Wanting in that self-respect
Which does virtue best protect.

All-endearing Cleanliness,
Virtue next to Godliness,
Easiest, cheapest, needful'st duty,
To the body health and beauty,
Who that's human would refuse it,
When a little water does it?

The Magnetic Lady To Her Patient
Percy Bysshe Shelley (1821)[10]

'Sleep, sleep on! forget thy pain;
My hand is on thy brow,
My spirit on thy brain;
My pity on thy heart, poor friend;
And from my fingers flow
The powers of life, and like a sign,
Seal thee from thine hour of woe;
And brood on thee, but may not blend
With thine.

---

[10]Written in 1821, first published in the *Athenaeum* magazine, 11 August 1832. In this poem, Shelley casts his intimate friend Jane Williams as a mesmerist or magnetizer, a healer who used hypnosis and other techniques to channel the vital fluid or internal magnetic forces of his or her patients.

'Sleep, sleep on! I love thee not;
But when I think that he
Who made and makes my lot
As full of flowers as thine of weeds,
Might have been lost like thee;
And that a hand which was not mine
Might then have charmed his agony
As I another's – my heart bleeds
For thine.

'Sleep, sleep, and with the slumber of
The dead and the unborn
Forget thy life and love;
Forget that thou must wake forever;
Forget the world's dull scorn;
Forget lost health, and the divine
Feelings which died in youth's brief morn;
And forget me, for I can never
Be thine.

'Like a cloud big with a May shower,
My soul weeps healing rain
On thee, thou withered flower!
It breathes mute music on thy sleep
Its odour calms thy brain!
Its light within thy gloomy breast
Spreads like a second youth again.
By mine thy being is to its deep
Possessed.

'The spell is done. How feel you now?'
'Better – Quite well,' replied
The sleeper. 'What would do
You good when suffering and awake?
What cure your head and side? –'
'What would cure, that would kill me, Jane:
And as I must on earth abide
Awhile, yet tempt me not to break
My chain.'

from *Miss Kilmansegg and her Precious Leg*
Thomas Hood (1840)

'As the twig is bent, the tree's inclined,'
Is an adage often recall'd to mind,
Referring to juvenile bias:

And never so well is the verity seen,
As when to the weak, warp'd side we lean,
While Life's tempests and hurricanes try us.

Even thus with Miss K. and her broken limb:
By a very, very remarkable whim,
She show'd her early tuition:
While the buds of character came into blow
With a certain tinge that served to show
The nursery culture long ago,
As the graft is known by fruition!

For the King's Physician, who nursed the case,
His verdict gave with an awful face,
And three others concurr'd to egg it;
That the Patient to give old Death the slip,
Like the Pope, instead of a personal trip,
Must send her Leg as a Legate.[11]

The limb was doom'd – it couldn't be saved!
And like other people the patient behaved,
Nay, bravely that cruel parting braved,
Which makes some persons so falter,
They rather would part, without a groan,
With the flesh of their flesh, and bone of their bone,
They obtain'd at St. George's altar.

But when it came to fitting the stump
With a proxy limb – then flatly and plump
She spoke, in the spirit olden;
She couldn't – she shouldn't – she wouldn't have wood!
Nor a leg of cork, if she never stood,
And she swore an oath, or something as good,
The proxy limb should be golden!

A wooden leg! what, a sort of peg,
For your common Jockeys and Jennies![12]
No, no, her mother might worry and plague –
Weep, go down on her knees, and beg,
But nothing would move Miss Kilmansegg!
She could – she would have a Golden Leg,
If it cost ten thousand guineas!

---

[11]Legate: a delegate of the Pope.
[12]Jennies are female donkeys.

Wood indeed, in Forest or Park,
With its sylvan honours and feudal bark,
Is an aristocratic article:
But split and sawn, and hack'd about town,
Serving all needs of pauper or clown,
Trod on! stagger'd on! Wood cut down
Is vulgar – fibre and particle!

And Cork! – when the noble Cork Tree shades
A lovely group of Castilian maids,
'Tis a thing for a song or sonnet! –
But cork, as it stops the bottle of gin,
Or bungs the beer – the *small* beer – in,
It pierced her heart like a corking-pin,
To think of standing upon it!

A Leg of Gold – solid gold throughout,
Nothing else, whether slim or stout,
Should ever support her, God willing!
She must – she could – she would have her whim,
Her father, she turn'd a deaf ear to him –
He might kill her – she didn't mind killing!
He was welcome to cut off her other limb –
He might cut her all off with a shilling!

All other promised gifts were in vain.
Golden Girdle, or Golden Chain,
She writhed with impatience more than pain,
And utter'd 'pshaws!' and 'pishes!'
But a Leg of Gold as she lay in bed,
It danced before her – it ran in her head!
It jump'd with her dearest wishes!

'Gold – gold – gold! Oh, let it be gold!'
Asleep or awake that tale she told,
And when she grew delirious:
Till her parents resolved to grant her wish,
If they melted down plate, and goblet, and dish,
The case was getting so serious.

So a Leg was made in a comely mould,
Of gold, fine virgin glittering gold,
As solid as man could make it –
Solid in foot, and calf, and shank,
A prodigious sum of money it sank;
In fact 'twas a Branch of the family Bank,
And no easy matter to break it.

All sterling metal – not half-and-half,
The Goldsmith's mark was stamp'd on the calf –
'Twas pure as from Mexican barter!
And to make it more costly, just over the knee,
Where another ligature used to be,
Was a circle of jewels, worth shillings to see,
A new-fangled Badge of the Garter!

'Twas a splendid, brilliant, beautiful Leg,
Fit for the Court of Scander-Beg,[13]
That Precious Leg of Miss Kilmansegg!
For, thanks to parental bounty,
Secure from Mortification's touch,
She stood on a Member that cost as much
As a Member for all the County!

Fragment, Probably Written During Illness
Thomas Hood (1862–63)

I'm sick of gruel, and the dietetics,[14]
I'm sick of pills, and sicker of emetics,[15]
I'm sick of pulses' tardiness or quickness,
I'm sick of blood, its thinness or its thickness,
In short, within a word, I'm sick of sickness.

Our Fathers of Old
Rudyard Kipling (1910)

Excellent herbs had our fathers of old –
Excellent herbs to ease their pain –
Alexanders and Marigold,
Eyebright, Orris, and Elecampane –
Basil, Rocket, Valerian, Rue,
(Almost singing themselves they run)
Vervain, Dittany, Call-me-to-you-
Cowslip, Melitot, Rose of the Sun,
Anything green that grew out of the mould
Was an excellent herb to our fathers of old.

Wonderful tales had our fathers of old –
Wonderful tales of the herbs and the stars –

---

[13]Skanderbeg was a fifteenth-century Albanian leader, who held off the Ottoman expansion into Europe.
[14]Dietetics concerns human nutrition and the regulation of the diet.
[15]Emetics are drugs administered to induce vomiting.

The Sun was Lord of the Marigold,
Basil and Rocket belonged to Mars.
Pat as a sum in division it goes –
(Every herb had a planet bespoke) –
Who but Venus should govern the Rose?
Who but Jupiter own the Oak?
Simply and gravely the facts are told
In the wonderful books of our fathers of old.

Wonderful little when all is said,
Wonderful little our fathers knew.
Half their remedies cured you dead –
Most of their teaching was quite untrue –
'Look at the stars when a patient is ill
(Dirt has nothing to do with disease),
Bleed and blister as much as you will,
Blister and bleed him as oft as you please.'
Whence enormous and manifold
Errors were made by our fathers of old.

Yet when the sickness was sore in the land,
And neither planets nor herbs assuaged
They took their lives in their lancet-hand
And, oh, what a wonderful war they waged !
Yes, when the crosses were chalked on the door –
(Yes when the terrible death-cart rolled!)
Excellent courage our fathers bore –
Excellent heart had our fathers of old.
None too learned but nobly bold
Into the fight went our fathers of old.

If it be certain, as Galen[16] says –
And sage Hippocrates[17] holds as much –
'That those afflicted by doubts and dismays
Are mightily helped by a dead man's touch,'
Then be good to us, stars above!
Then be good to us, herbs below!
We are afflicted by what we can prove,
We are distracted by what we know.
So – ah, so!
Down from your heaven or up from your mould,
Send us the hearts of our fathers of old!

---

[16]Galen of Pergamon (129–c.216 AD) was a prominent Greek physician, surgeon and philosopher.
[17]Hippocrates (c.460–370 BC) was a Greek physician and canonical figure in the history of medicine.

Appendectomy
Gottfried Benn (1912)[18]

Everything white and sterile and gleaming.
Under a sheet a moan and a stir.
Abdomen painted. Scalpels are gleaming.
'We are ready when you are, Sir.'

The first incision. Like cutting of bread.
'Clips!' A gusher of crimson red.
Deeper. The muscles flaming and fresh,
A garland of roses the vibrant flesh.

Is this pus that started to spurt?
Have the intestines perhaps been hurt?
'Doctor, if you stand in the light,
how can I keep that momentum in sight?

Anaesthetist, I cannot work,
The guy is making his belly jerk.'
Through the silence of mist and gore
The clatter of scissors dropped to the floor.

The patient nurse, with watchful eye,
Keeps sterile tampons in supply.
'I can't see a thing in all this rot!'
'Off with the mask! Blood starts to clot!'

'For Heaven's sake! Hey, Mister, please,
a little more pressure upon the knees!'
Everything tangled. Finally found.
'Cautery, nurse!' A hissing sound.

Boy, I should say you were fortunate.
The thing was about to perforate.
'See this green spot? Three hours, I guess,
and the mesentery would have been a mess.'

'Sutures! Bandage! Jolly good show.'
Everything closed. They wash up and go.
Raging, rattling her bony sword,
Death sneaks off to the cancer ward.

The Sanitary Three – a trio/song
James L. Halliday (c.1920)

We spray. We spray. We Spray. Every night and day
We chase the ubiquitous, little iniquitous, horrible germs away.

---

[18]Trans. Karl. F. Ross.

So if your head comes out in lumps,
Or father develops the measles or mumps,
Along we comes with our little pumps
To spray, spray, spray.

We spray. We spray. We Spray. We do the work for pay.
And send the bacteria causing diphtheria thousands of miles away.
We have not seen the germs as yet.
Nevertheless we turns the jet
Till the whole damned place is soaking wet
With spray, spray, spray.

We spray. We spray. We Spray. Oh hear our roundelay.
It looks so silly to hunt the bacilli, but then we knows the way.
We also deals with sundry smells
In schools, in slums and swish hotels.
All kinds of perfumes we dispels
With spray, spray, spray.

We spray. We spray. We Spray. The children shout 'hurray'.
When they watch our syringes destroying the chintzes, while mother looks on
in dismay.
So if a rat invades your house,
Or under the pillows you finds a mouse,
The vermin we will joyfully souse
And spray, spray, spray.

We spray. We spray. We Spray. When bugs come out to play,
We make a procession of our profession without a minute's delay.
And if anyone hasn't been washed for years
And potatoes are sprouting out of his ears,
We comes along (swish!) and the fruit disappears
In the spray, spray, spray.

We spray. We spray. We Spray. It is the only way
If the world's to be healthy and wise and wealthy and happy and snappy
and gay.
And if at the movies you have been
And the movies are not confined to the screen,
Just hold them down while they can be seen
Till we spray, spray, spray.

East Coker – Part IV
T. S. Eliot (1940)

The wounded surgeon plies the steel
That questions the distempered part;
Beneath the bleeding hands we feel

The sharp compassion of the healer's art
Resolving the enigma of the fever chart.

Our only health is the disease
If we obey the dying nurse
Whose constant care is not to please
But to remind of our, and Adam's curse,
And that, to be restored, our sickness must grow worse.

The whole earth is our hospital
Endowed by the ruined millionaire,
Wherein, if we do well, we shall
Die of the absolute paternal care
That will not leave us, but prevents us everywhere.

The chill ascends from feet to knees,
The fever sings in mental wires.
If to be warmed, then I must freeze
And quake in frigid purgatorial fires
Of which the flame is roses, and the smoke is briars.

The dripping blood our only drink,
The bloody flesh our only food:
In spite of which we like to think
That we are sound, substantial flesh and blood –
Again, in spite of that, we call this Friday good.

Faith Healing
Philip Larkin (1960)

Slowly the women file to where he stands
Upright in rimless glasses, silver hair,
Dark suit, white collar. Stewards tirelessly
Persuade them onwards to his voice and hands,
Within whose warm spring rain of loving care
Each dwells some twenty seconds. *Now, dear child,
What's wrong*, the deep American voice demands,
And, scarcely pausing, goes into prayer
Directing God about this eye, that knee.
Their heads are clasped abruptly; then, exiled

Like losing thoughts, they go in silence; some
Sheepishly stray, not back into their lives
Just yet; but some stay stiff, twitching and loud
With deep hoarse tears, as if a kind of dumb
And idiot child within them still survives
To re-awaken at kindness, thinking a voice

At last calls them alone, that hands have come
To lift and lighten; and such joy arrives
their thick tongues blort, their eyes squeeze grief, a crowd
Of huge unheard answers jam and rejoice –

What's wrong! Moustached in flowered frocks they shake:
By now, all's wrong. In everyone there sleeps
A sense of life lived according to love.
To some it means the difference they could make
By loving others, but across most it sweeps
As all they might have done had they been loved.
That nothing cures. An immense slackening ache,
As when, thawing, the rigid landscape weeps,
Spreads slowly through them – that, and the voice above
Saying *Dear child*, and all time has disproved.

Face Lift
Sylvia Plath (1961)

You bring me good news from the clinic,
Whipping off your silk scarf, exhibiting the tight white
Mummy-cloths, smiling: I'm all right.
When I was nine, a lime-green anaesthetist
Fed me banana-gas through a frog mask. The nauseous vault
Boomed with bad dreams and the Jovian[19] voices of surgeons.
Then mother swam up, holding a tin basin.
O I was sick.

They've changed all that. Traveling
Nude as Cleopatra in my well-boiled hospital shift,
Fizzy with sedatives and unusually humorous,
I roll to an anteroom where a kind man
Fists my fingers for me. He makes me feel something precious
Is leaking from the finger-vents. At the count of two,
Darkness wipes me out like chalk on a blackboard ...
I don't know a thing.

For five days I lie in secret,
Tapped like a cask, the years draining into my pillow.
Even my best friend thinks I'm in the country.
Skin doesn't have roots, it peels away easy as paper.
When I grin, the stitches tauten. I grow backward. I'm twenty,

---

[19]Jovian: characteristic of Jupiter, the god of thunder.

Broody and in long skirts on my first husband's sofa, my fingers
Buried in the lambswool of the dead poodle;
I hadn't a cat yet.

Now she's done for, the dewlapped lady
I watched settle, line by line, in my mirror –
Old sock-face, sagged on a darning egg.
They've trapped her in some laboratory jar.
Let her die there, or wither incessantly for the next fifty years,
Nodding and rocking and fingering her thin hair.
Mother to myself, I wake swaddled in gauze,
Pink and smooth as a baby.

The Operation
Anne Sexton (1964)

1.
After the sweet promise,
the summer's mild retreat
from mother's cancer, the winter months of her death,
I come to this white office, its sterile sheet,
its hard tablet, its stirrups, to hold my breath
while I, who must, allow the glove its oily rape,
to hear the almost mighty doctor over me equate
my ills with hers
and decide to operate.

It grew in her
as simply as a child would grow,
as simply as she housed me once, fat and female.
Always my most gentle house before that embryo
of evil spread in her shelter and she grew frail.
Frail, we say, remembering fear, that face we wear
in the room of the special smells of dying, fear
where the snoring mouth gapes
and is not dear.

There was snow everywhere.
Each day I grueled through
its sloppy peak, its blue-struck days, my boots
slapping into the hospital halls, past the retinue
of nurses at the desk, to murmur in cahoots
with hers outside her door, to enter with the outside
air stuck on my skin, to enter smelling her pride,
her upkeep, and to lie
as all who love have lied.

No reason to be afraid,
my almost mighty doctor reasons.
I nod, thinking that woman's dying
must come in seasons,
thinking that living is worth buying.
I walk out, scuffing a raw leaf,
kicking the clumps of dead straw
that were this summer's lawn.
Automatically I get in my car,
knowing the historic thief
is loose in my house
and must be set upon.

2.
Clean of the body's hair,
I lie smooth from breast to leg.
All that was special, all that was rare
is common here. Fact: death too is in the egg.
Fact: the body is dumb, the body is meat.
And tomorrow the O. R. Only the summer was sweet.

The rooms down the hall are calling
all night long, while the night outside
sucks at the trees. I hear limbs falling
and see yellow eyes flick in the rain. Wide eyed
and still whole I turn in my bin like a shorn lamb.
A nurse's flashlight blinds me to see who I am.

The walls color in a wash
of daylight until the room takes its objects
into itself again. I smoke furtively and squash
the butt and hide it with my watch and other effects.
The halls bustle with legs. I smile at the nurse
who smiles for the morning shift. Day is worse.

Scheduled late, I cannot drink
or eat, except for yellow pills
and a jigger of water. I wait and think
until she brings two mysterious needles: the skills
she knows she knows, promising, soon you'll be out.
But nothing is sure. No one. I wait in doubt.

I wait like a kennel of dogs
jumping against their fence. At ten
she returns, laughs and catalogues
my resistance to drugs. On the stretcher, citizen
and boss of my own body still, I glide down the halls
and rise in the iron cage toward science and pitfalls.

The great green people stand
over me; I roll on the table
under a terrible sun, following their command
to curl, head touching knee if I am able.
Next, I am hung up like a saddle and they begin.
Pale as an angel I float out over my own skin.

I soar in hostile air
over the pure women in labor,
over the crowning heads of babies being born.
I plunge down the backstair
calling *mother* at the dying door,
to rush back to my own skin, tied where it was torn.
Its nerves pull like wires
snapping from the leg to the rib.
Strangers, their faces rolling lilke hoops, require
my arm. I am lifted into my aluminum crib.

3.
Skull flat, here in my harness,
thick with shock, I call mother
to help myself, call toe to frog,
that woolly bat, that tongue of dog;
call God help and all the rest.
The soul that swam the furious water
sinks now in flies and the brain
flops like a docked fish and the eyes
are flat boat decks riding out the pain.

My nurses, those starchy ghosts,
hover over me for my lame hours
and my lame days. The mechanics
of the body pump for their tricks.
I rest on their needles, am dosed
and snoring amid the orange flowers
and the eyes of visitors. I wear,
like some senile woman, a scarlet
candy package ribbon in my hair.

Four days from home I lurk on my
mechanical parapet with two pillows
at my elbows, as soft as praying cushions.
My knees work with the bed that runs
on power. I grumble to forget the lie
I ought to hear, but don't. God knows
I thought I'd die – but here I am,

recalling mother, the sound of her
good morning, the odor of orange and jam.

All's well, they say. They say I'm better.
I lounge in frills or, picturesque,
I wear bunny pink slippers in the hall.
I read a new book and shuffle past the desk
to mail the author my first fan letter.
Time now to pack this humpty-dumpty
back the frightened way she came
and run along, Anne, and run along now,
my stomach laced like a football
for the game.

The Cure for Warts
Paul Muldoon (1973)

Had I been the seventh son of a seventh son
Living at the dead centre of a wood
Or at the dead end of a lane,
I might have cured by my touch alone
That pair of warts nippling at your throat,

Who had no faith in a snail rubbed on your skin
And spiked on a thorn like a king's head,
In my spittle on shrunken stone,
In bathing yourself at the break of dawn
In dew or the black cock's or the bull's blood,

In other such secrets told by way of a sign
Of the existence of one other god,
So I doubt if any woman's son
Could have cured by his touch alone
That pair of warts nibbling your throat.

Alive
Philip Appleman (1976)

Uncle Jimmie had a hunch that cancer,
the rat that gnawed away behind his ears,
was part of the warm earth and silver woods
and snowy meadows in the mountains. Surgeons
stabbed at the rat: scalpels sliced away
the ears one April dawn, as catbirds,
perched in the morning treetops, mocked the calling

of cardinals. Stabbed and missed – the rat survived.
The day they clipped out Uncle Jimmie's cheeks
and upper lip, he pondered artichokes,
truffles, and a certain Tuscan wine.
And when they snipped his nose, he wept for roses
and the fresh sea breeze – and thought a while, and played
his hunch: *Stop cutting*, Jimmie told them, *let
me go to earth and snow and silver trees.*
But the rat kept gnawing, and Auntie Flo went on
reading St. Paul *(The works of the flesh are uncleanness)*,
and praying, and paying the bills – and the surgeons huddled,
frowning at Jimmie's want of reverence
for faith and modern medicine. With skillful
suturing, they lifted out his tongue
and dropped the wagging muscle in a pail,
and Uncle Jim, who used to murmur quatrains
out of Omar,[20] kept his peace. Still, his eyes
kept pleading: *Stop the cutting, let me go
to earth and silver trees!* But Jimmie knew
the rat would work in just behind his eyes,
and Auntie Flo would go on reading Paul
(They that are Christ's have crucified the flesh)
and praying, and paying the bills – and the pale blue eyes
would have to go: one Sunday after Angelus, Jim began
his dark forgetting of the green
wheat fields, red hills in the sun,
and how the clouds drive storms across the sea.
Some Monday following, a specialist
trimmed away one-quarter of his brain
and left no last gray memory of Omar
or snowy fields or earth or silver trees.
But Uncle Jimmie lives: the rat lies quiet now,
and tubes lead in and out of Jimmie's veins
and vents. Auntie Flo comes every day
to read to bandages the Word Made Flesh,
and pray, and pay the bills, and watch with Jimmie,
whittled down like a dry stick, but living:
the heart, in its maze of tubes, pumps on,
while catbirds mock the calling of cardinals,
artichokes grow dusty green in sunshine,
butterflies dally with the roses,
and Uncle Jimmie is no part of these.

---

[20]*The Rubaiyat of Omar Khayyam.*

from *A Woman Dead in her Forties*
Adrienne Rich (1978)

1.
Your breasts/sliced-off   The scars
dimmed   as they would have to be
years later

All the women I grew up with are sitting
half-naked on rocks   in sun
we look at each other and
are not ashamed

and you too have taken off your blouse
but this was not what you wanted:

to show your scarred, deleted torso

I barely glance at you
as if my look could scald you
though I'm the one who loved you

I want to touch my fingers
to where your breasts had been
but we never did such things

You hadn't thought everyone
would look so perfect
unmutilated

you pull on
your blouse again: stern statement:

*There are things I will not share
with everyone*

2.
You send me back to share
my own scars   first of all
with myself

What did I hide from her
what have I denied her
what losses suffered

how in this ignorant body
did she hide

waiting for her release
till uncontrollable light began to pour

from every wound and suture
and all the sacred openings

7.
Time after time in dreams you rise
reproachful

once from a wheelchair pushed by your father
across a lethal expressway

Of all my dead it's you
who come to me unfinished

You left me amber beads
strung with turquoise from an Egyptian grave

I wear them wondering
How am I true to you?

I'm half-afraid to write poetry
for you   who never read it much

and I'm left laboring
with the secrets and the silence

In plain language   I never told you how I loved you
we never talked at your deathbed of your death

Grandfather at the Indian Health Clinic
Elizabeth Cook-Lynn (1983)

It's cold at last and cautious winds creep
softly into coves along the riverbank. At my insistence
he wears his denim cowboy coat high on his neck; averse to
an unceremonious world, he follows me through
hallways pushing down the easy rage he always has
with me, a youngest child, and smiles.
This morning the lodge is closed to the dance
and he reminds me these are not the men who
raise the bah above the painted marks; for the young
intern from New Jersey he bares his chest
but keeps a scarf tied on his steel-gray braids
and thinks of days that have no turning: he wore
yellow chaps and went as far as Canada to ride
Mad Dog and then came home to drive the Greenwood Woman's
cattle to his brother's place,
two hundred miles
along the timber line

the trees were bright
he turned his hat brim down in summer rain.

Now winter's here, he says, in this white lighted place
where lives are sometimes saved by
throwing blankets over spaces where the leaves are brushed away
and giving brilliant gourd-shell rattles
to everyone who comes.

Heart Test With An Echo Chamber
Margaret Atwood (1984)

Wired up at the ankles and one wrist,
a wet probe rolling over my skin,
I see my heart on a screen
like a rubber bulb or a soft fig, but larger,

enclosing a tentative double flutter,
the rhythm of someone out of breath
but trying to speak anyway; two valves opening
and shutting like damp wings
unfurling from a grey pupa.

This is the heart as television,
a softcore addiction
of the afternoon. The heart
as entertainment, out of date
in black and white.
The technicians watch the screen,
looking for something: a block, a leak,
a melodrama, a future
sudden death, clenching
of this fist which goes on
shaking itself at fate.
They say: It may be genetic.

(There you have it, from science,
that God has been whispering all along
through stones, madmen and birds' entrails:
hardness of the heart can kill you.)
They change the picture:
now my heart is cross-sectioned
like a slice of textbook geology.
They freeze-frame it, take its measure.

A deep breath, they say.
The heart gasps and plods faster.

It enlarges, grows translucent,
a glowing stellar
cloud at the far end
of a starscope. A pear
made of smoke and about to rot.
For once the blood and muscle
heart and the heart of pure
light are beating in unison,
visibly.

Dressing, I am diaphanous,
a mist wrapping a flare.
I carry my precarious
heart, radiant and already
fading, out with me
along the tiled corridors
into the rest of the world,
which thinks it is opaque and hard.
I am being very careful.
O heart, now that I know your nature,
who can I tell?

Metastasis[21]
Sandra M. Gilbert (1984)

At the cancer hotel, a lobby full of artificial plants,
leaves in the sane green shapes of health,
historical leaves mimicking the past –
and tubes blooming from groins, noses, armpits,
and starved faces in the dayroom
on every floor, thin images
reflecting the clean sheen of the ceiling...

'Just lie down, honey.' The nurse's aide,
indifferent as a bellboy, sells the new patient
on a quiet corner. This is it. The last resort.
'Here's your water. Here's your buzzer.'
The patient bobs, a courteous guest,
patient, never shows displeasure.
Looking east, over the river, her cousin

watches jets spurt toward Florida, California:
'Kennedy? LaGuardia?'[22] she wonders,

---

[21]Metastasis is the spread of a cancer from its primary site to other parts of the body.
[22]New York airports.

but the patient never turns, never answers.
Unpacking herself like a suitcase,
she sorts, plans, rearranges.
Here's the nightgown, there's the bathrobe.
When are the meals? Where's the soap?

Tomorrow she'll carry herself in a plastic bag,
sanitary, disposable, to the recreation room
at the end of the hall. The Magnavox[23]
will smile, a tour director,
and she'll gaze past sealed panes
at the roof of the children's wing
where roots of September flowers – 'autumn color' –

writhe in tubs, trying to get out,
and pigeons settle like insect swarms
among the swings and the deck chairs,
calm as travelers pretending not to see
the musty rugs, the infected
piazzas, the unsavory
kitchens of disease.

The Urine Specimen
Ted Kooser (1985)

In the clinic, a sun-bleached shell of stone
on the shore of the city, you enter
the last small chamber, a little closet
chastened with pearl – cool, white, and glistening,
and over the chilly well of the toilet
you trickle your precious sum in a cup.
It's as simple as that. But the heat
of this gold your body's melted and poured out
into a form begins to enthrall you,
warming your hand with your flesh's fevers
in a terrible way. It's like holding
an organ – spleen or fatty pancreas,
white, and glistening,
a lobe from your foamy brain still steaming
with worry. You know that just outside
a nurse is waiting to cool it into a gel
and slice it onto a microscope slide
for the doctor, who in it will read your future,

---

[23]Magnavox was a US electronics company, which manufactured televisions.

wringing his hands. You lift the chalice and toast
the long life of your friend there in the mirror,
who wanly smiles, but does not drink to you.

The Man Whose Smile Made Medical History
Lavinia Greenlaw (1993)

On dead afternoons my brother would borrow
rubber gloves and wellington boots
to chance the electrics of the ancient projector.

We would interrupt fifty-year-old summers where
a woman I now know in nappies and a walking frame
played leapfrog on a beach in West Wales

with a man whose smile made medical history.
The First World War revealed the infinite
possibilities of the human form,

so when in '16 he was sent back from France
without his top lip, the army doctors
decided to try and grow him a new one.

They selected the stomach as the ideal place
from which to tease a flap of skin
into a handle that could be stretched

and sewn to what was left of his mouth.
This additional feature was surgically removed
once it had fed the regeneration

of a thankfully familiar shape.
All I can find in my grandfather's face
to record the birth of plastic surgery

is the tight shyness he pulls into a grin,
unaware that scientific progress
which had saved his reflection could do nothing

to save his life. A doctor, aged thirty-four,
he died of viral pneumonia,
having recently heard of antibiotics.

Hands
SuAnne Doak (1994)

She looks at architecture
of bone, knuckle, skin,

the ballerina ease
of finger movement
and thinks of death,
that old lover, ally, enemy.
She's run after him
too many times,
razor in hand.
But, here's the same hand,
attached to this stubborn
engine, the body
with its chugging heart,
its veined pipeline
inside scarred wrists,
pumping blood –
that other familiar
she keeps digging up
to make sure it glistens
the same as it did on GIs[24]
in Da Nang,[25] and on her hands
that sealed veins dripping
red onto the floor,
picked out shrapnel
like metal-jacketed lice
from biceps, knees, ribs,
and her fists
that pounded failing chests,
her fingers entwined
with soldiers who lay
in pieces on the table,
her wrist strong against theirs
boneless as sand,
her lips inflating
their rubber mouths,
the respirator whump, whump
flattened to silence
as bodies cooled to gray.
Now she nurses
a bottle – puffs, blows
into it until it breathes back
bourbon, holds it
like it's alive.

---

[24]G.I. ('galvanized iron') is a nickname for US Army soldiers.
[25]Da Nang is one of the major port cities in Vietnam. During the Vietnam War, the city was home to a major airbase used by both the South Vietnamese and US Air Forces.

My Mammogram[26]
J. D. McClatchy (1994)

I.

In the shower, at the shaving mirror or beach,
For years I'd led... the unexamined life?
When all along and so easily within reach
(Closer even than the nonexistent wife)

Lay the trouble – naturally enough
Lurking in a useless, overlooked
Mass of fat and old newspaper stuff
About matters I regularly mistook

As a horror story for the opposite sex,
Nothing to do with what at my downtown gym
Are furtively ogled as The Guy's Pecs.

But one side is swollen, the too tender skin
Discolored. So the doctor orders an X-
Ray, and nervously frowns at my nervous grin.

II.

Mammography's on the basement floor.
The nurse has an executioner's gentle eyes.
I start to unbutton my shirt. She shuts the door.
Fifty, male, already embarrassed by the size

Of my 'breasts', I'm told to put the left one
Up on a smudged, cold, Plexiglas shelf,
Part of a robot half menacing, half glum,
Like a three-dimensional model of the Freudian self.

Angles are calculated. The computer beeps.
Saucers close on a flatness further compressed.
There's an ache near the heart neither dull nor sharp.

The room gets lethal. Casually the nurse retreats
Behind her shield. Anxiety as blithely suggests
I joke about a snapshot for my Christmas card.

III.

'No signs of cancer,' the radiologist swans
In to say – with just a hint in his tone
That he's done me a personal favour – whereupon
His look darkens. 'But what these pictures show ...

---

[26]Mammography is the process of using low-energy X-rays to examine the human breast, used as a diagnostic and screening tool for cancer.

Here, look, you'll notice the gland on the left's
Enlarged. See?' I see an aerial shot
Of Iraq, and nod. 'We'll need further tests,
Of course, but I'd bet that what *you've* got

Is a liver problem. Trouble with your estrogen[27]
Levels. It's time, my friend, to take stock.
It happens more often than you'd think to men.'

Reeling from its millionth Scotch on the rocks,
In other words, my liver's sensed the end.
Why does it come as something less than a shock?

IV.
The end of life as I've known it, that is to say –
Testosterone[28] sported like a power tie,
The matching set of drives and dreads that may
Now soon be plumped to whatever new designs

My apparently resentful, androgynous
Inner life has on me. Blind seer?
The Bearded Lady in some provincial circus?
Something that others both desire and fear.

Still, doesn't everyone *long* to be changed,
Transformed to, no matter, a higher or lower state,
To know the leathery D-Day hero's strange

Detachment, the queen bee's dreamy loll?
Oh, but the future each of blankly awaits
Was long ago written on the genetic wall.

V.
So suppose the breasts fill out until I look
Like my own mother... ready to nurse a son,
A version of myself, the infant understood
In the end as the way my own death had come.

Or will I in a decade be back here again,
The diagnosis this time not freakish but fatal?
The changes in one's later years all tend,
Until the last one, toward the farcical,

Each of us slowly turned into something that hurts,
Someone we no longer recognize.
If soul is the final shape I shall assume,

---

[27]Oestrogens, or estrogens, are the primary female sex hormones, though also present in males.
[28]Testosterone is the principal male sex hormone, secreted primarily by the testicles of males and, to a lesser extent, the ovaries and adrenal glands of females.

(– A knock at the door. Time to button my shirt
And head back out into the waiting room.)
Which of my bodies will have been the best disguise?

Plague Years
James Lasdun (1997)

> *'There is, it would seem, in the dimensional scale of the world, a kind of delicate*
> *meeting place between imagination and knowledge, a point, arrived at by*
> *diminishing large things and enlarging small ones, that is intrinsically artistic.'*
>
> – Vladimir Nabokov, *Speak Memory*

Sore throat, persistent cough... The campus doctor
Tells me 'just to be safe' to take the test.
The clinic protocol seems to insist
On an ironic calm. I hold my fear.
He draws a vial of blood for the City Lab,
I have to take it there, but first I teach
A class on Nabokov. Midway I reach
Into my bag for *Speak Memory*, and grab
The hot bright vial instead. I seem at once
Wrenched from the quizzical faces of my class
Into some silent anteroom of hell:
The 'delicate meeting place'; I feel it pounce;
Terror – my life impacted in the glass
My death enormous in its scarlet grail.

My Father's Hair
Deryn Rees-Jones (1998)

For it has stood up like a coxcomb before a fight.
For it is whiter than lace on a bobbin or snow on a bough.
For in his youth it was auburn, leading to blackness.
For it has a grave insouciance,
What they call in Sassoon's 'a natural air'.[29]
For it has resisted gels and lotions,
Brilliantine, mousses.
For it has been photographed, ridiculed,
Admired, swept back.
For it speaks the language of wild things, everywhere.
For it has suffered the barbary of barbers, and my mother.

---

[29]Vidal Sassoon (1928–2012) was a British hairdresser. Sassoon's refers to his hairdressing chain.

For it has been tamed with deerstalkers,
Baseball and camouflage caps.
For it is something of a pirate or an admiral.
It is a spark transmitter and a Special Constable,
It is Harrier, Jumpjet, parachute, Chinook.
For it is salt on an eyelash, fresh from the sea.
For it is loved by many women of the district,
And is piped aboard the sternest of vessels.
For it cannot be mentioned, the pot of *Vitalis*
She gave him on their honeymoon.
For its mind is as fast as light, the elastic stretch
Of a falling star. It is not anybody's servant.
For we will say nothing of Delilah and Seville.
It is both gravel path and skating rink.
It is velvet, it is epaulettes. It is sunrise, it is sunset.
O my father's hair! It is an unsung hero!
But because of the sickness, or the cure for the sickness,
It lies like an angel's on the pillow:
Long white strands, like wings, or long white wings, like hair.

Mastectomy
Alicia Ostriker (1998)

I shook your hand before I went.
Your nod was brief, your manner confident,
A ship's captain, and there I lay, a chart
Of the bay, no reefs, no shoals.
While I admired your boyish freckles,
Your soft green cotton gown with the oval neck,
The drug sent me away, like the unemployed.
I swam and supped with the fish, while you
Cut carefully in, I mean
I assume you were careful.
They say it took an hour or so.

I liked your freckled face, your honesty
That first visit, when I said
What's my odds on this biopsy[30]
And you didn't mince words,
One out of four it's cancer.
The degree on your wall shrugged slightly.
Your cold window onto Amsterdam

---

[30]A biopsy is a medical test involving sampling of cells or tissues for examination, to determine the presence
or extent of a disease.

Had seen everything, bums and operas.
A breast surgeon minces something other
Than language.
That's why I picked you to cut me.

Was I succulent? Was I juicy?
Flesh is grass, yet I dreamed you displayed me
In pleated paper like a candied fruit,
I thought you sliced me like green honeydew
Or like a pomegranate full of seeds
Tart as Persephone's,[31] those electric dots
That kept that girl in hell,
Those jelly pips that made her queen of death.
Doctor, you knifed, chopped, and divided it
Like a watermelon's ruby flesh
Flushed a little, serious
About your line of work
Scooped up the risk in the ducts
Scooped up the ducts
Dug out the blubber,
Spooned it off and away, nipple and all.
Eliminated the odds, nipped out
Those almost insignificant cells that might
Or might not have lain dormant forever.

The Lung Wash[32]
Michael Symmons Roberts (1999)

The first day, you cough up only water,
warm saline laced with vitamins and herbs.
Your lungs mistake healing for drowning,
they fetch up what tastes like the sea
into a white enamel bowl.
Your lungs mistake baptism for torture,
'O God. O my God. O God'.
You sought him out, like countless others
who speak too much and breathe too little,
you found the only doctor in the world
who washes lungs, and went to him.

---

[31]In Greek mythology, Persephone was abducted by Hades, god of the underworld, after he tricked her with a pomegranate. She was released from Hades by Hermes, but because she had tasted food in the underworld, she was obliged to spend each winter there.
[32]Lung lavage is used to treat a rare lung disease by washing away pulmonary alveolar proteinosis (accumulation of protein and lipids) from the lung air sacs, or alveoli.

The second day you know what comes –
'Breathe in Sir, now breathe out.'
The tube is pushed behind your voice
and water floods the hair's-breadth
channels of your lungs, you choke
'No no too much too much'
and phlegm rides up between the words,
coloured by the scent of home, and cigarettes.

By Wednesday the elegant office
with its dark red leather chairs
has won a terrifying fascination.
Sun streams through the window,
and the motes of dust light up
as if to show that air is only clean
when not seen for the carpet that it is.
Today you splutter up more phlegm,
with bonfires of your childhood,
other people's breath kissed into you,
incense and cooking smells
and long forgotten perfumes.
Then when all the phlegm is clear
the lighter, deeper hidden words begin
to bubble out into the room
'I always loved you, want to kill you,
be my life, come take my life.'

On Thursday morning you sleep in
and dream about a pulmonary specialist
in Venice with a plan, to counteract
the crumbling of his city with a thousand
human Venices, their lungs full
of the Grand Canal, but still you go.
'O Mama don't leave me. I'm hungry
I'm thirsty, I'm begging for some sleep'.
All the unsaid retches to be heard.
Il dottore with his bowl is ready to catch.

The last day you are growing into silence.
Four names from the bottom of your soul
were sobbed in sleep into the hot hotel room.
Morning brings a consciousness of breathing.
Coffee, or the smell of the lagoon
seem like a shot of meths.
Your chest is skinned and raw.
The still air of the clinic is like smelling salts,

The final treatment raises vowel sounds,
back to the first stirrings of your voice,
and then it stops.
That evening, eating shellfish in a café
full of idle conversation, you close
around your quietness. From now on
every word you use is plucked from nowhere.
Everything you say is sudden poetry.

Travels with John Hunter[33]
Les Murray (1999)

We who travel between worlds
lose our muscle and bone.
I was wheeling a barrow of earth
when agony bayoneted me.

I could not sit, or lie down,
or stand, in Casualty.
Stomach-calming clay caked my lips,
I turned yellow as the moon

and slid inside a CAT-scan wheel[34]
in a hospital where I met no-one
so much was my liver now my dire
preoccupation. I was sped down a road

of treetops and fishing-rod lightpoles
toward the three persons of God
and the three persons of John Hunter
Hospital.[35] Who said We might lose this one.

Twenty days or to the heat-death
of the Universe have the same duration:
vaguely half an hour. I awoke
giggling over a joke

about Paul Kruger[36] in Johannesburg
and missed the white court stockings

---

[33]John Hunter (1728–93), was a celebrated Scottish surgeon and anatomist.
[34]Computed axial tomography scans produce tomographic images (virtual 'slices') of specific areas of the body, allowing medics to see inside without cutting.
[35]The John Hunter Hospital is a principal hospital in New South Wales, Australia, with the busiest emergency department in the state.
[36]Paul Kruger (1825–1904), known as 'Oom Paul' or 'Uncle Paul', was the state president of the South African Republic (Transvaal). He gained international renown as the face of Boer resistance against the British during the South African or Second Boer War (1899–1902).

I half remembered from my prone
still voyage beyond flesh and bone.

I asked my friend who got new lungs
How long were you crazy, coming back?
Five days, he said. Violent and mad.
Fictive Afrikaner police were at him,

not unworldly Oom Paul Kruger.
Valerie, who had sat twenty days
beside me, now gently told me tales
of my time-warp. The operative canyon

stretched, stapled, with dry roseate walls
down my belly. Seaweed gel
plugged views of my pluck and offal.
Some accident had released flora

who live in us and will eat us
when we stop feeding them the earth.
I'd rehearsed the private office of the grave,
ceased excreting, made corpse gases

all while liana'd in tubes
and overseen by cockpit instruments
that beeped or struck up Beethoven's
Fifth at behests of fluid.

I also hear when I lay lipless
and far away I was anointed
first by a mild metaphoric church
then by the Church of no metaphors.

Now I said, signing a Dutch contract
in a hand I couldn't recognise,
let's go and eat Chinese soup
and drive to Lake Macquarie. Was I

not renewed as we are in Heaven?
In fact I could hardly endure
Earth gravity, and stayed weak and cranky
till the soup came, squid and vegetables,

pure Yang. And was sane thereafter.
It seemed I'd also travelled
in a Spring-in-Winter love-barque of cards,
of flowers and phone calls and letters,

concern I'd never dreamed was there
when black kelp boiled in my head.
I'd awoken amid my State funeral,
nevermore to eat my liver

or feed it to the Black Dog, depression
which the three Johns Hunter seem
to have killed with their scalpels:
it hasn't found its way home,

where I now dodder and mend
in thanks for devotion, for the ambulance
this time, for the hospital fork lift,
for pethidine, and this face of deity:

not the foreknowledge of death
but the project of seeing conscious life
rescued from death defines and will
atone for the human.

Dialysis[37]
Lucille Clifton (2000)

after the cancer, the kidneys
refused to continue.
they closed their thousand eyes.

blood fountains from the blind man's
arm and decorates the tile today.
somebody mops it up.

the woman who is over ninety
cries for her mother, if our dead
were here they would save us.

we are not supposed to hate
the dialysis unit. we are not
supposed to hate the universe.

this is not supposed to happen to me.
after the cancer the body refused

---

[37]Dialysis is a process for removing waste and excess water from the blood, used as an artificial replacement for lost kidney function in patients with renal failure.

to lose any more. even the poisons
were claimed and kept

until they threatened to destroy
the heart they loved. in my dream
a house is burning.

something crawls out of the fire
cleansed and purified.
in my dream i call it light.

after the cancer i was so grateful
to be alive. i am alive and furious.
Blessed be even this?

The Blister Test
Thomas Lux (2001)

They think you're dead but you're not. You're in a coma
or have a rare condition
that mimics death – you feel the pennies,
cool and heavy, on your eyelids,
you sense far-off weeping, but of the three people
here (the town priest, a quack doctor, and somewhat slow
Cousin Freddy) only Freddy *can* weep,
though rarely does so at deaths,
especially deaths in the family. As the doctor rifles
your pockets and the priest, using butter,
pulls a ring from your finger, you wish
Tanta Hedwig were here.
She's sharper than Freddy; she'd insist
(more out of superstition
than in real hope: Dead is dead, Tanta Hedwig
always said) on the blister test: a match
held to the sole
of the deceased's left foot. If it doesn't blister,
you're dead. If it does,
it means you live.
In the case of the former: you go to earth.
In the case of the latter: Mother's family
applies a balm of bark and pith,
which sometimes brings the sleeper back from 'the land between.'
Father's side
drains the blister
and keeps its fluid in a phial as antidote to dog bite
and complaints of the eye.

Insulin[38]
Joel Lane (2002)

It was 1979, a stark *Unknown*
Pleasures[39] riff of a year –
I was sixteen and burnt out,
creeping along the dry road,
pissing all night, drinking water
like it was air. My body was
a metaphor for capitalism:
glucose poisoning of the blood
while the tissues starved.
They put me on a drip,
rinsed out the sugar, gave me
a syringe full of daylight.
Too bright, at times. I got lost
between front door and hallway,
in moments that couldn't end.
Too much or not enough.

It's a chronic illness, of course,
like capitalism. Without a cure,
the state has to be managed.
Every few years, a new regime
to curb the extremes, protect
the vision. In the long run,
of course, it doesn't get easier.
But they say there's no body
these days: just holes that fill up
and empty, the insolvent organs
protesting the silence of their need.
The retina is corroding, but
we don't need care. We are new,
all skin and no blood, the users
of whatever reality we choose.
These days, only lies come free.

But the flesh has its message.
We need each other. What we share
is more precious than our blood.
The rage for survival kills us,

---

[38]Insulin is a pancreatic hormone that is vital in the production of sugar from carbohydrates for energy; it regulates blood sugar levels.
[39]*Unknown Pleasures* was the debut studio album by the English band Joy Division, 1979, Factory Records.

but we live by making contact.
The walls are permeable. We reach
to help each other stand, fallen
as we are, on private ground.

Gethsemane Day
Dorothy Molloy (2006)

They've taken my liver down to the lab,
left the rest of me here on the bed;
the blood I am sweating rubs off on the sheet,
but I'm still holding on to my head.

What cocktail is Daddy preparing for me?
What ferments in pathology's sink?
Tonight they will tell me, will proffer the cup,
and, like it or not, I must drink.

Theory of the Soul
Mark Doty (2008)

Ligustrum penicillium
three ragweeds, fusarium, marshelder, pollen of timothy, sweet vernal,
cocklebur and feathers, dog and tuna, dust mite, milk and yolk:

the allergist's assistant
pierces the skin of my back with ten clusters of needles,
each dipped in tinctures, and we wait to see which ones make me sick.

She says, You're okay, right?
and leaves the room. I'm a little tired, holding my face
in my hands, warm, leaning forward,

and then a doctor says,
How long ago did you give him that shot? A nurse says, Ten minutes.
A shot? Adrenaline, the doctor says, you had an allergic reaction

to the allergy test.
I thought if you blacked out you'd see it like a movie,
people gathering above your head, but of course I wasn't there

to know I was gone.
later, when I tell Claudia, she says, How can you know when you're not awake?
Ten minutes, no perception – just a little queasy,

then a jump cut
and I'm the hot center of a buzzing host afraid I'll sue them
because they've injected me with solutions of mouse hair, lobster and egg,

and left me to my own devices.
I tell Claudia this is what troubles me: I've been around enough dying
to trust that last breath wings out something more than air –

But where was I,
or that, if the self's embalmed by an injection of seafood and dust?
Animation, intelligence, the gathered weight of half a century

switched off like a lamp?
And then I tell her – well, Claudia isn't even in the room,
I'm talking to the Claudia I carry around in my head,

as I address our friends
in solitary moments, driving or walking uptown to the market –
I don't know why I tell her about the black kid

in the dingy passageway
to the L yesterday singing early Beatles with a radical purity,
everything distilled to a bright arcing liquid vulnerability

spilling over,
and the amaryllis bulbs in the florist's window flinging their bodies
forward in order to arrive at red, the single term of their arrival –

self made visible
in the reach for a form, breath in this body then
that, passed on or gone, and maybe that's why

we love to kiss,
because then we come closest to the exhaled quick.
We are what we make? Yeah, Claudia says,

all that. But where
is my work, while I'm prone on the allergist's floor?
The doctor who recommends, once I am breathing regularly,

that I avoid oysters,
and encourages me to call him again.

Operation at St Thomas' Hospital for Poor Women
Anna Robinson (2010)

I am moving yet tied down. I am blindfold
yet know they're here, feel their eyes
shame my body, not with lust but watchfulness.
These might be my last words and no one is listening.

I am cold in my fever. They wipe my forehead.
The sky is near yet I know this is a room,

can smell the dust. I think the roof is glass,
like the chapel in the workhouse.

They wipe my forehead. They cut.
Chest tears, bones scream *Oh* and *God*.
No pain is like this, not disease, not children.
They wipe my forehead. I am so tired.

There are stars, tiny and silver, and a pale
blue light washes me. I am leaving, I feel it.
Leaving through this gap in my chest
as if I am just what I breathe.

Intercession
Clare Best (2011)

Thoughts on a painting of Saint Agatha
by Fransisco de Zurbaran

Virgin martyr, protector
of valleys, wet nurses, bell founders –
invoked against breast disease,
earthquakes, eruptions of Mount Etna.
Agatha, whose breasts were excised[40]

with pincers by order of a jilted lover,
what do you make of these reconstructed
bodies? Muscle flaps. Tissue expanded
by balloon. Thigh and buttock flesh
ingeniously transposed. Do you admire

the silicone implants, the polished skin –
nipples grafted from earlobes and labia,
areolas tattooed? You stand there
serene, flat-chested, forever the girl,
bearing your breasts on a dish

and if people mistake the hemispheres
for handbells or perfect loaves of bread,
help them remember – each of us
has severed parts
we carry separately.

---

[40]Saint Agatha of Sicily (231–251 AD), is the patron saint of breast cancer patients, earthquakes and eruptions of Mount Etna, was portrayed as carrying her perfectly spherical breasts before her on a platter. Having dedicated her virginity to God, fifteen-year-old Agatha rejected the advances of the Roman prefect Quintianus, who then persecuted her by cutting off her breasts and sentencing her to be burnt at the stake. Saved by an earthquake, she was instead sent to prison where St. Peter the Apostle appeared to her and healed her wounds. She died in prison.

Account[41]
Clare Best (2011)

Four carriages stop in the street.
One last mouthful of wine
before I ascend the bed,
two nurses at my side.

Three chimes of the clock.
Seven men in black, seven
full glasses of claret.
Nine stacks of compresses, lint.

A cambric veil across my face,
the glitter of burnished steel
and backlit by sun,
a forearm over my chest.

The surgeon's index finger
describes a line, a circle, a cross.
Six incisions and he changes hands.
My screams, throughout.

Blood
Anthony Wilson (2012)

The nurse announces the cannula.
One *sharp scratch* and you're there,

vial after ochre vial,
unstoppable.

Cousin to tawny port
your sheen's a glossy russet.

You do not gush, you seep,
but would soak

the world
if you could.

You're not much to look at:
but, spun, you separate –

lymph, plasma
and marrow, the very core

---

[41]Author's note: In 1811, the writer Fanny Burney underwent a mastectomy, without anaesthetic, at her home near Paris. She later recorded the experience in her journal. See page 292–99.

of us, telling everything.
Famously salty

to the taste, you seem stable as mercury.
If only.

The Halving
Robin Robertson (2013)

Royal Brompton Hospital, 1986

General anaesthesia; a median sternotomy[42]
achieved by sterna saw; the ribs
held aghast by retractor; the tubes
and cannulae drawing the blood
to the reservoir, and its bubbler;
the struggling aorta
cross-clamped, the heart
chilled and stopped and left to dry.
The incompetent bicuspid valve[43] excised,
the new one – a carbon-coated disc, housed
expensively in a cage of tantalum[44] –
is broken from its sterile pouch
then heavily implanted into the native heart,
bolstered, seated with sutures,
the aorta freed, the heart re-started.
The blood allowed back
after its time abroad
circulating in the machine.
The rib-spreader relaxed
and the plumbing removed, the breast-bone
lashed with sterna wires, the incision closed.

Four hours I'd been away: out of my body.
Made to die then jerked back to the world.
The distractions of delirium
came and went and then,
as the morphine drained, I was left with a split
chest that ground and grated on itself.
Over the pain, a blackness rose and swelled;

---

[42]Median sternotomy is a surgical procedure in which a vertical cut is made along the sternum, which is then 'cracked', providing access to the heart and lungs for surgery.
[43]The bicuspid valve, or mitral valve, controls blood flow between the left atrium and the left ventricle.
[44]Named after the mythical Tantalus, who is eternally punished in Tartarus, tantalum is a rare, highly corrosion resistant metal.

'pump-head' is what some call it
– debris from the bypass machine
migrating to the brain – but it felt
more interesting than that.
Halved and unhelmed,
I have been away, I said to the ceiling,
and now I am not myself.

MEDICAL WRITING:

Gonosologium Novum
John Marten (1709)

But a day or two ago, the following letter was brought, of a case and management, which, the better to show the fallacy of such that pretend to what they do not understand, I shall so far trespass upon the reader's patience as to insert it, and is this:

Dear Sir,

I crave your patience and leisure to read the following relation, and then your skilful and sagacious judgment.

About seven weeks ago I unhappily got a *Clap*,[45] for cure of which I apply'd my self having met with one of his bills, to the *German* or *Dutch Quack*, at the *Hand and Urinal* in *High-Holborn*, who told me, between stammering and speaking, oh! He would cure me presently, and gave me purges for five or six times, and then some medicines he called Strengtheners; insomuch, that in about three weeks, I heard no more of my *Running Nag*, and paid him, and as he assur'd me, thought myself well, and away I went well satisfy'd; but in about three weeks time after, I began to be in pain all over me, and grew upon me more and more, that I could scarce walk; every one call'd it a rheumatism. I had a physician who came to me, and enquiring into my condition, whisper'd me in the ear that it was the *pox*; but I forgot to tell you that when the pains encreas'd, I was advis'd to sweat, which I did with *Venice Treacle*, etc. whereupon I had blotches all over me that turn'd to white mealy scabs, which my physician said were *pocky* ones, and order'd me something for the present, which set me upon my legs a little, that I made a shift to go in a coach to that d*****d *quack* that *poxt* me, to show him how I was, who, a P**gue take him, told me I had got it a-fresh, and that I must drink his *Royal Decoction*, as he call'd it, which would cure me, but I d****d his ignorance and knavery, and with a few hardy c**ses, God forgive me, I left him, wishing him to have my distemper. The next day I saw my physician again, to whom I told the whole story, as I have now done to you, who laugh'd at my folly, as well he might, that I should be drawn in, and bubled by one of the most notorious *quacks* of the town, which, he says, he and every one knows him to be, he knowing him to be such many years: But upon enquiring of my physician what

---

[45]Clap, or gonorrhea.

I must do to be well, he told me I must be salivated out of hand, and advis'd me to you; telling me that you lately cur'd a very good friend of his, a knight, that he recommended to you, who no body else could cure, and that you was a man of judgment and honour, and would do me justice. I therefore having told you the whole story, desire you, good Sir, to consider of my case against this night, when, about seven a clock, I will wait of you at your house, and beg of you by all that is sacred, you would put me in a proper method, and finish my cure with all the expedition you can, for which you shall be honourably and gratefully rewarded; but you must excuse me, dear Sir, that I am oblig'd to desire you never to enquire, who or what I am, or the physician's name that advis'd me to you, because by that means I shall come to be known, for whatever you must have, I will pay you down before-hand, to avoid your suspecting me. I hope, Sir, for all what my doctor says, it may be done without salivation,[46] but when I wait of you, you will know better. Why do you and others of the profession, suffer such a dog to live under your noses? Send him packing with a P*x to him to his own country, to kill the people there with his d****d *Turpentine* and *devilish Decoction*, for I have been told since that he has spoil'd several. Good Sir, don't fail being in the way at seven at night; in the interim favour me with a line by this porter whether you receiv'd my letter, fairly seal'd in three places; and one more thing I have to request of you, that you would not let this be seen by any, but burn it as soon as you have read it, my hand being remarkable, and thousands of this town know it. I beg your pardon for this tedious scroll, and am, dear Sir,

Your must humble and most obedient
(tho' unknown) Servant.

This letter sufficiently shows the ignorance of the man in those cases, and how it can be thought or imagin'd by any, he should be otherways than ignorant, who, for all his Life-time, as far as I know, at least for many years, has got his living by *casting of piss*, and *telling of fortunes*, as we are told by an advertisement lately publish'd in the news-papers; and which, it seems, will be demonstrated in a book preparing for the press by one Dr *Fitcherton*, a regular physician; as also that a book of that disease set forth by that *quack*, is all other men's works. So far I know myself of it, having run it over, that great part of it is my Book of the *Venereal Disease* abridg'd, he having transcrib'd in many places, the very words and sentences, and dispos'd many of the paragraphs in the same order as mine are, which is such plagiary, that I have directed some hints to that worthy gentleman that is answering his book, which I hope he will so far favour me as to incert. Such is the ill nature of foreign audacious *QUACKS*, who care not what they do, who they steal from, or who they ruin, so they get but the mony, which is all their aim and design; but 'tis hop'd by the methods now a taking to suppress all foreign and domestick *quacks*, *mountebanks*, *fortune-tellers*, etc. which are the very pest of the nation, he, who is one of the tribe, will be silenc'd, and shown beter manners than has been taught him in his own country and made to know, that tho' the mob may for a while, yet the wise part of the people of *England* are not to be so abus'd by strangers.

---

[46]Salivation was a very unpleasant treatment with mercury.

From this very *quack*, sometime since, came a gentleman to me, who by taking his drink, which he calls the *Royal Decoction*, has brought into an involuntary emission of urine, had such a propensity as that he could not hold it a minute, but would come away in his breeches, insomuch that he was difficultly sav'd from a *Diabetes*: He was from a plump fleshy man, brought by drinking that *Decoction*, into a thin, wasting, declining condition, and tho' he went through his method for thirty days, was so far from being cur'd of his indisposition (which that *quack* told him was the *pox*, which I aver, and can make it appear, was nothing of that disease) that he was render'd much worse, even to the endangering a *consumption* as well as a *diabetes*, which might have cost him his life. I undertook him and cur'd him, and he had twenty guineas for my pains. These relations afore spoken of, I aver and can prove to be fact; as also others under the same *quack*'s hands, taken notice of in my Book of *Venereal Disease*, Sixth Edition, to which I refer the reader for further satisfaction; and have besides, divers other well attested relations and accounts of his managing venereal people, which as opportunity offers, may be made public by, John Marten.

Letter on Smallpox in Turkey
Lady Mary Wortly Montagu (1717)[47]

A propos of distempers, I am going to tell you a thing, that will make you wish yourself here. The small-pox, so fatal, and so general amongst us, is here entirely harmless, by the invention of engrafting, which is the term they give it. There is a set of old women, who make it their business to perform the operation, every autumn, in the month of September, when the great heat is abated. People send to one another to know if any of their family has a mind to have the small-pox; they make parties for this purpose, and when they are met (commonly fifteen or sixteen together) the old woman comes with a nut-shell full of the matter of the best sort of small-pox, and asks what vein you please to have opened. She immediately rips open that you offer to her, with a large needle (which gives you no more pain than a common scratch) and puts into the vein as much matter as can lie upon the head of her needle, and after that, binds up the little wound with a hollow bit of shell, and in this manner opens four or five veins. The Grecians have commonly the superstition of opening one in the middle of the forehead, one in each arm, and one on the breast, to mark the sign of the Cross; but this has a very ill effect, all these wounds leaving little scars, and is not done by those that are not superstitious, who chuse to have them in the legs, or that part of the arm that is concealed. The children or young patients play together all the rest of the day, and are in perfect health to the eighth. Then the fever begins to seize them, and they keep their beds two days, very seldom three. They have very rarely above twenty or thirty in their faces, which never mark, and in eight days time they are as well as before their illness. Where they

---

[47]In 1715, Lady Montagu suffered from, and was left scarred by, smallpox. In 1717, Lady Montagu and her British ambassador husband were living in the Ottoman Empire. She observed that the local practice of inoculation – deliberately introducing a mild form of the disease to the body – that gave people resistance to the disease. By the end of the eighteenth century, the English physician Edward Jenner had developed vaccination – using cattle-pox serum – to render humans immune, which led to the worldwide eradication of the illness.

are wounded, there remains running sores during the distemper, which I don't doubt is a great relief to it. Every year, thousands undergo this operation, and the French Ambassador says pleasantly, that they take the small-pox here by way of diversion, as they take the waters in other countries. There is no example of any one that has died in it, and you may believe I am well satisfied of the safety of this experiment, since I intend to try it on my dear little son. I am patriot enough to take the pains to bring this useful invention into fashion in England, and I should not fail to write to some of our doctors very particularly about it, if I knew any one of them that I thought had virtue enough to destroy such a considerable branch of their revenue, for the good of mankind. But that distemper is too beneficial to them, not to expose to all their resentment, the hardy wight that should undertake to put an end to it. Perhaps if I live to return, I may, however, have courage to war with them. Upon this occasion, admire the heroism in the heart of

Your friend, etc. etc.

An Historical Account of the Small-Pox Inoculated in New England
Zabdiel Boyston (1726)

June the 26th, 1721.

I inoculated my son Thomas, of about six, my Negro man, Jack, thirty six, and Jackey, two and a half years old. They all complained on the 6th day; upon the 7th, the two children were a little hot, dull and sleepy, Thomas (only) had twitchings and started in his sleep. The 8th, the children's fevers continued, Tommy's twitchings and startings in sleep increased; and though the fever was gentle and his senses bright, yet as the practice was new, and the clamour, or rather rage of the people against it so violent that I was put into a very great fright; and not having any directions from Dr Timonius and Pyllarinus[48] concerning this practice, I had nothing to have recourse to but patience, and therefore waited upon nature for a crisis (neither my fears nor the symptoms abating) until the 9th; when early in the morning I have him a vomit, upon which the symptoms went off, and the same day, upon him and the black child, a kind and favourable small-pox came out, of about an hundred a piece; after which their circumstances became easy, our trouble was over, and they soon were well.

Jack's complaints, in two or three days were over, and though he had but a few pustles about one of his inoculations, I am inclined to think he had had the small-pox before.

It was plain and easy to see, (even in these two) with pleasure, the difference between having small-pox this way, and that of having it in the natural way.

...

And pray let us consider what this method, [inoculation], in procuring the distinct small-pox, does prevent: it prevents the confluent, which, in itself is a plague, and that in a high degree; some of the bad symptoms attending which, are as follows:

---

[48]The Boston physician Cotton Mather tried to convince his peers to inoculate by sharing the findings of Drs Timonius and Pyllarinus, who had successfully inoculated in the Levant. It seems only Boyston was convinced.

purple spots, the bloody and parchment pox, hemorahages of blood at the mouth, nose, fundament, and privities; ravings and delriums; convulsions, and other fits; violent inflammations and swellings in the eyes and throat; so that they cannot see or scarcely breathe, or swallow anything, to keep them from starving. Some looking as black as the stock, others as white as a sheet; in some, the pock runs into blisters, and the skin stripping off, leaves the flesh raw, like creatures flea'd. Some have a burning, others a smarting pain, as if in the fire, or scalded with boiling water: some have insatiable thirsts, others greedy appetites, and will crave food when dying. Some have been filled with loathsome ulcers; others have had deep, and fistulous ulcers in their bodies, or in their limbs or joints; with rottenness of the ligaments and bones: some who live are cripples, others idiots, and many blind all their days; beside the other deformities it brings upon many, in their faces, limbs, or body, with many more grievous symptoms, which the world has had too great experience of, as being the attendants of that fatal distemper called the confluent small-pox.

What this humour of the small-pox, in us, is, or when, and how it is communicated to us, the Learned have not yet informed us. ... However otherways it may be this is certain, that as it is a most loathsome, painful, and destructive distemper, so Providence has wisely and mercifully ordered it, that once only, in our lives, we shall be distressed by it and has now, in greater goodness, discovered to us a way or method how to moderate that distemper and to render the small-pox, inoculated, no further dangerous than a common intermittent fever. ... And shall not the world gratefully accept and thankfully make use of such a method, (when known) and especially Great Britain, which has had so much experience of its good effects, and that for five years following? Shall not they come fully into and take the benefit of it? And shall not the physicians, who are the medicinal guides, with the surgeons, recommend and bring it to greater esteem and practice?

An Inquiry Into the Causes and Effects of the Variolæ Vaccinæ, Or Cow-Pox
Edward Jenner (1798)

The deviation of man from the state in which he was originally placed by nature seems to have proved to him a prolific source of diseases. From the love of splendour, from the indulgences of luxury, and from his fondness for amusement he has familiarised himself with a great number of animals, which may not originally have been intended for his associates.

...

In this dairy country a great number of cows are kept, and the office of milking is performed indiscriminately by men and maid servants. One of the former having been appointed to apply dressings to the heels of a horse affected with the grease, and not paying due attention to cleanliness, incautiously bears his part in milking the cows, with some particles of the infectious matter adhering to his fingers. When this is the case, it commonly happens that a disease is communicated to the cows, and from the cows to the dairymaids, which spreads through the farm until the most of the cattle and domestics feel its unpleasant consequences. This disease has obtained the name of the cow-pox. It appears on the nipples of the cows in the form of irregular pustules. At their first appearance they are commonly of a palish blue, or rather of a colour somewhat approaching to livid, and are surrounded by an erysipelatous inflammation.[49] These pustules, unless a timely remedy be applied, frequently degenerate into phagedenic ulcers,[50] which prove extremely troublesome. The animals become indisposed, and the secretion of milk is much lessened. Inflamed spots now begin to appear on different parts of the hands of the domestics employed in milking, and sometimes on the wrists, which quickly run on to suppuration, first assuming the appearance of the small vesications produced by a burn. Most commonly they appear about the joints of the fingers and at their extremities; but whatever parts are affected, if the situation will admit, these superficial suppurations put on a circular form, with their edges more elevated than their centre, and of a colour distantly approaching to blue. Absorption takes place, and tumours appear in each axilla.[51] The system becomes affected – the pulse is quickened; and shiverings, succeeded by heat, with general lassitude and pains about the loins and limbs, with vomiting, come on. The head is painful, and the patient is now and then even affected with delirium. These symptoms, varying in their degrees of violence, generally continue from one day to three or four, leaving ulcerated sores about the hands, which, from the sensibility of the parts, are very troublesome, and commonly heal slowly, frequently becoming phagedenic, like those from whence they sprung. The lips, nostrils, eyelids, and other parts of the body are sometimes affected with sores; but these evidently arise from their being heedlessly rubbed or scratched with the patient's infected fingers. No eruptions on the skin have followed the decline of the feverish symptoms in any instance that has come under my inspection, one only excepted, and in this case a very few appeared on the arms: they were very minute, of a vivid red colour, and soon died away without advancing to maturation; so that I cannot determine whether they had any connection with the preceding symptoms.

Thus the disease makes its progress from the horse to the nipple of the cow, and from the cow to the human subject.

Morbid matter of various kinds, when absorbed into the system, may produce effects in some degree similar; but what renders the cow-pox virus so extremely singular is that the person who has been thus affected is forever after secure from the infection of the small-pox; neither exposure to the variolous effluvia, nor the insertion of the matter into the skin, producing this distemper.

...

CASE VI. It is a fact so well known among our dairy farmers that those who have had the smallpox either escape the cow-pox or are disposed to have it slightly, that as soon as the complaint shows itself among the cattle, assistants are procured, if possible, who are thus rendered less susceptible of it, otherwise the business of the farm could scarcely go forward.

In the month of May, 1796, the cow-pox broke out at Mr Baker's, a farmer who lives near this place. The disease was communicated by means of a cow which was purchased in an infected state at a neighbouring fair, and not one of the farmer's

---

[49]Erysipelas is a bacterial infection of the skin, which becomes red and swollen.
[50]Phagedenic ulcers: painful, weeping lesions of the skin.
[51]The axilla is the armpit, or the equivalent, of an animal.

cows (consisting of thirty) which were at that time milked escaped the contagion. The family consisted of a man servant, two dairymaids, and a servant boy, who, with the farmer himself, were twice a day employed in milking the cattle. The whole of this family, except Sarah Wynne, one of the dairymaids, had gone through the smallpox. The consequence was that the farmer and the servant boy escaped the infection of the cow-pox entirely, and the servant man and one of the maid servants had each of them nothing more than a sore on one of their fingers, which produced no disorder in the system. But the other dairymaid, Sarah Wynne, who never had the smallpox, did not escape in so easy a manner. She caught the complaint from the cows, and was affected with the symptoms... in so violent a degree that she was confined to her bed, and rendered incapable for several days of pursuing her ordinary vocations in the farm.

March 28th, 1797, I inoculated this girl and carefully rubbed the variolous matter into two slight incisions made upon the left arm. A little inflammation appeared in the usual manner around the parts where the matter was inserted, but so early as the fifth day it vanished entirely without producing any effect on the system.

Account from Paris of a Terrible Operation
Fanny Burney (1812)[52]

A Physician was now called in, Dr Moreau, to hear if he could suggest any new means: but Dr Larrey had left him no resources untried. A formal consultation now was held, of Larrey, Ribe, and Moreau – and, in fine, I was formally condemned to an operation by all Three.[53] I was as much astonished as disappointed – for the poor breast was no where discoloured, and not much larger than its healthy neighbour. Yet I felt the evil to be deep, so deep, that I often thought if it could not be dissolved, it could only with life be extirpated. I called up, however, all the reason I possessed, or could assume, and told them that – if they saw no other alternative, I would not resist their opinion and experience: – the good Dr Larrey, who, during his long attendance had conceived for me the warmest friendship, had now tears in his Eyes; from my dread he had expected resistance. He proposed again calling in M. Dubois.[54] No, I told him, if I could not by himself be saved, I had no sort of hope elsewhere, and, if it must be, what I wanted in courage should be supplied by Confidence. The good man was now dissatisfied with himself, and declared that I ought to have the First and most eminent advice his Country could afford; 'Vous êtes si considerée, Madame,' said he, 'ici, que le public même

---

[52]Journal Letter to Esther Burney, 22 March–June, 1812. See Clare Best's poem earlier in this section.
[53]Jacques-Louis Moreau de la Sarthe (1771–1826) was a French surgeon and anatomist. Baron Dominique-Jean Larrey (1766–1842) was a celebrated French army surgeon. François Ribes (1765–1845) was a French anatomist, surgeon and colleague of Baron Larrey.
[54]Antoine Dubois (1756–1837) was a celebrated French surgeon, anatomist and obstetrician, who attended the Empress Marie Louise.

sera mecontent si vous n'avez pas tout le secour que nous avons à vous offrir.'[55] Yet this modest man is premier chirugien de la Garde Imperiale,[56] and had been lately created a Baron for his eminent services! M. Dubois, he added, from his super-skill and experience, might yet, perhaps, suggest some cure. This conquered me quickly, ah – Send for him! Send for him! I cried – and Dr Moreau received the commission to consult with him. – What an interval was this! Yet my poor M. d'Arblay[57] was more to be pitied than myself, though he knew not the terrible idea I had internally annexed to the trial – but Oh what he suffered! – and with what exquisite tenderness he solaced all that I had to bear! My poor Alex I kept as much as possible, and as long, ignorant of my situation. – M. Dubois behaved extremely well, no pique intervened with the interest he had professed in my well-doing, and his conduct was manly and generous. It was difficult still to see him, but he appointed the earliest day in his power for a general and final consultation. I was informed of it only on the Same day, to avoid any useless agitation. He met here Drs Larrey, Ribe, and Moreau. The case, I saw, offered uncommon difficulties, or presented eminent danger, but the examination over, they desired to consult together. I left them – what an half hour I passed alone! – M. d'Arblay was at his office. Dr Larrey then came to summon me. He did not speak, but looked very like my dear Brother James, to whom he has a personal resemblance that has struck M. d'Arblay as well as myself. I came back, and took my seat, with what calmness I was able. All were silent, and Dr Larrey, I saw, hid himself nearly behind my Sofa. My heart beat fast: I saw all hope was over. I called upon them to speak. M. Dubois then, after a long and unintelligible harangue, from his own disturbance, pronounced my doom. I now saw it was inevitable, and abstained from any further effort. They received my formal consent, and retired to fix a day.

All hope of escaping this evil now at an end, I could only console or employ my Mind in considering how to render it less dreadful to M. d'Arblay. M. Dubois had pronounced 'il faut s'attendre à souffrir, Je ne veux pas vous tromper – Vous Souffrirez – vous souffrirez *beaucoup*! –'[58] M. Ribe had *charged* me to cry! to withhold or restrain myself might have seriously bad consequences, he said. M. Moreau, in echoing this injunction, enquired whether I had cried or screamed at the birth of Alexander – Alas, I told him, it had not been possible to do otherwise; Oh then, he answered, there is no fear! – What terrible inferences were here to be drawn! I desired, therefore, that M. d'Arblay might be kept in ignorance of the day till the operation should be over. To this they agreed, except M. Larrey, with high approbation: M. Larrey looked dissentient, but was silent. M. Dubois protested he would not undertake to act, after what he had seen of the agitated spirits of M. d'Arblay if he were present: nor would he suffer me to know the time myself over

---

[55]'You are so esteemed here, Madam, that the public itself would be unhappy if you did not receive all the help that we have to offer.'
[56]First surgeon of the Imperial Guard.
[57]In 1793, aged 42, she married a French exile, General Alexandre D'Arblay. They had one child, a son, Alexander, who was born in 1794.
[58]'You must expect to suffer, I do not want to deceive you – you will suffer – you will suffer *very much*!–'

night; I obtained with difficulty a promise of 4 hours warning, which were essential to me for sundry regulations.

From this time, I assumed the best spirits in my power, *to meet the coming blow*; – and support my too sympathising Partner. They would let me make no preparations, refusing to inform me what would be necessary; I have known, since, that Mme de Tessé,[59] an admirable old friend of M. d'Arblay, now mine, equally, and one of the first of her sex, in any country, for uncommon abilities, and nearly universal knowledge, had insisted upon sending me all that might be necessary, and of keeping me in ignorance. M. d'Arblay filled a Closet with Charpie,[60] compresses, and bandages. All that to me was owned, as wanting, was an arm Chair and some Towels. Many things, however, joined to the depth of my pains, assured me the business was not without danger. I therefore made my Will – unknown, to this moment, to M. d'Arblay, and entrusted it privately to M. La Tour Maubourg,[61] without even letting my friend his Sister, Mme de Maisonneuve, share the secret. M. de Maubourg conveyed it for me to Maria's excellent M. Gillet, from whom M. de Maubourg brought me directions. As soon as I am able to go out I shall reveal this clandestine affair to M. d'Arblay. Till then, it might still affect him. Mme de Maisonneuve desired to be present at the operation; but I would not inflict such pain. Mme de Chastel belle soeur[62] de Mme de Boinville, would also have sustained the shock; but I secured two Guards, one of whom is known to my two dear Charlottes,[63] Mme Soubiren, portiere[64] de l'Hotel Marengo: a very good Creature, who often amuses me by repeating '*ver. vell, Mawm;*' which she tells me she learnt of Charlotte the younger, whom she never names but with rapture, the other is a workman whom I have often employed. The kindnesses I received at this period would have made me for-ever love France, had I hitherto been hard enough of heart to hate it – but Mme d'Henin[65] – the tenderness she showed me surpasses all description. Twice she came to Paris from the Country, to see, watch and sit with me; there is nothing that can be suggested of use or comfort that she omitted. She loves me not only from her kind heart, but also from her love of Mrs. Lock, often, often, exclaiming 'Ah! si votre Angelique amie étoit ici! –'[66] But I must force myself from these episodes, though my dearest Esther will not think them *de trop.*[67]

After sentence thus passed, I was in hourly expectation of a summons to execution; judge, then to my surprise to be suffered to on full 3 Weeks in the same state! M. Larrey from time to time visited me, but pronounced nothing, and was always melancholy. At length, M d'Arblay was told that he waited himself for a Summons! and that, a formal one, and in writing! *I* could not give one. A *consent*

---

[59]Adrienne-Catherine, comtesse de Tessé (1741–1813).

[60]Charpie is linen for surgical dressings.

[61]César, comte de Latour-Marbourg (1757–1831).

[62]Sister-in-law.

[63]The two Charlottes are Burney's sister and niece.

[64]*Portiere:* Doorkeeper.

[65]Former Princesse d'Henin, who had been one of Marie-Antoinette's ladies-in-waiting.

[66]'Ah! if your angelic friend were here!' (referring to her friend Amelie Beck).

[67]*De trop:* excessive.

was my utmost effort. But poor M. d'Arblay wrote a desire that the operation, if necessary, might take place without further delay. In my own mind, I had all this time been persuaded there were hopes of a cure: why else, I thought, let me know my doom thus long? But here I must account for this apparently useless, and therefore cruel measure, though I only learnt it myself 2 months afterwards. M. Dubois had given his opinion that the evil was too far advanced for any remedy; that the cancer was already internally declared; that I was inevitably destined to that most frightful of deaths, and that an operation would but accelerate my dissolution. Poor M. Larrey was so deeply affected by this sentence that, – as he has lately told me, he regretted to his Soul ever having known me, and was upon the point of demanding a commission to the furthest end of France in order to force me into other hands. I had said, however, he remembered, once, that I would far rather suffer a quick end without, than a lingering life with this dreadfullest of maladies: he finally, therefore, considered it might be possible to save me by the trial, but that without it my case was desperate, and resolved to make the attempt. Nevertheless, the responsibility was too great to rest upon his own head entirely; and therefore he waited the formal summons. – In fine, One morning – the last of September, 1811, while I was in Bed, and M. d'Arblay was arranging some papers for his office, I received a Letter written by M. de Lally to a Journalist, in vindication of the honoured memory of his Father against the assertions of Mme du Deffand.[68] I read it aloud to My Alexanders, with tears of admiration and sympathy, and then sent it by Alex to its excellent Author, as I had promised the preceding evening.

I then dressed, aided, as usual for many months, by my maid, my right arm being condemned to total inaction; but not yet was the grand business over, when another Letter was delivered to me – another, indeed! – 'twas from M. Larrey, to acquaint me that at 10 o'clock he should be with me, properly accompanied, and to exhort me to rely as much upon his sensibility & his prudence, as upon his dexterity and his experience; he charged to secure the absence of M. d'Arblay, and told me that the young Physician who would deliver me this *announce*, would prepare for the operation, in which he must lend his aid: and also that it had been the decision of the consultation to allow me but two hours' notice. – Judge, my Esther, if I read this unmoved! – Yet I had to disguise my sensations and intentions from M. d'Arblay! – Dr Aumont,[69] the Messenger and terrible Herald, was in waiting; M. d'Arblay stood by my bedside; I affected to be long reading the Note, to gain time for forming some plan, and such was my terror of involving M. d'Arblay in the unavailing wretchedness of witnessing what I must go through, that it conquered every other, and gave me the force to act as if I were directing some third person. The detail would be too *Wordy*, as James says, but the *wholesale* is, I called Alex to my Bedside, and sent him to inform M. Barbier Neuville, chef du division du Bureau de M. d'Arblay[70] that *the*

---

[68]In 1766, Marie du Deffand wrote to Horace Walpole in favour of the decision to execute the comte de Lally, Tolenadal's father for treason. De Lally, who likely learned this from the 1811 edition of du Deffand's letters to Walpole, responded by writing the vindicating letter.
[69]Philippe-Éléonore-Godefroy Aumond.
[70]Divisional head of d'Arblay's office.

moment was come, and I entreated him to write a summons upon urgent business for M. d'Arblay and to detain him till all should be over. Speechless and appalled, off went Alex, and, as I have since heard, was forced to sit down and sob in executing his commission. I then, by the maid, sent word to the young Dr Aumont that I could not be ready till one o'clock: and I finished my breakfast and – not with much appetite, you will believe! forced down a crust of bread, and hurried off, under various pretences, M. d'Arblay. He was scarcely gone, when M Du Bois arrived: I renewed my request for one o'clock: the rest came; all were fain to consent to the delay, for I had an apartment to prepare for my banished Mate. This arrangement, and those for myself, occupied me completely. Two engaged nurses were out of the way – I had a bed, Curtains, and heaven knows what to prepare – but business was good for my nerves. I was obliged to quit my room to have it put in order: – Dr Aumont would not leave the house; he remained in the Salon, folding linen! He had demanded 4 or 5 old and fine left off under Garments – I glided to our Book Cabinet: sundry necessary works and orders filled up my time entirely till One O'clock when all was ready – but Dr Moreau then arrived, with news that M. Dubois could not attend till three. Dr Aumont went away, and the Coast was clear. This, indeed, was a dreadful interval. I had no longer anything to do – I had only to think –Two Hours thus spent seemed never-ending. I would fain have written to my dearest Father – to You, my Esther – to Charlotte James – Charles – Amelia Lock – but my arm prohibited me: I strolled to the Salon – I saw it fitted with preparations, and I recoiled – But I soon returned; to what effect disguise from myself what I must so soon know? – yet the sight of the immense quantity of bandages, compresses, sponges, lint – Made me a little sick: – I walked backwards and forwards till I quieted all emotion, and became, by degrees, nearly stupid – torpid, without sentiment or consciousness; – and thus I remained till the Clock struck three. A sudden spirit of exertion then returned, – I defied my poor arm, no longer worth sparing, and took my long banished pen to write a few words to M. d'Arblay, and a few more for Alex, in case of a fatal result. These short billets I could only deposit safely, when the Cabriolets[71] – one, two, three, four – succeeded rapidly to each other in stopping at the door. Dr Moreau instantly entered my room, to see if I were alive. He gave me a wine cordial, and went to the Salon. I rang for my Maid and Nurses, – but before I could speak to them, my room, without previous message, was entered by 7 Men in black, Dr Larry, M. Dubois, Dr Moreau, Dr Aumont, Dr Ribe, and a pupil of Dr Larry, and another of M. Dubois. I was now awakened from my stupor – and by a sort of indignation – Why so many? and without leave? – But I could not utter a syllable.

M. Dubois acted as Commander in Chief. Dr Larry kept out of sight; M. Dubois ordered a Bed stead into the middle of the room. Astonished, I turned to Dr Larry, who had promised that an Arm Chair would suffice; but he hung his head, and would not look at me. Two *old mattresses* M. Dubois then demanded, and an old Sheet. I now began to tremble violently, more with distaste and horror of the preparations even than of the pain. These arranged to his liking, he desired me

---

[71]Cabriolet: a one-horse carriages.

to mount the Bed stead. I stood suspended, for a moment, whether I should not abruptly escape – I looked at the door, the windows – I felt desperate – but it was only for a moment, my reason then took the command, and my fears and feelings struggled vainly against it. I called to my maid – she was crying, and the two Nurses stood, transfixed, at the door. 'Let those women all go!' cried M. Dubois. This order recovered me my Voice – 'No,' I cried, 'let them stay! *qu'elles restent!*'[72] This occasioned a little dispute, that re-animated me – The Maid, however, and one of the nurses ran off – I charged the other to approach, and she obeyed. M. Dubois now tried to issue his commands *en militaire*, but I resisted all that were resistable – I was compelled, however, to submit to taking off my long robe de Chambre,[73] which I had meant to retain. Ah, then, how did I think of My Sisters! – Not one, at so dreadful an instant, at hand, to protect – adjust – guard me – I regretted that I had refused Mme de Maisonneuve – Mme Chastel – no one upon whom I could rely – my departed Angel![74] How did I think of her! How did I long, long for my Esther, my Charlotte! – My distress was, I suppose, apparent, though not my Wishes, for M. Dubois himself now softened, and spoke soothingly. 'Can *You*,' I cried, 'feel for an operation that, to *You*, must seem so trivial?' – 'Trivial?' he repeated, taking up a bit of paper, which he tore, unconsciously, into a million of pieces, '*oui – c'est peu de chose   mais –*'[75] he stammered, and could not go on. No one else attempted to speak, but I was softened myself, when I saw even M. Dubois grow agitated, while Dr Larry kept always aloof, yet a glance showed me he was pale as ashes. I knew not, positively, then, the immediate danger, but every thing convinced me danger was hovering about me, and that this experiment could alone save me from its jaws. I mounted, therefore, unbidden, the Bed stead – and M. Dubois placed me upon the mattress, and spread a cambric handkerchief upon my face. It was transparent, however, and I saw, through it, that the Bed stead was instantly surrounded by the 7 men and my nurse. I refused to be held; but when, Bright through the cambric, I saw the glitter of polished Steel – I closed my Eyes. I would not trust to convulsive fear the sight of the terrible incision. A silence the most profound ensued, which lasted for some minutes, during which, I imagine, they took their orders by signs, and made their examination – Oh what a horrible suspension! – I did not breathe, and M. Dubois tried vainly to find any pulse. This pause, at length, was broken by Dr Larry, who in a voice of solemn melancholy, said 'Qui me tiendra ce sein?'[76]

No one answered; at least not verbally; but this aroused me from my passively submissive state, for I feared they imagined the whole breast infected – feared it too justly – for, again through the Cambric, I saw the hand of M. Dubois held up, while his forefinger first described a straight line from top to bottom of the breast, secondly a Cross, and thirdly a circle; intimating that the Whole was to be taken off. Excited by this idea, I started up, threw off my veil, and, in answer to the demand

---

[72]'Let them stay.'
[73]*Robe de Chambre:* dressing gown.
[74]The departed Angel is her younger sister Susanna Phillips (née Burney).
[75]'Yes – it's a small thing, but ....'
[76]'Who will hold this breast for me?'

'Qui me tiendra ce sein?' cried 'C'est moi, Monsieur!'[77] and I held My hand under it, and explained the nature of my sufferings, which all sprang from one point, though they darted into every part. I was heard attentively, but in utter silence, and M. Dubois then re-placed me as before, and, as before, spread my veil over my face. How vain, alas, my representation! immediately again I saw the fatal finger describe the Cross, and the circle. Hopeless, then, desperate, and self-given up, I closed once more my Eyes, relinquishing all watching, all resistance, all interference, and sadly resolute to be wholly resigned.

My dearest Esther, and all my dears to whom she communicates this doleful ditty, will rejoice to hear that this resolution once taken, was firmly adhered to, in defiance of a terror that surpasses all description, and the most torturing pain. Yet – when the dreadful steel was plunged into the breast – cutting through veins – arteries – flesh – nerves – I needed no injunctions not to restrain my cries. I began a scream that lasted unintermittingly during the whole time of the incision – and I almost marvel that it rings not in my Ears still! so excruciating was the agony. When the wound was made, and the instrument was withdrawn, the pain seemed undiminished, for the air that suddenly rushed into those delicate parts felt like a mass of minute but sharp and forked poniards, that were tearing the edges of the wound – but when again I felt the instrument – describing a curve – cutting against the grain, if I may so say, while the flesh resisted in a manner so forcible as to oppose and tire the hand of the operator, who was forced to change from the right to the left, then, indeed, I thought I must have expired. I attempted no more to open my Eyes, – they felt as if hermetically shut, and so firmly closed, that the Eyelids seemed indented into the Cheeks. The instrument this second time withdrawn, I concluded the operation over, – Oh no! presently the terrible cutting was renewed – and worse than ever, to separate the bottom, the foundation of this dreadful gland from the parts to which it adhered – Again all description would be baffled – yet again all was not over, – Dr Larry rested, but his own hand, and – Oh Heaven! – I then felt the Knife rackling against the breast bone – scraping it! This performed, while I yet remained in utterly speechless torture, I heard the Voice of Mr Larry, (all others guarded a dead silence) in a tone nearly tragic, desire everyone present to pronounce if anything more remained to be done; or if he thought the operation complete. The general voice was Yes, – but the finger of Mr Dubois, which I literally *felt* elevated over the wound, though I saw nothing, and though he touched nothing, so indescribably sensitive was the spot – pointed to some further requisition, and again began the scraping! – and, after this, Dr Moreau thought he discerned a peccant atom[78] – and still, and still, M. Dubois demanded atom after atom. – My dearest Esther, not for days, not for Weeks, but for Months I could not speak of this terrible business without nearly again going through it! I could not *think* of it with impunity! I was sick, I was disordered by a single question – even now, 9 months after it is over,[79] I have a headache from going

---

[77]'I will, Sir!'
[78]Peccant atom: refers to traces of diseased breast tissue.
[79]June, 1812.

on with the account! and this miserable account, which I began 3 Months ago, at least, I dare not revise, nor read, the recollection is still so painful.

To conclude, the evil was so profound, the case so delicate, and the precautions necessary for preventing a return so numerous, that the operation, including the treatment and the dressing, lasted 20 minutes! a time, for sufferings so acute, that was hardly supportable – However, I bore it with all the courage I could exert, and never moved, nor stopt them, nor resisted, nor remonstrated, nor spoke – except once or twice, during the dressings, to say 'Ah Messieurs! que je vous plains!'[80] for indeed I was sensible to the feeling concern with which they all saw what I endured, though my speech was principally – *very* principally meant for Dr Larry. Except this, I uttered not a syllable, save, when so often they re-commenced, calling out 'Avertissez moi, Messieurs! Avertissez moi! –'[81] Twice, I believe, I fainted; at least, I have two total chasms in my memory of this transaction, that impede my tying together what passed. When all was done, and they lifted me up that I might be put to bed, my strength was so totally annihilated, that I was obliged to be carried, and could not even sustain my hands and arms, which hung as if I had been lifeless; while my face, as the Nurse has told me, was utterly colourless. This removal made me open my Eyes, and I then saw my good Dr Larry, pale nearly as myself, his face streaked with blood, and its expression depicting grief, apprehension, and almost horror.

Illustrations of the Antiseptic System of Treatment in Surgery
Joseph Lister (1867)

Decomposition or putrefaction has long been known to be a source of great mischief in surgery, and antiseptic applications have for several years been employed by many surgeons. But the full extent of the evil, and the paramount importance of adopting effectual measures against it, are far from being generally recognized.

It is now six years since I first publicly taught in the University of Glasgow that the occurrence of suppuration in a wound under ordinary circumstances, and its continuance on a healthy granulating sore treated with water dressing, are determined simply by the influence of decomposing organic matter. The subject has since received a large share of my attention, resulting in the system of treatment which I have been engaged for the last three years in elaborating. The benefits which attend this practice are so remarkable that I feel it incumbent upon me to do what I can to diffuse them; and with this view I propose to present to the readers of *The Lancet* a series of illustrative cases, prefacing them with a short notice of the principles which it is essential to bear in mind in order to attain success.

The cases in which this treatment is most signally beneficial are divisible into three great classes – incised wounds, of whatever form; contused or lacerated wounds, including compound fractures; and abscesses, acute or chronic – a list,

---

[80]'Ah Sirs! how I pity you!'
[81]'Warn me, Sirs! warn me!'

indeed, which comprises the greater part of surgery. In each of these groups our aim is simply to prevent the occurrence of decomposition in the part, in order that its reparatory powers may be left undisturbed by the irritating and poisoning influence of putrid materials. In pursuing this object we are guided by the 'germ theory', which supplies us with a knowledge of the nature and habits of the subtle foe we have to contend with; and without a firm belief in the truth of that theory, perplexity and blunders must be of frequent occurrence. The facts upon which it is based appear sufficiently convincing. We know from the researches of Pasteur[82] that the atmosphere does contain among its floating particles the spores of minute vegetations and infusoria, and in greater numbers where animal and vegetable life abound, as in crowded cities or under the shade of trees, than where the opposite conditions prevail, as in unfrequented caves or on Alpine glaciers. Also, it appears that the septic energy of the air is directly proportioned to the abundance of the minute organisms in it, and is destroyed entirely by means calculated to kill its living germs – as, for example, by exposure for a while to a temperature of 212° Fahr. or a little higher, after which it may be kept for an indefinite time in contact with putrescible substances, such as urine, milk, or blood, without producing any effect upon them. It has further been shown, and this is particularly striking, that the atmosphere is deprived of its power of producing decomposition as well as organic growth by merely passing in a very gentle stream through a narrow and tortuous tube of glass, which, while it arrests all its solid particles, cannot possibly have any effect upon its gases; while conversely, 'air-dust' collected by filtration rapidly gives rise simultaneously to the development of organisms and the putrefactive changes. Lastly, it seems to have been established that the character of the decomposition which occurs in a given fermentable substance is determined by the nature of the organism that develops in it. Thus the same saccharine solution may be made to undergo either the vinous or the butyric fermentation, according as the yeast plant or another organism, described by Pasteur, is introduced into it. Hence we cannot, I think, refuse to believe that the living beings invariably associated with the various fermentative and putrefactive changes are indeed their causes. And it is peculiarly in harmony with the extraordinary powers of self-diffusion and penetration exhibited by putrefaction that the chief agents in this process appear to be 'vibrios' endowed with the faculty of locomotion, so that they are able to make their way speedily along a layer of fluid such as serum or pus.

Admitting, then, the truth of the germ theory, and proceeding in accordance with it, we must, when dealing with any case, destroy in the first instance once for all any septic organisms which may exist within the part concerned; and after this has been done, our efforts must be directed to the prevention of the entrance of others into it. And provided that these indications are really fulfilled, the less the antiseptic agent comes in contact with the living tissues the better, so that unnecessary disturbance from its irritating properties may be avoided.

---

[82]The French microbiologist Louis Pasteur (1822–95) is renowned for his world-changing discoveries concerning vaccination, germ theory, pasteurization and the causes and preventions of many diseases. Pasteur's vinous or butyric fermentation that Lister mentions in this paragraph refers, respectively, to the fermentation that produces alcohol and fermentation as a result of decomposition.

On a New Kind of Rays, December 28, 1895
W. C. Röntgen (1895)[83]

A discharge from a large induction coil is passed through a Hittorf's vacuum tube, or through a well-exhausted Crookes' or Lenard's tube. Glass tubes were used in the production of X-ray pictures. The tube is surrounded by a fairly close-fitting shield of black paper; it is then possible to see, in a completely darkened room, that paper covered on one side with barium platinocyanide lights up with brilliant fluorescence when brought into the neighbourhood of the tube, whether the painted side or the other be turned towards the tube. The fluorescence is still visible at two metres distance. It is easy to show that the origin of the fluorescence lies within the vacuum tube.

It is seen, therefore, that some agent is capable of penetrating black cardboard which is quite opaque to ultra-violet light, sunlight, or arc-light. It is therefore of interest to investigate how far other bodies can be penetrated by the same agent. It is readily shown that all bodies possess this same transparency, but in very varying degrees. For example, paper is very transparent; the fluorescent screen will light up when placed behind a book of a thousand pages; printer's ink offers no marked resistance. Similarly the fluorescence shows behind two packs of cards; a single card does not visibly diminish the brilliancy of the light. So, again, a single thickness of tinfoil hardly casts a shadow on the screen; several have to be superposed to produce a marked effect. Thick blocks of wood are still transparent. Boards of pine two or three centimetres thick absorb only very little. A piece of sheet aluminium, 15 mm. thick, still allowed the X-rays (as I will call the rays, for the sake of brevity) to pass, but greatly reduced the fluorescence. Glass plates of similar thickness behave similarly; lead glass is, however, much more opaque than glass free from lead. Ebonite several centimetres thick is transparent. If the hand be held before the fluorescent screen, the shadow shows the bones darkly, with only faint outlines of the surrounding tissues.

Water and several other fluids are very transparent. Hydrogen is not markedly more permeable than air. Plates of copper, silver, lead, gold, and platinum also allow the rays to pass, but only when the metal is thin. Platinum .2 mm. thick allows some rays to pass; silver and copper are more transparent. Lead 1.5 mm. thick is practically opaque. If a square rod of wood 20 mm. in the side be painted on one face with white lead, it casts little shadow when it is so turned that the painted face is parallel to the X-rays, but a strong shadow if the rays have to pass through the painted side. The salts of the metals, either solid or in solution, behave generally as the metals themselves.

...

The justification of the term 'rays', applied to the phenomena, lies partly in the regular shadow pictures produced by the interposition of a more or less permeable body between the source and a photographic plate or fluorescent screen.

---

[83]This 1933 translation (by Otto Glasser) of Röntgen's first communication varies somewhat from the original translation, by G. F. Barker in 1896.

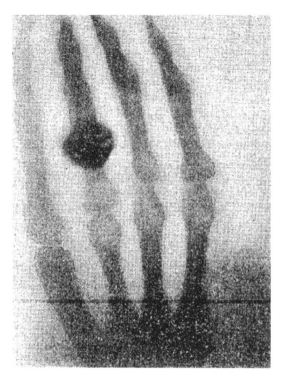

FIGURE 3a: X-ray Photograph of the bones in the fingers of a living human hand. The third finger has a ring upon it.

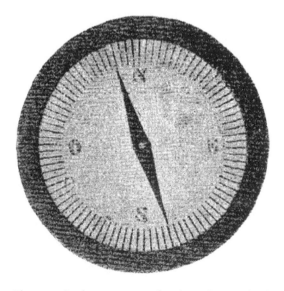

FIGURE 3b: X-ray Photograph of a compass card and needle completely enclosed in a metal case.

I have observed and photographed many such shadow pictures. Thus, I have an outline of part of a door covered with lead paint; the image was produced by placing the discharge-tube on one side of the door, and the sensitive plate on the other. I have also a shadow of the bones of the hand (Figure 3a), of a wire wound upon a bobbin, of a set of weights in a box, of a compass card and needle completely enclosed in a metal case (Figure 3b), of a piece of metal where the X-rays show the want of homogeneity, and of other things. For the rectilinear propagation of the rays, I have a pin-hole photograph of the discharge apparatus covered with black paper. It is faint but unmistakable.

Of Medicine and Poetry
William Carlos Williams (1948)

When they ask me, as of late they frequently do, how I have for so many years continued an equal interest in medicine and the poem, I reply that they amount for me to nearly the same thing. Any worth-this-salt physician knows that no one is 'cured'. We recover from some somatic, some bodily 'fever' whereas observers we have seen various engagements between our battalions of cells playing at this or that lethal maneuver with other natural elements. It has been interesting. Various sewers or feed-mains have given way here or there under pressure: various new patterns have been thrown up for us upon the screen of our knowledge. But a cure is absurd, as absurd as calling these deployments 'diseases'. Sometimes the home team wins, sometimes the visitors. Great excitement. It is noteworthy that the sulfonamids, penicillin, came in about simultaneously with Ted Williams, Ralph Kiner[84] and the rubber ball. We want home runs, antibiotics to 'cure' man with a single shot in the buttocks.

But after you've knocked the ball into center-field bleachers and won the game, you still have to go home to supper. So what? The ball park lies empty-eyed until the next game, the next season, the next bomb. Peanuts.

Medicine, as an art, never had much attraction for me, though it fascinated me, especially the physiology of the nervous system. That's something. Surgery always seemed to me particularly unsatisfying. What is there to cut off or out that will 'cure' us? And to stand there for a lifetime sawing away! You'd better be a chef, if not a butcher. There is joy in it, I realize, to know that you've really cut the cancer out and that the guy will come in to score, but I never wanted to be a surgeon. Marvelous men – I take off my hat to them. I knew one once who whenever he'd get into a malignant growth would take a hunk of it and rub it into his armpit afterward. Never knew why. It never hurt him, and he lived to a great old age. He had imagination, curiosity and a sense of humor, I suppose.

---

[84]Ted Williams (1918–2002) and Ralph Kiner (1922–2014) were American Major League Baseball players.

The cured man, I want to say, is no different from any other. It is a trivial business unless you add the zest, whatever that is, to the picture. That's how I came to find writing such a necessity, to relieve me from such a dilemma. I found by practice, by trial and error, that to treat a man as something to which surgery, drugs, and hoodoo applied was an indifferent matter; to treat him as material for a work of art made him somehow come alive to me.

What I wanted to do with him (or her, or it) fascinated me. And it didn't make any difference, apparently, that he was in himself distinguished or otherwise. It wasn't that I wanted to save him because he was a good and useful member of society. Death had no respect for him for that reason, neither does the artist, neither did I. As far as I can tell that kind of 'use' doesn't enter into it; I am myself curious as to what I do find. The attraction is bizarre.

Thus I have said 'the mind'. And the mind? I can't say that I have ever been interested in a completely mindless person. But I have known one or two that are close to mindless, certainly useless, even fatal to their families, or what remains of their families, whom yet I find far more interesting than plenty of others whom I serve.

...

This immediacy, the thing, as I went on writing, living as I could, thinking a secret life I wanted to tell openly – if only I could – how it lives, secretly about us as much now as ever. It is the history, the anatomy of this, not subject to surgery, plumbing or cures, that I wanted to tell. I don't know why. Why tell that which no one wants to hear? But I saw that when I was successful in portraying something, by accident, of that secret world of perfection, that they did want to listen. Definitely. And my 'medicine' was the thing which gained me entrance to these secret gardens of the self. It lay there, another world, in the self. I was permitted by my medical badge to follow the poor, defeated body into those gulfs and grottos. And the astonishing thing is that at such times and in such places – foul as they may be with the stinking ischio-rectal abscesses of our comings and goings – just there, the thing, in all its greatest beauty, may for a moment be freed to fly for a moment guiltily about the room. In illness, in the permission I as a physician have had to be present at deaths and births, at the tormented battles between daughter and diabolic mother, shattered by a gone brain – just there – for a split second – from one side or the other, it has fluttered before me for a moment, a phrase which I quickly write down on anything at hand, any piece of paper I can grab.

It is an identifiable thing, and its characteristic, its chief character is that it is sure, all of a piece and, as I have said, instant and perfect: it comes, it is there, and it vanishes. But I have seen it, clearly I have seen it. I know it because there it is. I have been possessed by it just as I was in the fifth grade – when she leaned over the back of the seat before me and greeted me with some obscene remarks – which I cannot repeat even if made by a child forty years ago, because no one would or could understand what I am saying that then, there, it had appeared.

The great world never much interested me (except at the back of my head) since its effects, from what I observed, were so disastrously trivial – other than in their bulk; smelled the same as most public places. As Bob McAlmon said after the well-dressed Spanish woman passed us in Juarez (I had said, 'Wow! there's perfume for you!'):

'You mean that?' he said. 'That's not perfume, I just call that whores.'

CHAPTER SIX

Hospitals, Practitioners and Professionals

To Dr William Hunter[1]
Hugh Downman (1781)

> Hunter, than whom (bless'd with peculiar art)
> With equal clearness to the eyes of youth,
> None e'er demonstrated the Human Frame;
> To which, to Surgery how dear thy name!
> Whose penetrative mind & feeling heart
> Smit with the love of nature and of Truth,
> Following their dictates, spite of Envy's Race,
> Have perfected the just Obstetric Plan;
> Whence rescued from the gloomy gates of *Death*
> What crowds survive, still more to spread thy fame
> The Matron's, and her offspring's grateful breath
> Whose Thoughts e'en late Posterity, embrace,
> Intent to them thy useful stores I impart;
> These Numbers with thy wonted Kindness scan!

An Oration which Might have been Delivered to Students of Anatomy on the Late Rupture
Francis Hopkinson (1789)[2]

> Friends and associates! lend a patient ear,
> Suspend intestine broils and reason hear.
> Ye followers of F— your wrath forbear –
> Ye sons of S— your invectives spare;

---

[1]William Hunter (1718–83), was a Scottish anatomist, physician and one of the most renowned obstetricians of the late eighteenth century. Hugh Downman (c.1765–1858) was a blind poet and physician who practiced in Exeter, Devon. He inscribed this poem on the flyleaf of a copy of his 1781 *Poems to Thespia*, which was sent to Hunter.

[2]The ostensible impetus for this poem was the longstanding rivalry (or what Hopkinson describes, in a letter to Thomas Jefferson, as a 'ridiculous quarrel') between Philadelphia's rivaling faculties of medicine (the University of Pennsylvania and the College of Philadelphia). The poem addresses the students loyal to 'F' (Lecturer in anatomy and obstetrics, Dr John Foulke) and his rival 'S' (Professor of Anatomy, Dr William Shippen).

The fierce dissension your high minds pursue
Is sport for others – ruinous to you.

Surely some fatal influenza reigns,
Some epidemic *rabies* turns your brains;
Is this a time for brethren to engage
In public contest and in party rage?
Fell discord triumphs in your doubtful strife,
And, smiling, whets her anatomic knife;
Prepared to cut our precious limbs away
And leave the bleeding body to decay.

Seek ye for foes? alas, my friends, look round,
In every street, see numerous foes abound!
Methinks I hear them cry, in varied tones,
'Give us our father's – brother's – sister's bones.'
Methinks I see a mob of sailors rise –
'Revenge! – revenge!' they cry, and damn their eyes –
Revenge for comrade Jack, whose flesh they say,
You minced to morsels and then threw away.
Methinks I see a black infernal train –
The genuine offspring of accursed *Cain* –[3]
Fiercely on you their angry looks are bent,
They grin and gibber dangerous discontent,
And seem to say – 'Is there not meat enough?
Ah! massa cannibal, why eat poor CUFF?'
Even hostile watchmen stand in strong array,
And o'er our heads their threatening staves display:
Howl hideous discord through the noon of night,
And shake their dreadful lanthorns in our sight.

Say, are not these sufficient to engage
Your high wrought souls eternal war to wage?
Combine your strength these monsters to subdue,
No friends of science and sworn foes to you;
On these – on these, your wordy vengeance pour,
And strive our fading glory to restore.

Ah! think how, late, our mutilated rites
And midnight orgies, were by sudden frights

---

[3] In the Book of Genesis, the first son of Adam and Eve, Cain is a farmer who, jealous of God's preference for his shepherd brother Abel, commits the first murder by killing Abel. In this stanza, Hopkinson alludes to a series of incidents: a 1765 'Sailor's Mob' stormed Dr. William Shippen's anatomy class and his home; a 1788 'Doctor's Mob' formed against anatomy classes in New York City; and the reference to cannibalism and 'Cuff' in the next lines likely refers to the 1788 protest of African-American citizens against graverobbing at the Negro Burying Ground in New York.

And loud alarms profan'd – the sacrifice,
Stretch'd on a board before our eager eyes,
All naked lay – even when our chieftain stood
Like a high priest, prepared for shedding blood;
Prepared, with wonderous skill to cut or slash,
The gentle sliver or the deep drawn gash;
Prepar'd to plunge ev'n elbow deep in gore,
Nature and nature's secrets to explore –
Then a tumultuous cry – a sudden fear –
Proclaim'd the foe – the enraged foe is near –
In some dark hole the hard-got corpse was laid,
And we, in wild confusion, fled dismay'd.

Think how, like brethren, we have shar'd the toil,
When in the Potter's field[4] we sought for spoil,
Did midnight ghosts and death and horror brave –
To delve for science in the dreary grave.
Shall I remind you of that awful night
When our compacted hand maintained the fight
Against an armed host? – fierce was the fray,
And yet we bore our sheeted prize away.
Firm on a horse's back the corpse was laid,
High blowing winds the winding sheet display'd;
Swift flew the steed – but still his burthen bore –
Fear made him fleet, who ne'er was fleet before;
O'er tombs and sunken graves he cours'd around,
Nor ought respected consecrated ground.
Meantime the battle rag'd – so loud the strife,
The dead were almost frighten'd into life –
Though not victorious, yet we scorn'd to yield,
Retook our prize, and left the doubtful field.

In this degenerate age, alas! how few
The paths of science with true zeal pursue?
Some trifling contest, some delusive joy
Too oft the unsteady minds of youth employ.
For me – whom Esculapius hath inspir'd –
I boast a soul with love of science fir'd;
By one great object is my heart possess'd –
One ruling passion quite absorbs the rest –
In this bright point my hopes and fears unite;
And one pursuit alone can give delight.

---

[4]Author's note: Potter's Field is 'the Negro burial ground'.

To me things are not as to vulgar eyes,
I would all nature's works anatomize –
This world a living monster seems, to me,
Rolling and sporting in the aerial sea;
The soil encompasses her rocks and stones
As flesh in animals encircles bones.
I see vast ocean, like a heart in play,
Pant *systole* and *diastole*[5] every day,
And by unnumbered *venous* streams supply'd
Up her broad river force the *arterial* tide.
The world's great lungs, monsoons and tradewinds show
From east to west, from west to east they blow
Alternate respiration –
The hills are pimples which earth's face defile,
And burning Ætna, an eruptive boil:
On her high mountains *hairy* forests grow,
And *downy* grass o'erspreads the vales below;
From her vast body perspirations rise,
Condense in clouds and float beneath the skies:
Thus fancy, faithful servant of the heart,
Transforms all nature by her magic art.

Even mighty love, whose power all power controls;
Is not, in me, like love in other souls –
Yet I have loved – and Cupid's subtle dart
Hath through my *pericardium* pierced my heart.
Brown CADAVERA did my soul ensnare,
Was all my thought by night and daily care –
I long'd to clasp, in her transcendant charms,
A living skeleton within my arms.

Long, lank, and lean, my CADAVERA stood,
Like the tall pine, the glory of the wood –
Oft times I gaz'd, with learned skill to trace
The sharp edg'd beauties of her bony face –
There rose *os frontis*[6] prominent and bold,
In deep sunk *orbits* two large eye-balls roll'd,
Beneath those eye-balls, two arch'd bones were seen
Whereon two flabby cheeks hung loose and lean;
Beneath those cheeks, proturberant arose,
In form triangular, her lovely nose,
Like Egypt's pyramid it seem'd to rise,
Scorn earth, and bid defiance to the skies;

---

[5]Systole and diastole are the names for the phases of dilation and contraction of the heart respectively.
[6]Os frontis: the forehead.

Thin were her lips, and of a sallow hue,
Her open'd mouth expos'd her teeth to view;
Projecting strong, protuberant and wide
Stood *incisores* – and on either side
The *canine* rang'd, with many a beauteous flaw,
And last the *grinders*, to fill up the jaw –
All in their *alveoli* fix'd secure,
Articulated by *gomphosis*[7] sure.
Around her mouth, perpetual smiles had made
Wrinkles wherein the loves and graces play'd;
There, stretch'd and rigid by continual strain,
Appear'd the *zygomatic*[8] muscles plain,
And broad *montanus* o'er her peaked chin
Extended to support the heavenly grin.
In amorous dalliance oft I strok'd her arm,
Each rising muscle was a rising charm.
O'er the *flexores* my fond fingers play'd,
I found instruction with delight convey'd –
There *carpus, cubitus* and *radius* too
Were plainly felt and manifest to view.
No muscles on her lovely hand were seen,
But only bones envelop'd by a skin.
Long were her fingers and her knuckles bare,
Much like the claw-foot of a walnut chair.
So plain was complex *metacarpus*[9] shown
It might be fairly counted bone by bone.
Her slender *phalanxes*[10] were well defin'd
And each with each by *ginglymus*[11] combin'd.
Such were the charms that did my fancy fire,
And love – chaste, scientific love inspire.

The Surgeon's Warning
Robert Southey (1799)

The Doctor whisper'd to the Nurse,
And the Surgeon knew what he said;
And he grew pale at the Doctor's tale,
And trembled in his sick-bed.

'Now fetch me my brethren, and fetch them with speed,'
The Surgeon affrighted said;

---

[7]Gomphosis: a peg-and-socket joint, as in teeth.
[8]Zygomatic refers to the cheekbone.
[9]The metacarpus is the intermediate part of the hand.
[10]The phalanges are the finger bones.
[11]The ginglymus is a hinge joint.

'The Parson and the Undertaker,
Let them hasten or I shall be dead.'

The Parson and the Undertaker
They hastily came complying,
And the Surgeon's Prentices ran up stairs
When they heard that their Master was dying.

The Prentices all they enter'd the room,
By one, by two, by three;
With a sly grin came Joseph in,
First of the company.

The Surgeon swore as they enter'd his door,
'Twas fearful his oaths to hear ...
'Now send these scoundrels out of my sight,
I beseech ye, my brethren dear!'

He foam'd at the mouth with the rage he felt,
And he wrinkled his black eye-brow,
'That rascal Joe would be at me, I know,
But zounds, let him spare me now!'

Then out they sent the Prentices,
The fit it left him weak,
He look'd at his brothers with ghastly eyes,
And faintly struggled to speak.

'All kinds of carcases I have cut up,
And now my turn will be;
But, brothers, I took care of you,
So pray take care of me.

I have made candles of dead men's fat,
The Sextons have been my slaves,
I have bottled babes unborn, and dried
Hearts and livers from rifled graves.

And my Prentices now will surely come
And carve me bone from bone,
And I who have rifled the dead man's grave
Shall never have rest in my own.

Bury me in lead when I am dead,
My brethren, I entreat,
And see the coffin weigh'd, I beg,
Lest the plumber should be a cheat.

And let it be solder'd closely down,
Strong as strong can be, I implore;

And put it in a patent coffin,
That I may rise no more.

If they carry me off in the patent coffin,
Their labour will be in vain;
Let the Undertaker see it bought of the maker,
Who lives by St. Martin's Lane.

And bury me in my brother's church,
For that will safer be;
And I implore, lock the church door,
And pray take care of the key.

And all night long let three stout men
The vestry watch within;
To each man give a gallon of beer,
And a keg of Holland's gin;

Powder and ball and blunderbuss,
To save me if he can,
And eke five guineas if he shoot
A Resurrection Man.[12]

And let them watch me for three weeks,
My wretched corpse to save;
For then I think that I may stink
Enough to rest in my grave.'

The Surgeon laid him down in his bed,
His eyes grew deadly dim,
Short came his breath, and the struggle of death
Did loosen every limb.

They put him in lead when he was dead,
And with precaution meet,
First they the leaden coffin weigh,
Lest the plumber should be a cheat.

They had it solder'd closely down,
And examin'd it o'er and o'er,
And they put it in a patent coffin
That he might rise no more.

For to carry him off in a patent coffin,
Would, they thought, be but labour in vain,
So the Undertaker saw it bought of the maker.
Who lives by St. Martin's Lane.

---

[12] In the eighteenth and nineteenth centuries, resurrectionists exhumed the recently buried dead and sold them to anatomists for dissection.

In his brother's church they buried him,
That safer he might be;
They lock'd the door, and would not trust
The Sexton with the key.

And three men in the vestry watch
To save him if they can,
And should he come there to shoot they swear
A Resurrection Man.

And the first night by lanthorn light
Through the church-yard as they went,
A guinea of gold the Sexton show'd
That Mister Joseph sent.

But conscience was tough, it was not enough,
And their honesty never swerved,
And they bade him go with Mister Joe
To the Devil as he deserved.

So all night long by the vestry fire
They quaff'd their gin and ale,
And they did drink, as you may think,
And told full many a tale.

The Cock he crew cock-a-doodle-doo,
Past five! the watchmen said;
And they went away, for while it was day
They might safely leave the dead.

The second night by lanthorn light
Through the church-yard as they went,
He whisper'd anew, and show'd them two
That Mister Joseph sent.

The guineas were bright and attracted their sight,
They look'd so heavy and new,
And their fingers itch'd as they were bewitch'd,
And they knew not what to do.

But they waver'd not long, for conscience was strong
And they thought they might get more,
And they refused the gold, but not
So rudely as before.

So all night long by the vestry fire
They quaff'd their gin and ale,
And they did drink, as you may think,
And told full many a tale.

The third night as by lanthorn light
Through the church-yard they went,
He bade them see, and show'd them three
That Mister Joseph sent.

They look'd askaunce with greedy glance,
The guineas they shone bright,
For the Sexton on the yellow gold
Let fall his lanthorn light.

And he look'd sly with his roguish eye,
And gave a well-timed wink,
And they could not stand the sound in his hand,
For he made the guineas chink.

And conscience, late that had such weight,
All in a moment fails,
For well they knew that it was true
A dead man tells no tales.

And they gave all their powder and ball,
And took the gold so bright,
And they drank their beer and made good cheer,
Till now it was midnight.

Then, though the key of the church-door
Was left with the Parson, his brother,
It open'd at the Sexton's touch...
Because he had another.

And in they go with that villain Joe,
To fetch the body by night,
And all the church look'd dismally
By his dark-lanthorn light.

They laid the pick-axe to the stones,
And they moved them soon asunder;
They shovell'd away the hard-prest clay,
And came to the coffin under.

They burst the patent coffin first,
And they cut through the lead;
And they laugh'd aloud when they saw the shroud,
Because they had got at the dead.

And they allow'd the Sexton the shroud,
And they put the coffin back;
And nose and knees they then did squeeze
The Surgeon in a sack.

The watchmen as they past along
Full four yards off could smell,
And a curse bestow'd upon the load
So disagreeable.

So they carried the sack a-pick-a-back,
And they carved him bone from bone,
But what became of the Surgeon's soul
Was never to mortal known.

from *The Borough: Professions – Physic*
George Crabbe (1810)

Helpers of men they're call'd, and we confess
Theirs the deep study, theirs the lucky guess;
We own that numbers join with care and skill,
A temperate judgment, a devoted will:
Men who suppress their feelings, but who feel
The painful symptoms they delight to heal;
Patient in all their trials, they sustain
The starts of passion, the reproach of pain;
With hearts affected, but with looks serene,
Intent they wait through all the solemn scene;
Glad if a hope should rise from nature's strife,
To aid their skill and save the lingering life;
But this must virtue's generous effort be,
And spring from nobler motives than a fee:
To the Physician of the Soul, and these,
Turn the distress'd for safety, hope, and ease.
But as physicians of that nobler kind
Have their warm zealots, and their sectaries blind;
So among these for knowledge most renowned,
Are dreamers strange, and stubborn bigots found:
Some, too, admitted to this honourd name,
Have, without learning, found a way to fame;
And some by learning – young physicians write,
To set their merit in the fairest light;
With them a treatise in a bait that draws
Approving voices – 'tis to gain applause,
And to exalt them in the public view,
More than a life of worthy toil could do.
When 'tis proposed to make the man renown'd,
In every age, convenient doubts abound;
Convenient themes in every period start,
Which he may treat with all the pomp of art;
Curious conjectures he may always make,

And either side of dubious questions take;
He may a system broach, or, if he please,
Start new opinions of an old disease:
Or may some simple in the woodland trace,
And be its patron, till it runs its race;
As rustic damsels from their woods are won,
And live in splendour till their race be run;
It weighs not much on what their powers be shown,
When all his purpose is to make them known.
To show the world what long experience gains,
Requires not courage, though it calls for pains;
But at life's outset to inform mankind
Is a bold effort of a valiant mind.
The great, good man, for noblest cause displays
What many labours taught, and many days;
These sound instruction from experience give,
The others show us how they mean to live.
That they have genius, and they hope mankind
Will to its efforts be no longer blind.
There are, beside, whom powerful friends advance,
Whom fashion favours, person, patrons, chance:
And merit sighs to see a fortune made
By daring rashness or by dull parade.
But these are trifling evils; there is one
Which walks uncheck'd, and triumphs in the sun:
There was a time, when we beheld the Quack,
On public stage, the licensed trade attack;
He made his laboured speech with poor parade,
And then a laughing zany lent him aid:
Smiling we pass'd him, but we felt the while
Pity so much, that soon we ceased to smile;
Assured that fluent speech and flow'ry vest
Disguised the troubles of a man distress'd –
But now our Quacks are gamesters, and they play
With craft and skill to ruin and betray;
With monstrous promise they delude the mind,
And thrive on all that tortures human-kind.
Void of all honour, avaricious, rash,
The daring tribe compound their boasted trash –
Tincture of syrup, lotion, drop, or pill;
All tempt the sick to trust the lying bill;
And twenty names of cobblers turn'd to squires,
Aid the bold language of these blushless liars.
There are among them those who cannot read,
And yet they'll buy a patent, and succeed;
Will dare to promise dying sufferers aid,

For who, when dead, can threaten or upbraid?
With cruel avarice still they recommend
More draughts, more syrup, to the journey's end:
'I feel it not;' – 'Then take it every hour:'
'It makes me worse;' – 'Why then it shows its power;'
'I fear to die;' – 'Let not your spirits sink,
You're always safe, while you believe and drink.'
How strange to add, in this nefarious trade,
That men of parts are dupes by dunces made:
That creatures, nature meant should clean our streets,
Have purchased lands and mansions, parks and seats:
Wretches with conscience so obtuse, they leave
Their untaught sons their parents to deceive;
And when they're laid upon their dying bed,
No thought of murder comes into their head,
Nor one revengeful ghost to them appears,
To fill the soul with penitential fears.
Yet not the whole of this imposing train
Their gardens, seats, and carriages obtain:
Chiefly, indeed, they to the robbers fall,
Who are most fitted to disgrace them all;
But there is hazard – patents must be bought,
Venders and puffers for the poison sought;
And then in many a paper through the year,
Must cures and cases, oaths and proofs appear;
Men snatch'd from graves, as they were dropping in,
Their lungs cough'd up, their bones pierced through their skin
Their liver all one schirrus,[13] and the frame
Poison'd with evils which they dare not name;
Men who spent all upon physicians' fees,
Who never slept, nor had a moment's ease,
Are now as roaches sound, and all as brisk as bees,
If the sick gudgeons to the bait attend,
And come in shoals, the angler gains his end:
But should the advertising cash be spent,
Ere yet the town has due attention lent,
Then bursts the bubble, and the hungry cheat
Pines for the bread he ill deserves to eat;
It is a lottery, and he shares perhaps
The rich man's feast, or begs the pauper's scraps.
From powerful causes spring th' empiric's gains,
Man's love of life, his weakness, and his pains;
These first induce him the vile trash to try,
Then lend his name, that other men may buy:

---

[13] A schirrus is a hard, dense, cancerous growth.

This love of life, which in our nature rules,
To vile imposture makes us dupes and tools;
Then pain compels th' impatient soul to seize
On promised hopes of instantaneous ease;
And weakness too with every wish complies,
Worn out and won by importunities.
Troubled with something in your bile or blood,
You think your doctor does you little good;
And grown impatient, you require in haste
The nervous cordial, nor dislike the taste;
It comforts, heals, and strengthens; nay, you think
It makes you better every time you drink;
'Then lend your name' you're loth, but yet confess
Its powers are great, and so you acquiesce:
Yet think a moment, ere your name you lend,
With whose 'tis placed, and what you recommend;
Who tipples brandy will some comfort feel,
But will he to the med'cine set his seal?
Wait, and you'll find the cordial you admire
Has added fuel to your fever's fire:
Say, should a robber chance your purse to spare,
Would you the honour of the man declare?
Would you assist his purpose? swell his crime?
Besides, he might not spare a second time.
Compassion sometimes sets the fatal sign,
The man was poor, and humbly begg'd a line;
Else how should noble names and titles back
The spreading praise of some advent'rous quack?
But he the moment watches, and entreats
Your honour's name – your honour joins the cheats;
You judged the med'cine harmless, and you lent
What help you could, and with the best intent;
But can it please you, thus to league with all
Whom he can beg or bribe to swell the scrawl?
Would you these wrappers with your name adorn
Which hold the poison for the yet unborn?
No class escapes them – from the poor man's pay,
The nostrum takes no trifling part away:
See! those square patent bottles from the shop,
Now decoration to the cupboard's top;
And there a favourite hoard you'll find within,
Companions meet! the julep and the gin.
Time too with cash is wasted; 'tis the fate
Of real helpers to be call'd too late;
This find the sick, when (time and patience gone)
Death with a tenfold terror hurries on.

Spurzheim and Lavater[14]
Anonymous (c.1819)

Lavater was once quite 'the go'
And noses and eyes were the plan,
By which all the wise ones would know
The talents and thoughts of a man:
As for noses, I know not I vow,
What they really mean or import,
But all who read Sterne[15] must allow
That a long one's preferr'd to a short.

But oh! 'tis a glance of the eye –
'Tis the radiance its flashes impart,
Gives the light that I love to read by,
When I study the Head or the Heart:
And who is so sightless or dull
But could learn much more by one look
Of what passes within heart or skull,
Than by studying Spurzheim's whole book.

Craniology[16]
Thomas Hood (1827)

'Tis strange how like a very dunce,
Man – with his bumps upon his sconce,
Has lived so long, and yet no knowledge he
Has had, till lately, of Phrenology[17] –
A science that by simple dint of
Head-combing he should find a hint of,
When scratching o'er those little poll-hills,
The faculties throw up like mole-hills;
A science that, in very spite
Of all his teeth, ne'er came to light,
For though he knew his skull had *grinders*,
Still there turned up no *organ* finders,

---

[14]Johann Casper Lavater (1741–1801) was a Swiss theologian and writer, whose *Essays on Physiognomy* was widely translated and reprinted. Physiognomy was the practice of reading human character and intelligence from the features of the face. Johann Gaspar Spurzheim (1776–1832) was a German physician who became one of the chief proponents of phrenology, which posited that character, thoughts and emotions were located in specific parts of the brain, 'readable' by the shape of the bones of the skull.

[15]In Laurence Sterne's novel *The Life and Opinions of Tristram Shandy* (1759), the title character has his nose crushed by forceps during delivery.

[16]Craniology is a form of anthropometry, the measuring of the human skull to identify human physical variation and, in paleoanthropology, to correlate physical with racial, psychological, and sociological traits.

[17]See footnote 14 to previous poem above.

Still sages wrote, and ages fled,
And no man's head came in his head –
Not even the pate of Erra Pater,[18]
Knew aught about its pia mater.[19]
At last great Dr. Gall bestirs him –
I don't know but it might be Spurzheim[20] –
Tho' native of a dull and slow land,
And makes partition of our Poll-land;
At our Acquisitiveness guesses,
And all those necessary *nesses*
Indicative of human habits,
All burrowing in the head like rabbits.
Thus Veneration, he made known,
Had got a lodging at the Crown;
And Music (see Deville's example)
A set of chambers in the Temple;
That Language taught the tongues close by,
And took in pupils through the eye,
Close by his neighbor Computation,
Who taught the eyebrows numeration.

The science thus – to speak in fit
Terms – having struggled from its nit,
Was seized on by a swarm of Scotchmen
Those scientifical hotch-potch men,
Who have at least a penny dip,
And wallop in all doctorship,
Just as in making broth they smatter
By bobbing twenty things in water:
These men, I say, made quick appliance
And close, to phrenologic science;
For of all learned themes whatever,
That schools and colleges deliver,
There's none they love so near the bodles,[21]
As analysing their own noddles;
Thus in a trice each northern blockhead
Had got his fingers in his shock head,
And of his bumps was babbling yet worse

---

[18]Erra Pater was the assumed name of the author of an astrological almanac first published in 1535, and referred to by Samuel Butler in *Hudibras* (I.i), and by William Congreve in *Love for Love*.
[19]The *pia mater*, from the Latin meaning 'tender mother', is the delicate innermost layer of the meninges, the membranes surrounding the brain and spinal cord.
[20]Franz Joseph Gall (1758–1828) was a German neuroanatomist, physiologist and early phrenologist. On his colleague Johann Spurzheim, see previous poem.
[21]A small Scottish coin worth about one sixth of an English penny.

Than poor Miss Capulet's dry wet-nurse[22];
Till having been sufficient rangers
Of their own heads, they took to strangers'.
And found in Presbyterians' polls[23]
The things they hated in their souls!
For Presbyterians hear with passion
Of organs joined with veneration.
No kind there was of human pumpkin
But at its bumps it had a bumpkin;
Down to the very lowest gullion,
And oiliest skull of oily scullion.
No great man died but this they *did* do,
They begged his cranium of his widow:
No murderer died by law disaster,
But they took off his sconce in plaster;
For thereon they could show depending,
'The head and front of his offending':
How that his philanthropic bump
Was mastered by a baser lump;
For every bump (these wags insist)
Has its direct antagonist,
Each striving stoutly to prevail,
Like horses knotted tail to tail!
And many a stiff and sturdy battle
Occurs between these adverse cattle,
The secret cause, beyond all question,
Of aches ascribed to indigestion –
Whereas 'tis but two knobby rivals
Tugging together like sheer devils,
Till one gets mastery, good or sinister,
And comes in like a new prime-minister.

Each bias in some master node is: –
What takes M'Adam where a road is,
To hammer little pebbles less?
His organ of Destructiveness.
What makes great Joseph so encumber
Debate? a lumping lump of Number:
Or Malthas[24] rail at babies so?

---

[22]In Shakespeare's *Romeo and Juliet,* the Nurse is Juliet's confidante.
[23]Presbyterianism is a branch of the Reformed Protestant Church, which typically emphasizes the sovereignty of God, the authority of the scriptures and the necessity of grace through faith in Christ.
[24]Reverend Thomas Robert Malthus (1766–1834), was an English political economist, whose *Essay on the Principle of Population* (1798) posits that human population is naturally checked by famine and disease.

The smallness of his Philopro –[25]
What severs man and wife? a simple
Defect of the Adhesive pimple[26]:
Or makes weak women go astray?
Their bumps are more in fault than they.

These facts being found and set in order
By grave M. D.'s[27] beyond the Border,
To make them for some months eternal,
Were entered monthly in a journal,
That many a northern sage still writes in,
And throws his little Northern Lights in,
And proves and proves about the phrenos,
A great deal more than I or he knows:
How Music suffers, *par exemple*,
By wearing tight hats round the temple;
What ills great boxers have to fear
From blisters put behind the ear;
And how a porter's Veneration
Is hurt by porter's occupation;
Whether shillelaghs[28] in reality
May deaden Individuality;
Or tongs and poker be creative
Of alterations in th' Amative;
If falls from scaffolds make us less
Inclined to all Constructiveness[29]:
With more such matters, all applying
To heads – and therefore *head-ifying*.

The Stethoscope Song: A Professional Ballad
Oliver Wendell Holmes (1848)

There was a young man in Boston town,
He bought him a stethoscope nice and new,
All mounted and finished and polished down,
With an ivory cap and a stopper too.

It happened a spider within did crawl,
And spun him a web of ample size,

---

[25]Philoprogenitiveness is the love of offspring, and according to the principles of phrenology, this organ is located at the back of the skull.
[26]Adhesiveness, a term introduced by the phrenologist Johann Spurzheim (1776–1832), refers to the faculty of human attachment.
[27]Doctors of Medicine.
[28]A shillelagh is a type of Irish walking stick, with club.
[29]In phrenology, constructiveness refers to the faculty of initiative, invention and creativity. The craniological location is on the temples.

Wherein there chanced one day to fall
A couple of very imprudent flies.

The first was a bottle-fly, big and blue,
The second was smaller, and thin and long;
So there was a concert between the two,
Like an octave flute and a tavern gong.

Now being from Paris but recently,
This fine young man would show his skill;
And so they gave him, his hand to try,
A hospital patient extremely ill.

Some said that his liver was short of bile,
And some that his heart was over size,
While some kept arguing, all the while,
He was crammed with tubercles[30] up to his eyes.

This fine young man then up stepped he,
And all the doctors made a pause;
Said he, The man must die, you see,
By the fifty-seventh of Louis's laws.

But since the case is a desperate one,
To explore his chest it may be well;
For if he should die and it were not done,
You know the autopsy would not tell.

Then out his stethoscope he took,
And on it placed his curious ear;
Mon Dieu! said he, with a knowing look,
Why, here is a sound that's mighty queer!

The bourdonnement[31] is very clear –
Amphoric buzzing, as I'm alive!
Five doctors took their turn to hear;
Amphoric buzzing, said all the five.

There's empyema[32] beyond a doubt
We'll plunge a trocar[33] in his side.
The diagnosis was made out –
They tapped the patient; so he died.

---

[30]Round nodules or outgrowths found on bones or skin or, in cases of tuberculosis, in the lungs.
[31]*Bourdonnement*: buzzing.
[32]Empyema refers to a collection of pus within an anatomical cavity.
[33]A trocar is a sharp instrument, used to puncture the skin and withdraw fluids from the body.

Now such as hate new-fashioned toys
Began to look extremely glum;
They said that rattles were made for boys,
And vowed that his buzzing was all a hum.

There was an old lady had long been sick,
And what was the matter none did know:
Her pulse was slow, though her tongue was quick;
To her this knowing youth must go.

So there the nice old lady sat,
With phials and boxes all in a row;
She asked the young doctor what he was at,
To thump her and tumble her ruffles so.

Now, when the stethoscope came out,
The flies began to buzz and whiz:
Oh, ho! the matter is clear, no doubt;
An aneurism[34] there plainly is.

The bruit de râpe and the bruit de scie
And the bruit de diable[35] are all combined;
How happy Bouillaud[36] would be,
If he a case like this could find!

Now, when the neighboring doctors found
A case so rare had been descried,
They every day her ribs did pound
In squads of twenty; so she died.

Then six young damsels, slight and frail,
Received this kind young doctor's cares;
They all were getting slim and pale,
And short of breath on mounting stairs.

They all made rhymes with 'sighs' and 'skies,'
And loathed their puddings and buttered rolls,
And dieted, much to their friends' surprise,
On pickles and pencils and chalk and coals.

---

[34]An aneurism is a bulge in the wall of a blood vessel.

[35]*Bruit de rape*: harsh, rasping murmurs. *Bruit de scie*: harsh 'sawing' heart sound heard in systole and diastole. *Bruit de diable*: 'Devil's noise' or a 'venous hum' in the upper chest that can be heard through a stethoscope.

[36]Jean-Baptiste Bouillaud (1796–1881) was a French physician who studied heart sounds and heart diseases; he identified links between rheumatism and heart disease ('Bouillaud's disease').

So fast their little hearts did bound,
The frightened insects buzzed the more;
So over all their chests he found
The râle sifflant and the râle sonore.[37]

He shook his head. There's grave disease –
I greatly fear you all must die;
A slight post-mortem, if you please,
Surviving friends would gratify.

The six young damsels wept aloud,
Which so prevailed on six young men
That each his honest love avowed,
Whereat they all got well again.

This poor young man was all aghast;
The price of stethoscopes came down;
And so he was reduced at last
To practise in a country town.

The doctors being very sore,
A stethoscope they did devise
That had a rammer to clear the bore
With a knob at the end to kill the flies.

Now use your ears, all you that can,
But don't forget to mind your eyes,
Or you may be cheated, like this young man,
By a couple of silly, abnormal flies.

from *An Epistle Containing the Strange Medical Experience of Karshish, the Arab Physician*[38]
Robert Browning (1855)

Karshish, the picker-up of learning's crumbs,
The not-incurious in God's handiwork
(This man's-flesh He hath admirably made,
Blown like a bubble, kneaded like a paste,
To coop up and keep down on earth a space
That puff of vapour from His mouth, man's soul)
– To Abib, all-sagacious in our art,

---

[37]Rales: more terms for rattles and sounds within the chest cavity.
[38]A poem 'letter' written in the voice of Karshish, an Arab physician, traveling around Jerusalem to gather medical knowledge, c.67–69 AD, a generation after the death of Jesus. The intended recipient of the letter is Abib, also a physician, and a mentor to Karshish. The letter tells the story of Karshish's encounter with Lazarus, whom Jesus is supposed to have raised from the dead, but Karshish casts doubts on Lazarus's story.

Breeder in me of what poor skill I boast,
Like me inquisitive how pricks and cracks
Befall the flesh through too much stress and strain,
Whereby the wily vapour fain would slip
Back and rejoin its source before the term, –
And aptest in contrivance (under God)
To baffle it by deftly stopping such: –
The vagrant Scholar to his Sage at home
Sends greeting (health and knowledge, fame with peace)
Three samples of true snakestone – rarer still,
One of the other sort, the melon-shaped,
(But fitter, pounded fine, for charms than drugs)
And writeth now the twenty-second time.

My journeyings were brought to Jericho:
Thus I resume. Who studious in our art
Shall count a little labour unrepaid?
I have shed sweat enough, left flesh and bone
On many a flinty furlong of this land.
Also, the country-side is all on fire
With rumours of a marching hitherward –
Some say Vespasian[39] cometh, some, his son.
A black lynx snarled and pricked a tufted ear;
Lust of my blood inflamed his yellow balls:
I cried and threw my staff and he was gone.
Twice have the robbers stripped and beaten me,
And once a town declared me for a spy;
But at the end, I reach Jerusalem,
Since this poor covert where I pass the night,
This Bethany,[40] lies scarce the distance thence
A man with plague-sores at the third degree
Runs till he drops down dead. Thou laughest here!
'Sooth, it elates me, thus reposed and safe,
To void the stuffing of my travel-scrip
And share with thee whatever Jewry yields.
A viscid choler[41] is observable
In tertians,[42] I was nearly bold to say;
And falling-sickness hath a happier cure
Than our school wots of: there's a spider here

---

[39]Vespasian (9–79 AD) was Roman Emperor from 69–79 AD and founder of the Flavian dynasty.
[40]In the Bible, Bethany is the name of a village near Jerusalem, the site of the miracle in which Jesus raised Lazarus from the dead.
[41]Viscid choler, or angry, irritable bile.
[42]Tertian fever, malaria.

Weaves no web, watches on the ledge of tombs,
Sprinkled with mottles on an ash-grey back;
Take five and drop them... but who knows his mind,
The Syrian runagate[43] I trust this to?
His service payeth me a sublimate[44]
Blown up his nose to help the ailing eye.
Best wait: I reach Jerusalem at morn,
There set in order my experiences,
Gather what most deserves, and give thee all –
Or I might add, Judæa's gum-tragacanth[45]
Scales off in purer flakes, shines clearer-grained,
Cracks 'twixt the pestle and the porphyry,
In fine exceeds our produce. Scalp-disease
Confounds me, crossing so with leprosy –
Thou hadst admired one sort I gained at Zoar –
But zeal outruns discretion. Here I end.

Surgeons must be very careful
Emily Dickinson (1856)

Surgeons must be very careful
When they take the knife!
Underneath their fine incisions
Stirs the culprit, – Life!

Enter Patient
William Earnest Henley (1875)

The morning mists still haunt the stony street;
The northern summer air is shrill and cold;
And lo, the Hospital, gray, quiet, old,
Where Life and Death like friendly chafferers meet.
Through the loud spaciousness and draughty gloom
A small, strange child – so agèd yet so young! –
Her little arm besplinted and beslung,
Precedes me gravely to the waiting-room.
I limp behind, my confidence all gone.
The gray-haired soldier-porter waves me on,
And on I crawl, and still my spirits fail:
A tragic meanness seems so to environ
These corridors and stairs of stone and iron,
Cold, naked, clean – half-workhouse and half-jail.

---

[43]A runagate is a deserter, a renegade or an apostate.
[44]Sublimate: condensed vapours.
[45]A natural gum derived from certain shrubs.

The Wound-Dresser
Walt Whitman (1881–82)

An old man bending I come among new faces,
Years looking backward resuming in answer to children,
Come tell us old man, as from young men and maidens that love me,
(Arous'd and angry, I'd thought to beat the alarum, and urge relentless war,
But soon my fingers fail'd me, my face droop'd and I resign'd myself,
To sit by the wounded and soothe them, or silently watch the dead;)
Years hence of these scenes, of these furious passions, these chances,
Of unsurpass'd heroes, (was one side so brave? the other was equally brave;)
Now be witness again, paint the mightiest armies of earth,
Of those armies so rapid so wondrous what saw you to tell us?
What stays with you latest and deepest? of curious panics,
Of hard-fought engagements or sieges tremendous what deepest remains?

O maidens and young men I love and that love me,
What you ask of my days those the strangest and sudden your talking recalls,
Soldier alert I arrive after a long march cover'd with sweat and dust,
In the nick of time I come, plunge in the fight, loudly shout in the rush of
    successful charge,
Enter the captur'd works – yet lo, like a swift-running river they fade,
Pass and are gone they fade – I dwell not on soldiers' perils or soldiers' joys,
(Both I remember well – many the hardships, few the joys, yet I was content.)

But in silence, in dreams' projections,
While the world of gain and appearance and mirth goes on,
So soon what is over forgotten, and waves wash the imprints off the sand,
With hinged knees returning I enter the doors, (while for you up there,
Whoever you are, follow without noise and be of strong heart.)

Bearing the bandages, water and sponge,
Straight and swift to my wounded I go,
Where they lie on the ground after the battle brought in,
Where their priceless blood reddens the grass the ground,
Or to the rows of the hospital tent, or under the roof'd hospital,
To the long rows of cots up and down each side I return,
To each and all one after another I draw near, not one do I miss
An attendant follows holding a tray, he carries a refuse pail,
Soon to be fill'd with clotted rags and blood, emptied, and fill'd again.

I onward go, I stop,
With hinged knees and steady hand to dress wounds,
I am firm with each, the pangs are sharp yet unavoidable,
One turns to me his appealing eyes – poor boy! I never knew you,
Yet I think I could not refuse this moment to die for you, if that would
    save you.

On, on I go, (open doors of time! open hospital doors!)
The crush'd head I dress, (poor crazed hand tear not the bandage away,)
The neck of the cavalry-man with the bullet through and through I examine,
Hard the breathing rattles, quite glazed already the eye, yet life struggles hard,
(Come sweet death! be persuaded O beautiful death!
In mercy come quickly.)

From the stump of the arm, the amputated hand,
I undo the clotted lint, remove the slough, wash off the matter and blood,
Back on his pillow the soldier bends with curv'd neck and side-falling head,
His eyes are closed, his face is pale, he dares not look on the bloody stump,
And has not yet look'd on it.

I dress a wound in the side, deep, deep,
But a day or two more, for see the frame all wasted and sinking,
And the yellow-blue countenance see.

I dress the perforated shoulder, the foot with the bullet-wound,
Cleanse the one with a gnawing and putrid gangrene, so sickening, so offensive,
While the attendant stands behind aside me holding the tray and pail.

I am faithful, I do not give out,
The fractur'd thigh, the knee, the wound in the abdomen,
These and more I dress with impassive hand, (yet deep in my breast a fire,
     a burning flame).

Thus in silence in dreams' projections,
Returning, resuming, I thread my way through the hospitals,
The hurt and wounded I pacify with soothing hand,
I sit by the restless all the dark night, some are so young,
Some suffer so much, I recall the experience sweet and sad,
(Many a soldier's loving arms about this neck have cross'd and rested,
Many a soldier's kiss dwells on these bearded lips.)

The Sons of Science
George Barlow (1884)

I sometimes with a horror past all speech
Shrink from the hands of those we fondly call
Truth-seeking sons of Science. God help all
Whose hapless bodies come within their reach!
Lies are their daily food, and lies they preach
From house to house, in school or lecture hall.
Their coarse foul fleshly blood-tinged hands appal:
Love they disdain, and mercy they impeach.

England is blinded, hood-winked once again.
'Cancer research!' Unutterable crime.

No truth that saves the race, no gift sublime
Was ever wrenched from out the hideous pain
Of writhing rabbits. Mankind will not climb
To heaven through Vivisection's hell-deep drain.

Waiting
William Ernest Henley (1888)

A square squat room (a cellar on promotion),
Drab to the soul, drab to the very daylight;
Plasters astray in unnatural-looking tinware;
Scissors and lint and apothecary's jars.

Here, on a bench a skeleton would writhe from,
Angry and sore, I wait to be admitted:
Wait till my heart is lead upon my stomach,
While at their ease two dressers do their chores.

One has a probe – it feels to me a crowbar.
A small boy sniffs and shudders after bluestone.[46]
A poor old tramp explains his poor old ulcers.
Life is (I think) a blunder and a shame.

Man and Woman Go through the Cancer Ward
Gottfried Benn (1912)[47]

The man:
Here in this row are wombs that have decayed,
and in this row are breasts that have decayed.
Bed beside stinking bed. Hourly the sisters change.
Come, quietly lift up this coverlet.
Look, this great mass of fat and ugly humours
was precious to a man once, and
meant ecstasy and home.
Come, now look at the scars upon this breast.
Do you feel the rosary of small soft knots?
Feel it, no fear. The flesh yields and is numb.
Here's one who bleeds as though from thirty bodies.
No one has so much blood.
They had to cut a child from this one, from her cancerous womb.
They let them sleep. All day, all night. They tell
the newcomers: here sleep will make you well. But Sundays

---

[46]Bluestone: copper sulfate used as an emetic (to induce vomiting).
[47]Trans. Babette Deutsch.

one rouses them a bit for visitors.
They take a little nourishment. Their backs
are sore. You see the flies. Sometimes
the sisters wash them. As one washes benches.
Here the grave rises up about each bed.
And flesh is leveled down to earth. The fire
Burns out. And sap prepares to flow. Earth calls.

To Madame Curie[48]
Alice Moore Dunbar-Nelson (1921)

Oft have I thrilled at deeds of high emprise,
And yearned to venture into realms unknown,
Thrice blessed she, I deemed, whom God had shown
How to achieve great deeds in woman's guise.
Yet what discov'ry by expectant eyes
Of foreign shores, could vision half the throne
Full gained by her, whose power fully grown
Exceeds the conquerors of th' uncharted skies?
So would I be this woman whom the world
Avows its benefactor; nobler far,
Than Sybil, Joan, Sappho, or Egypt's queen.[49]
In the alembic forged her shafts and hurled
At pain, diseases, waging a humane war;
Greater than this achievement, none, I ween.

Doctors
Rudyard Kipling (1923)

Man dies too soon, beside his works half-planned.
His days are counted and reprieve is vain:
Who shall entreat with Death to stay his hand;
Or cloke the shameful nakedness of pain?

Send here the bold, the seekers of the way –
The passionless, the unshakeable of soul,
Who serve the inmost mysteries of man's clay,
And ask no more than leave to make them whole.

---

[48]Marie Skłodowska-Curie (1867–1934) was a Polish, naturalized French physicist and chemist who conducted pioneering research on radioactivity. She was the first woman to win a Nobel Prize.
[49]In ancient Greece, the Sibyls were oracular women believed to possess prophetic powers. Joan of Arc (c.1412–1431) was a French national heroine. Sappho (born c.630–612 BC) was a Greek lyric poet from Lesbos. 'Egypt's Queen' was Cleopatra.

In the Theatre (A true incident)
Dannie Abse (1938)

'Only a local anaesthetic was given because of the blood pressure problem. The
patient, thus, was fully awake throughout the operation. But in those days – in
1938, in Cardiff, when I was Lambert Rogers' dresser[50] – they could not locate a
brain tumour with precision. Too much normal brain tissue was destroyed as the
surgeon searched for it, before he felt the resistance of it ... all somewhat hit and
miss. One operation I shall never forget ...'

Dr Wilfred Abse

Sister saying – 'Soon you'll be back in the ward,'
sister thinking – 'Only two more on the list,'
the patient saying – 'Thank you, I feel fine';
small voices, small lies, nothing untoward,
though, soon, he would blink again and again
because of the fingers of Lambert Rogers,
rash as a blind man's, inside his soft brain.

If items of horror can make a man laugh
then laugh at this: one hour later, the growth
still undiscovered, ticking its own wild time;
more brain mashed because of the probe's braille path;
Lambert Rogers desperate, fingering still;
his dresser thinking, 'Christ! Two more on the list,
a cisternal puncture and a neural cyst.'[51]

Then, suddenly, the cracked record in the brain,
a ventriloquist voice that cried, 'You sod,
leave my soul alone, leave my soul alone,' –
the patient's dummy lips moving to that refrain,
the patient's eyes too wide. And, shocked,
Lambert Rogers drawing out the probe
with nurses, students, sister, petrified.

'Leave my soul alone, leave my soul alone,'
that voice so arctic and that cry so odd
had nowhere else to go – till the antique
gramophone wound down and the words began
to blur and slow, '...leave...my...soul...alone...'
to cease at last when something other died.
And silence matched the silence under snow.

---

[50]A dresser assisted the surgeon in operations.
[51]A cisternal puncture is made at the base of the skull to obtain cerebrospinal fluid; a neural cyst or Tarlov
cyst, is a fluid-filled sac that forms on nerves at the base of the spine.

Interne at Provident
Langston Hughes (1946)

White coats
White aprons
White dresses
White shoes
Pain and a learning
To take away to Alabama.
Practice on a State Street cancer,
Practice on a stockyards rupture,
Practice on the small appendix
Of 26-girl at the corner,
Learning skills of surgeons
Brown and wonderful with longing
To cure ills of Africa,
Democracy,
And mankind,
Also ills quite common
Among all who stand on two feet.

Brown hands
Black hands
Golden hands in white coat,
Nurses' hands on suture.
Miracle maternity:
Pain on hind legs rising,
Pain tamed and subsiding
Like a mule broke to the halter.

Charity's checked money
Aids triumphant entry squalling
After bitter thrust of bearing
Chocolate and blood:

Projection of a day!

Tears of joy
And Coca-Cola
Twinkle on the rubber gloves
He's wearing.
A crown of sweat
Gleams on his forehead.

In the white moon
Of the amphitheatre
Magi are staring.

The light on the Palmolive Building
Shines like a star in the East.

Nurses turn glass doorknobs
Opening into corridors.

A mist of iodine and ether
Follows the young doctor,
Cellophanes his long stride,
Cellophanes his future.

The Cottage Hospital
John Betjeman (1958)

At the end of a long-walled garden in a red provincial town,
A brick path led to a mulberry – scanty grass at its feet.
I lay under blackening branches where the mulberry leaves hung down
Sheltering ruby fruit globes from a Sunday-tea-time heat.
Apple and plum espaliers basked upon bricks of brown;
The air was swimming with insects, and children played in the street.

Out of this bright intentness into the mulberry shade
Musca domestica (housefly) swung from the August light
Slap into slithery rigging by the waiting spider made
Which spun the lithe elastic till the fly was shrouded tight.
Down came the hairy talons and horrible poison blade
And none of the garden noticed that fizzing, hopeless fight.

Say in what Cottage Hospital whose pale green walls resound
With the tap upon polished parquet of inflexible nurses' feet
Shall I myself be lying when they range the screens around?
And say shall I groan in dying, as I twist the sweaty sheet?
Or gasp for breath uncrying, as I feel my senses drown'd
While the air is swimming with insects and children play in the street?

The Hospital in Winter
Roy Fisher (1959)

A dark bell leadens the hour,
        the three-o'-clock
light falls amber across a tower.

Below, green-railed within a wall
        of coral brick,
stretches the borough hospital

monstrous with smells that cover death,
   white gauze tongues,
cold-water-pipes of pain, glass breath,

porcelain, blood, black rubber tyres;
   and in the yards
plane trees and slant telephone wires.

On benches squat the afraid and cold
   hour after hour.
Chains of windows snarl with gold.

Far off, beyond the engine-sheds,
   motionless trucks
grow ponderous, their rotting reds

deepening towards night; from windows
   bathrobed men
watch the horizon flare as the light goes.

Smoke whispers across the town,
   high panes are bleak;
pink of coral sinks to brown;
a dark bell brings the dark down.

The Examination
W. D. Snodgrass (1959)

Under the thick beams of that swirly smoking light,
The black robes are huddled in together.
Hunching their shoulders, they spread short, broad sleeves like night –
Black grackles' wings; then they reach bone-yellow leather-

Y fingers, each to each. And are prepared. Each turns
His single eye – or since one can't discern their eyes,
That reflective, single, moon-pale disc which burns
Over each brow – to watch this uncouth shape that lies

Strapped to their table. One probes with his ragged nails
The slate-sharp calf, explores the thigh and the lean thews
Of the groin. Others raise, red as piratic sails,
His wings, stretching, trying the pectoral sinews.

One runs his finger down the whet of that cruel
Golden beak, lifts back the horny lids from the eyes,
Peers down in one bright eye malign as a jewel
And steps back suddenly. 'Is he anesthetize-

D?' 'He is. He is. He is.' The tallest of them, bent
Down by the head rises: 'This drug possesses powers
Sufficient to still all gods in this firmament.
This is Garuda[52] who was fierce. He's yours for hours.

'We shall continue, please.' Now, once again, he bends
To the skull, and its clamped tissues; into the cran-
Ial cavity, he plunges both of his hands
Like obstetric forceps and lifts out the great brain,

Holds it aloft, then gives it to the next who stands
Beside him. Each, in turn, accepts it, although loath,
Turns it this way, that way, feels it between his hands
Like a wasp's nest or some sickening outsized growth.

They must decide what thoughts each part of it must think.
They tap at, then listen beside, each suspect lobe;
Next, with a crow's quill dipped into India ink,
Mark on its surface, as if on a map or globe,

Those dangerous areas which need to be excised.
They rinse it, then apply antiseptics to it;
Now silver saws appear which, inch by inch, slice
Through its ancient folds and ridges, like thick suet.

It's rinsed, dried, and daubed with thick salves. The smoky saws
Are scrubbed, resterilized, and polished till they gleam.
The brain is repacked in its case. Pinched in their claws,
Glimmering needles stitch it up, that leave no seam.

Meantime, one of them has set blinders to the eyes,
Inserted light packing beneath each of the ears,
And caulked the nostrils in. One, with thin twine, ties
Up the heart. With long wooden-handled shears,

Another chops pinions out of the scarlet wings.
It's hoped that with disuse, he will forget the sky
Or, at least, in time, learn, among other things,
To fly no higher than his superiors fly.

Well, that's a beginning. The next time, they can split
His tongue and teach him to talk correctly, can give
Him opinions on fine books and choose clothing fit
For the integrated area where he'll live.

---

[52]In Hinduism and Buddhism, Garuda is a large human-like bird, who serves as the mount of Lord Vishnu.

Their candidate may live to give them thanks one day.
He might recover and may hope for such success
He might return to rejoin their ranks. Bowing away,
They nod, whispering, 'One of ours; one of ours. Yes. Yes.'

Two Views of a Cadaver Room
Sylvia Plath (1959)

1.

The day she visited the dissecting room
They had four men laid out, black as burnt turkey,
Already half unstrung. A vinegary fume
Of the death vats clung to them;
The white-smocked boys started working.
The head of his cadaver had caved in,
And she could scarcely make out anything
In that rubble of skull plates and old leather.
A sallow piece of string held it together.

In their jars the snail-nosed babies moon and glow.
He hands her the cut-out heart like a cracked heirloom.

2.

In Brueghel's panorama of smoke and slaughter[53]
Two people only are blind to the carrion army:
He, afloat in the sea of her blue satin
Skirts, sings in the direction
Of her bare shoulder, while she bends,
Fingering a leaflet of music, over him,
Both of them deaf to the fiddle in the hands
Of the death's-head shadowing their song.
These Flemish lovers flourish; not for long.

Yet desolation, stalled in paint, spares the little country
Foolish, delicate, in the lower right hand corner.

The Surgeon at 2 a.m.
Sylvia Plath (1961)

The white light is artificial, and hygienic as heaven.
The microbes cannot survive it.
They are departing in their transparent garments, turned aside
From the scalpels and the rubber hands.
The scalded sheet is a snowfield, frozen and peaceful.
The body under it is in my hands.

---

[53]This second stanza is based on *The Triumph of Death*, a painting by Pieter Bruegel the Elder, painted c.1562 (Museo del Prado, Madrid).

As usual there is no face. A lump of Chinese white
With seven holes thumbed in. The soul is another light.
I have not seen it; it does not fly up.
Tonight it has receded like a ship's light.

It is a garden I have to do with – tubers and fruit
Oozing their jammy substances,
A mat of roots. My assistants hook them back.
Stenches and colors assail me.
This is the lung-tree.
These orchids are splendid. They spot and coil like snakes.
The heart is a red bell-bloom, in distress.
I am so small
In comparison to these organs!
I worm and hack in a purple wilderness.

The blood is a sunset. I admire it.
I am up to my elbows in it, red and squeaking.
Still it seeps up, it is not exhausted.
So magical! A hot spring
I must seal off and let fill
The intricate, blue piping under this pale marble.
How I admire the Romans –
Aqueducts, the Baths of Caracella,[54] the eagle nose!
The body is a Roman thing.
It has shut its mouth on the stone pill of repose.

It is a statue the orderlies are wheeling off.
I have perfected it.
I am left with and arm or a leg,
A set of teeth, or stones
To rattle in a bottle and take home,
And tissues in slices – a pathological salami.
Tonight the parts are entombed in an icebox.
Tomorrow they will swim
In vinegar like saints' relics.
Tomorrow the patient will have a clean, pink plastic limb.

Over one bed in the ward, a small blue light
Announces a new soul. The bed is blue.
Tonight, for this person, blue is a beautiful color.
The angels of morphia have borne him up.
He floats an inch from the ceiling,
Smelling the dawn drafts.
I walk among sleepers in gauze sarcophagi.

---

[54]The Baths of Caracalla (*Terme di Caracalla*) in Rome, Italy, are the second largest Roman public baths.

The red night lights are flat moons. They are dull with blood.
I am the sun, in my white coat,
Grey faces, shuttered by drugs, follow me like flowers.

Ambulances
Philip Larkin (1961)

Closed like confessionals, they thread
Loud noons of cities, giving back
None of the glances they absorb.
Light glossy grey, arms on a plaque,
They come to rest at any kerb:
All streets in time are visited.

Then children strewn on steps or road,
Or women coming from the shops
Past smells of different dinners, see
A wild white face that overtops
Red stretcher-blankets momently
As it is carried in and stowed,

And sense the solving emptiness
That lies just under all we do,
And for a second get it whole,
So permanent and blank and true.
The fastened doors recede. *Poor soul*
They whisper at their own distress;

For borne away in deadened air
May go the sudden shut of loss
Round something nearly at an end,
And what cohered in it across
The years, the unique random blend
Of families and fashions, there

At last begin to loosen. Far
From the exchange of love to lie
Unreachable inside a room
The traffic parts to let go by
Brings closer what is left to come,
And dulls to distance all we are.

Surgical Ward
W. H. Auden (1971)

They are and suffer; that is all they do;
A bandage hides the place where each is living,

His knowledge of the world restricted to
The treatment that the instruments are giving.

And lie apart like epochs from each other
– Truth in their sense is how much they can bear;
It is not talk like ours, but groans they smother –
And are remote as plants; we stand elsewhere.

For who when healthy can become a foot?
Even a scratch we can't recall when cured,
But are boist'rous in a moment and believe

In the common world of the uninjured, and cannot
Imagine isolation. Only happiness is shared,
And anger, and the idea of love.

The Building[55]
Philip Larkin (1972)

Higher than the handsomest hotel
The lucent comb shows up for miles, but see,
All round it close-ribbed streets rise and fall
Like a great sigh out of the last century.
The porters are scruffy; what keep drawing up
At the entrance are not taxis; and in the hall
As well as creepers hangs a frightening smell.

There are paperbacks, and tea at so much a cup,
Like an airport lounge, but those who tamely sit
On rows of steel chairs turning the ripped mags
Haven't come far. More like a local bus.
These outdoor clothes and half-filled shopping-bags
And faces restless and resigned, although
Every few minutes comes a kind of nurse

To fetch someone away: the rest refit
Cups back to saucers, cough, or glance below
Seats for dropped gloves or cards. Humans, caught
On ground curiously neutral, homes and names
Suddenly in abeyance; some are young,
Some old, but most at that vague age that claims
The end of choice, the last of hope; and all

Here to confess that something has gone wrong.
It must be error of a serious sort,

---

[55] Hull Royal Infirmary.

For see how many floors it needs, how tall
It's grown by now, and how much money goes
In trying to correct it. See the time,
Half-past eleven on a working day,
And these picked out of it; see, as they climb

To their appointed levels, how their eyes
Go to each other, guessing; on the way
Someone's wheeled past, in washed-to-rags ward clothes:
They see him, too. They're quiet. To realise
This new thing held in common makes them quiet,
For past these doors are rooms, and rooms past those,
And more rooms yet, each one further off

And harder to return from; and who knows
Which he will see, and when? For the moment, wait,
Look down at the yard. Outside seems old enough:
Red brick, lagged pipes, and someone walking by it
Out to the car park, free. Then, past the gate,
Traffic; a locked church; short terraced streets
Where kids chalk games, and girls with hair-dos fetch

Their separates from the cleaners – O world,
Your loves, your chances, are beyond the stretch
Of any hand from here! And so, unreal
A touching dream to which we all are lulled
But wake from separately. In it, conceits
And self-protecting ignorance congeal
To carry life, collapsing only when

Called to these corridors (for now once more
The nurse beckons –). Each gets up and goes
At last. Some will be out by lunch, or four;
Others, not knowing it, have come to join
The unseen congregations whose white rows
Lie set apart above – women, men;
Old, young; crude facets of the only coin

This place accepts. All know they are going to die.
Not yet, perhaps not here, but in the end,
And somewhere like this. That is what it means,
This clean-sliced cliff; a struggle to transcend
The thought of dying, for unless its powers
Outbuild cathedrals nothing contravenes
The coming dark, though crowds each evening try

With wasteful, weak, propitiatory flowers.

Hospital Window
Allen Ginsberg (1975)

At gauzy dusk, thin haze like cigarette smoke
ribbons past Chrysler Building's silver fins
tapering delicately needletopped, Empire State's
taller antenna filmed milky lit amid blocks
black and white apartmenting veil'd sky over Manhattan,
offices new built dark glassed in bluish heaven – The East
50s & 60s covered with castles & watertowers, seven storied
tar-topped house-banks over York Avenue, late may-green trees
surrounding Rockefellers' blue domed medical arbour –
Geodesic science at the waters edge – Cars running up
East River Drive, & parked at N. Y. Hospital's oval door
where perfect tulips flower the health of a thousand sick souls
trembling inside hospital rooms. Triboro bridge steel-spiked
penthouse orange roofs, sunset tinges the river and in a few
Bronx windows, some magnesium vapor brilliances're
spotted five floors above E 59th St under grey painted bridge
trestles. Way downstream along the river, as Monet saw Thames
100 years ago, Con Edison smokestacks 14th street,
& Brooklyn Bridge's skeined dim in modern mists –
Pipes sticking up to sky nine smokestacks huge visible –
U.N. Building hangs under an orange crane, & red lights on
vertical avenues below the trees turn green at the nod
of a skull with a mild nerve ache. Dim dharma,[56] I return
to this spectacle after weeks of poisoned lassitude, my thighs
belly chest & arms covered with poxied welts,
head pains fading back of the neck, right eyebrow cheek
mouth paralyzed – from taking the wrong medicine, sweated
too much in the forehead helpless, covered my rage from
gorge to prostate with grinding jaw and tightening anus
not released the weeping scream of horror at robot Mayaguez[57]
World self ton billions metal grief unloaded
Pnom Penh to Nakon Thanom, Santiago & Tehran.
Fresh warm breeze in the window, day's release
from pain, cars float downside the bridge trestle
and uncounted building-wall windows multiplied a mile
deep into ash-delicate sky beguile
my empty mind. A seagull passes alone wings
spread silent over roofs.

---

[56]In Buddhism, dharma refers to 'cosmic law and order' and 'phenomena'.
[57]The *Mayaguez* incident took place between Cambodia and the United States from 12 to 15 May 1975, less than a month after the Khmer Rouge took control of the capital Phnom Penh, ousting the US-backed Khmer Republic. It was the last official battle of the Vietnam War.

The Art of Healing
W. H. Auden (1976)

In Memoriam David Protetch, M. D.

Most patients believe
dying is something they do,
not their physician,
that white-coated sage,
never to be imagined
naked or married.

Begotten by one,
I should know better. 'Healing,'
Papa would tell me,
'is not a science,
but the intuitive art
of wooing Nature.

Plants, beasts, may react
according to the common
whim of their species,
but all humans have
prejudices of their own
which can't be foreseen.

To some, ill-health is
a way to be important,
others are stoics,
a few fanatics,
who won't feel happy until
they are cut open.'

Warned by him to shun
the sadist, the nod-crafty,
and the fee-conscious,
I knew when we met,
I had found a consultant
who thought as he did,

yourself a victim
of medical engineers
and their arrogance,
when they atom-bombed
your sick pituitary[58]
and over-killed it.

---

[58]The pituitary gland is the endocrine gland controlling growth, blood pressure, metabolism, kidney function, temperature and many other bodily functions.

'Every sickness
is a musical problem,'
so said Novalis,[59]
'and every cure
a musical solution':
You knew that also.

Not that in my case
you heard any shattering
discords to resolve:
to date my organs
still seem pretty sure of their
self-identity.

For my small ailments
you, who were mortally sick,
prescribed with success:
my major vices,
my mad addictions, you left
to my own conscience.

Was it your very
predicament that made me
sure I could trust you,
if I were dying,
to say so, not insult me
with soothing fictions?

Must diabetics
all contend with a nisus
to self-destruction?
One day you told me:
'It is only bad temper
that keeps me going.'

But neither anger
nor lust are omnipotent,
nor should we even
want our friends to be
superhuman. Dear David,
dead one, rest in peace,

having been what all
doctors should be, but few are,
and, even when most

---

[59]Novalis is the pseudonym of Georg Philipp Friedrich Freiherr von Hardenberg (1772–1801), a German poet, author and philosopher of early German Romanticism.

difficult, condign
of our biased affection
and objective praise.

Parish Doctor
Sterling A. Brown (1980)

> They come to him for subscriptions
> They resent examination, investigation
> They tell *him* what is wrong with them,
>   They *know*.
>
> It is pus on de heart, hole in de head
> The maul is open, they got stummatache,
> Somebody let some night air in the battens.
> They want him only to subscribe,
> The *medcins*: bitter-bitter is the best.
>
> 'Docteur, I doan b'leeve you can do nottin
>   fuh me
>
> I got a snake in me. I know, me, I been
>   spelled.
>
> You laugh, mon? I tell you son, a snake he in
>   my inside.'
>
> He tells them he's the best conjuh doctor, best
>   for roots and herbs,
>
> North of New Orleans. They pop their eyes;
>
> 'You tink he know dose ting for true?'
>
> They drink the boiled juices of a jit black hen
> For diarrhea, for consumption[60]
> They kill a jit black dog, bury him three days,
>   then cook him
>
> And oil the ailing person with the grease;
> For rheumatism they kill a turkey buzzard,
> Dry him up; rub the stiff jints with the mess.
> But jit black dogs and *caranchos* are none
>   too plentiful.
> They come to see their docteur, when these fail.

---

[60]Consumption is the archaic name for tuberculosis.

They like him; young, good-looking, easy laugher,
As brown as they and one of theirs forever.
The women call him *cher*: tender but embarrassed.
Their good men pass sly glances at his
                clipped moustache.

They think he lies about the conjuh knowledge
But still he got sharp eyes, you never know.
They pay him off with garden truck and cane
                   juice.

One auntie brought him six hens tied together
Squawking and screaming enough to wake a
                 graveyard.

One hen was jit-black to help him fix his
                 medcins.

One night, past midnight, we jolted twelve miles to
                 a cabin

It seemed as if the Lord would never make it.
'Tank Gawd, you'se here. I tole'em you would
                 get here.

He's hurted bad. He caught a bullet in his laig.
Tank Gawd, you'se come.' In the dull light of
                 the lamp.

I watched his skillful probing for the slug.
Outside the ring of light, dark faces watched us,
His fingers were deft and gentle. The woman's
                 sobbing

Quieted; the man on the table lay there
                 sweating

Breathing heavily, but trusting; his eyes rolled
                 Following the hands.

Their Bodies
David Wagoner (1983)

To the students of anatomy at Indiana University

That gaunt old man came first, his hair as white
As your scoured tables. Maybe you'll recollect him
By the scars of steelmill burns on the backs of his hands,
On the nape of his neck, on his arms and sinewy legs,

And her by the enduring innocence
Of her face, as open to all of you in death
As it would have been in life: she would memorize
Your names and ages and pastimes and hometowns
If she could, but she can't now, so remember her.

They believed in doctors, listened to their advice,
And followed it faithfully. You should treat them
One last time as they would have treated you.
They had been kind to others all their lives
And believed in being useful. Remember somewhere
Their son is trying hard to believe you'll learn
As much as possible from them, as *he* did,
And will do your best to learn politely and truly.

They gave away the gift of those useful bodies
Against his wish. (They had their own ways
Of doing everything, always.) If you're not certain
Which ones are theirs, be gentle to everybody.

The Anatomy Lesson of Dr. Nicolaas Tulp: Amsterdam, 1632[61]
Linda Bierds (1988)

High winter. All canals
clogged with an icy marrow. And the flax –
just a blue wash in the mind of
the painter who puffs up the tower stairs.
It is the time for festival – Aris Kindt
is hanged. And soon

up through these same stairs, up
to the slope-seated deal and chestnut
Theatrum Anatomicum, the surgeons will come:
Mathys and Hartman, Frans, Adriaan,
three Jacobs, then the bleeders and barbers,
the wheelwrights, needle-makers, goldsmiths,
the potters and sculptors, two
thin-chested harehounds. A lesson!
A dissection! All the reverent, mercantile faces
peering off through the scaffolds

that are now just empty,
just a deal and chestnut funnel tapered down

---

[61]This is the title of a 1632 oil painting by Rembrandt (Mauritshuis Museum, The Hague). In it, Dr Nicolaes Tulp dissects and explains the musculature of the arm to medical professionals. The body is that of Aris Kindt (alias of Adriaan Adriaanszoon), who was convicted for armed robbery and sentenced to death by hanging.

to a corpse:

Aris Kindt. Quiver-maker.
One necklace of rope-lace curled under his ears –
while over his body, the shadow of a painter's hat
circles, re-circles, like a moth at a candle.

So this is fresh death, its small, individual teeth.

Rembrandt walks past the breechcloth, then the forearm
soon to split to a stalk that would be grotesque
but for its radiance: rhubarb tendons
on a backdrop of winter. He swallows,
feels the small dimplings of lunch pork

drop away. And here will be Tulp,
his tweezers and white ruff. And here,
perhaps Hartman, perhaps the shadow of
a violet sleeve closing over the death-face.
It is commissioned: eight faces
Forever immortal, and one – slightly waxen –
Locked in mortality! He smiles.
How perfect the ears, and the pale eyelids

drawn up from the sockets
like the inner lids of pheasants. Just outside a window,
the day has climbed down to the amber color
of this candlelit room. Rembrandt turns,
crosses out the sponges and vessels.
There is the sputter of wagon wheels through a fresh ice,
and in all the storefronts
torches hang waiting for a pageant –

scarlet blossoms for a new spring.

His room has turned cold with the slow evening.
Far off in a corner
is a canvas clogged with the glue-skin of rabbits – a wash
of burnt umber, and the whites
built up, layer by layer.
Now a fire, the odor of beets.
And here, where the whites buckle, will be Tulp,
perhaps Mathys, their stunned
contemplation of death. He touches a spoon,

then a curve of plump bread. All across his shoulders
and into his hairline winds a little chill,
thin and infinite, like a thread-path
through the stars:

there will be umber

and madder root, yellow ochre, bone-black,
the scorch of sulfur, from
the oils of walnut and linseed – all things of the earth –
that forearm, that perfect ear.

What the Doctor Said
Raymond Carver (1989)

He said it doesn't look good
he said it looks bad in fact real bad
he said I counted thirty-two of them on one lung before
I quit counting them
I said I'm glad I wouldn't want to know
about any more being there than that
he said are you a religious man do you kneel down
in forest groves and let yourself ask for help
when you come to a waterfall
mist blowing against your face and arms
do you stop and ask for understanding at those moments
I said not yet but I intend to start today
he said I'm real sorry he said
I wish I had some other kind of news to give you
I said Amen and he said something else
I didn't catch and not knowing what else to do
and not wanting him to have to repeat it
and me to have to fully digest it
I just looked at him
for a minute and he looked back it was then
I jumped up and shook hands with this man who'd just given me
something no one else on earth had ever given me
I may have even thanked him habit being so strong

Knowing Our Place
Carole Satyamurti (1990)

Class is irrelevant in here.
We're part of a new scale
– mobility is all one way
and the least respected
are envied most.

First, the benigns,
in for a night or two,
nervous, but unappalled;
foolishly glad their bodies
don't behave like *that*.

Then the exploratories;
can't wait to know, but have to.
Greedy for signs, they swing
from misery to confidence,
or just endure.

The primaries are in
for surgery – what kind? What then?
Shocked, tearful perhaps;
things happening too fast.
Still can't believe it, really.

The reconstructions are survivors,
experienced, detached.
They're bent on being almost normal;
don't want to think
of other possibilities.

Secondaries (treatment)
are often angry – with doctors, fate...
– or blame themselves.
They want to tell their stories,
not to feel so alone.

Secondaries (palliative)
are admitted swathed in pain.
They become gentle, grateful,
they've learned to live
one day at a time.

Terminals are royalty,
beyond the rest of us.
they lie in side-rooms
flanked by exhausted relatives,
sans everything.

We learn the social map
fast. Beneath the ordinary chat,
jokes, kindnesses, we're scavengers,
gnawing at each other's histories
for scraps of hope.

The Doctor's Stone
Maurice Riordan (1995)

The Doc, in slippers and samite gown,
serves warmed milk and honey,
rashers, wads of blood pudding,

to cure a night on whiskey.
He's telling of a trip to Achill –[62]
how, as he squatted on the sand,
he saw beyond the ocean's rim
the bright tips of a palm forest.
He never found the spot again
but knows he glimpsed Hy Brazil.[63]
And he takes from a leather case
a stone, the size of a wren's egg,
that three days ago was lodged
inside his kidney. He traces
its passage to the bladder
down the urinary tract
into the palm of his hand.
Gives me the stone to hold.
It is so light and real
it could well be the one
I all but wrested from a dream.

The Old Operating Theatre, London, All Souls Night
Thomas Lynch (1998)

To rooms like this old resurrectionists
returned the bodies they had disinterred –
fresh corpses so fledging anatomists
could study Origin and Insertion points
of deltoids, pecs, trapezius and count
the vertebrae, the ball & socket joints.
And learn the private parts and Latin names
by which the heart becomes a myocardium,
the high cheek bone as zygoma, the brain,
less prone to daydream as a cerebellum.

And squirming in their stiff, unflinching seats,
apprentice surgeon witnessed, in the round,
new methods in advanced colostomy,
the amputation of gangrenous limbs
and watched as Viennese lobotomists
banished the ravings of a raving man
but left him scarred and drooling in a way
that made them wonder was he much improved?

---

[62]Achill: the largest island off the (west) coast of Ireland.
[63]Hy Brazil is a phantom island said to lie in the Atlantic Ocean west of Ireland. In Irish myth, it was said to be cloaked in mist, except for one day every seven years, when it became visible but still impossible to reach.

But here the bloodied Masters taught dispassionate
incisions – how to suture and remove.

In the rooms like this, the Greeks and Romans staged
their early dramas. Early Christians knelt
and hummed the liturgies when it was held
that prayer and penance were the only potions.
Ever since Abraham, guided by God,
first told his tribesman of the deal he made –
their foreskins for the ancient Covenant –
good medicine's meant letting human blood.
Good props include the table and the blade.
Good theatre is knowing where to cut.

At the Nurses' Station
Aidan Matthews (1998)

To property:
One three-quarter-length cavalry overcoat,
Sand-coloured pine-needle corduroy trousers
And a pair of desert-boots soled with odour-eaters.
Veteran leather briefcase (contents: one skipping rope);
Keys on a key-ring with the metal capital A.

To pharmacy:
Tricyclic anti-depressant capsules (forty),
Muscle relaxants, major tranquilizers (*ditto* approx.),
Non-prescription mixed analgesics (*circa* one hundred),
And two additional Ventolin inhalers which may be stored
Pro tem at the nurses' station on the closed male ward.

To laundry:
Shirt (worn at collar and cuffs on admission); all underwear –
Argyll socks, medium Y-fronts, one St Michael's vest –
And a lady's handkerchief that may/may not be heirloom,
therefore advise possible dryclean? Please provide
Interim toiletries. He is convinced that he smells.

Miscellaneous (Cellaneous? Anneous? Miss?):
Wristwatch, wedding-ring and miraculous medal Mary,
Hair from a sweetheart and/or saint in cellophane,
Nicotine pastilles, a multiple-organ donor-card,
Polaroid of a child touching an elephant's trunk,
Plus a pocket-diary that stinks of roll-on deodorant.

Its pages for the next sixteen months are already
Black and blue with commitments that cannot be broken.

A Ballad for Apothecaries
Anne Stevenson (2000)

> Being a Poem to Honour the Memory of
> Nicholas Culpeper, Gent.
> Puritan, Apothecary, Herbalist, Astrologer
> Who in the year of our Lord 1649
> Did publish A PHYSICAL DIRECTORY
> A translation from the Latin of the London Despensatory
> made by the College of Physicians
> 'Being that Book by which all Apothecaries are strictly
> commanded to make all their Physicke.'

In sixteen-hundred-and-sixteen
(The year Will Shakespeare died),
Earth made a pact with a curious star,
And a newborn baby cried.

Queen Bess's bright spring was over,
James Stuart frowned from the throne;
A more turbulent, seditious people
England had never known.

Now, Nick was a winsome baby,
And Nick was a lively lad,
So they gowned him and sent him to Cambridge
Where he went, said the priests, to the bad.

For though he excelled in Latin
And could rattle the Gospels in Greek,
He thought to himself, there's more to be said
Than the ancients knew how to speak.

He was led to alchemical studies
Through a deep Paracelsian text.
He took up the art of astrology first,
And the science of botany next.

To the theories of Galen he listened,
And to those of Hippocrates, too,
But he said to himself, there's more to be done
Than the ancients knew how to do.

For though Dr Tradition's a rich man,
He charges a rich man's fee.
Dr Reason and Dr Experience
Are my guides in philosophy.

The College of Learned Physicians
prescribes for the ruling class:
Physick for the ills of the great, they sneer,
Won't do for the vulgar mass.

But I say the heart of a beggar
Is as true as the heart of a king,
And the English blood in our English veins
Is of equal valuing.

Poor Nick fell in love with an heiress,
But en route to their desperate tryst,
The lady was struck down by lightning
Before they'd embrased or kissed.

So our hero consulted the Heavens
Where he saw he was fated to be
A friend to the sick and the humble
But the Great World's enemy.

Nick packed up his books in Cambridge
And came down without a degree
To inspirit Red Lion Street Spitalfields,
With his fiery humanity.

As a reckless, unlicensed physician,
He was moved to disseminate
Cures for the ills of the body
With cures for the ills of the state.

Who knows what horrors would have happened
To Nicholas Culpeper, Gent.,
If the king hadn't driven his kingdom
Into war with Parliament.

In the ranks of the New Model Army
Nick fought with the medical men,
Till a Royalist bullet at Newbury
Shot him back to his thundering pen.

'Scholars are the people's jailors,
And Latin's their jail,' he roared,
'Our fates are in thrall to knowledge;
Vile men would have knowledge obscured!'

When they toppled King Charles's head off
Nick Culpeper cried, 'Amen!'
It's well that he died before the day
they stuck it on again.

Still, English tongues won their freedom
In those turbulent years set apart;
And the wise, they cherish Nick's courage
While the cheer his compassionate heart.

So whenever you stop in a chemist's
For an aspirin or salve for a sore,
Give a thought to Nicholas Culpeper
Who dispensed to the London poor.

For cures for the ills of the body
Are cures for the ills of the mind;
And a welfare state is a sick state
When the dumb are led by the blind.[64]

What I Would Give
Rafael Campo (2002)

What I would like to give them for a change
is not the usual prescription with
its hubris of the power to restore,
to cure; what I would like to give them, ill
from not enough of laying in the sun

---

[64]Author's note: In a series of prefaces to this best-selling manual in English (reprinted at least fourteen times before 1718), Culpeper denounced the College of Physicians who secured their monopoly by keeping the secrets of medicine in the Latin language – just as Rome's priests, before the Reformation, had maintained power by preserving the mysteries of the Bible in Latin. Culpeper's translation, he declared, was made 'out of pure pity to the commonality of England ... many of whom to my knowledge have perished either for want of money to fee a physician or want of knowledge of a remedy happily growing in their garden.'

When the victory of the Parliamentarian Army was still in doubt, Culpeper was branded by the Royalist *Mercurious Pragmaticus* as an Anabaptist 'who had arrived at the battlement of an Absolute Atheist, and by two years drunken labour hath Gallimawfred the apothecaries book into nonsense, mixing every receipt therein with some scruples at least of rebellion or atheism, besides the danger of poisoning men's bodies. And (to supply his drunkenness and lechery with a thirty-shilling award) endeavoured to bring into obloquy the famous Societies of Apothecaries and Chyrugeons.' Such abuses, all of them unfounded, were levelled by his political opponents. Even during the Cromwellian interregnum, a broadside appeared (1652) entitled 'A farm in Spittlefields where all the knick-knacks of astrology are exposed to open sale, where Nicholas Culpeper brings under his velvet jacket: 1. His chalinges against the Doctors of Physick, 2. A Pocket Medicine. 3. An Abnormal Circle.'

Culpeper's *London Dispensary*, however, together with a *Directory for Midwives* and others of his seventy-nine books and pamphlets, continued to sell in large numbers. In 1652–3, he brought out his celebrated herbal under the title of *The English Physitian: or, an Astrological-Physical Discourse of the Vulgar Herbs of this Nation, Being a Compleat Method of Physick, whereby a man may preserve his Body in Health, or cure himself, being sick, for three pence charge, with such things as grow in England, they being most fit for English Bodies.*

Though Culpeper may have been in some ways a charlatan, his *Dispensary* remained in print into the eighteenth century and his *English Physitian* continues to be the most celebrated of English herbals even today. Sadly, Culpeper's remedies, praised and prized by the London poor, were not able to prevent his death at thirty-eight (from an old wound received while he was fighting in the Parliamentarian Army), nor the deaths of six of his seven children who predeceased him.

not caring what the onlookers might think
while feeding some banana to their dogs –
what I would like to offer them is this,
not reassurance that their lungs sound fine,
or that the mole they've noticed change is not
a melanoma, but instead of fear
transfigured by some doctorly advice
I'd like to give them my astonishment
at sudden rainfall like the whole world weeping,
and how ridiculously gently it
slicked down my hair; I'd like to give them that,
the joy I felt while staring in your eyes
as you learned epidemiology
(the science of disease in populations),
the night around our bed like timelessness,
like comfort, like what I would give to them.

Anatomy Class
Sasha Dugdale (2003)

First day at medical school.
I hold my instruments and brace myself for lessons
In the long hall of cadavers. They lie in wait,
They lie in state – six hundred yellowing bags of gut.

I've been unwell. I looked pale in the mirror
When I washed, but here I look like life itself.
The bodies regard me with their royal eyelids,
Their nose bones, their pursed regretful lips.

The great ship hulks of their pelvic regions,
The gently undulating sand dunes of their chests,
The open softness of the elbow, once pulsed through,
All of it before me on the slab.

Unrolling the leather tool bag I discover
I am equipped with a needle and a nail file,
A velvet pincushion made at school,
A measuring tape and a souvenir penknife.

The fear of sudden exposure makes me dizzy:
The others are all cutting out to pattern.
But how to slice and flay precisely,
When you have no scalpel and no practice,

Is not a question I ever asked myself.
So I start by trimming nails. Twenty in all.

Cutting nose hairs and measuring the ears.
Then I take the pins and one by one

Insert them gently into flesh
Around the shoulder joint and down the arms.
Marching down in pairs like tiny pylons
Straddling the dried up tide path of the veins.

And in the bated breath of concentration
The exact measuring, placing, trimming,
I absorb myself so utterly that time
Lies still before me and the world

Turns more slowly than it's used to.
And all around the soft clatter of the scalpel,
The slicing skin, as if a tailor cut the cloth,
The ticking of the clock and muted voices.

And I wonder if I couldn't be a doctor
And pursue science with a sewing kit
And pin and stitch and splice the broken bodies
And decorate the dead for what comes after.

But most of all I think of nothing,
I'm doodling, idling out the living hours,
As close to death as anyone could wish.
As far from death as I will ever be.

Hand-Washing Technique – Government Guidelines
Simon Armitage (2006)

i.m. Dr David Kelly[65]

1 Palm to palm.
2 Right palm over left dorsum and left palm over right dorsum.
3 Palm to palm fingers interlaced.
4 Backs of fingers to opposing palms with fingers interlocked.
5 Rotational rubbing of right thumb clasped in left palm and vice versa.
6 Rotational rubbing, backwards and forwards with clasped fingers of right
   hand in left palm and vice versa.

---

[65]David Christopher Kelly, CMG (1944–2003), was a British scientist and authority on biological warfare, employed by the British Ministry of Defence. Formerly a UN weapons inspector in Iraq, he came to public attention in July 2003 when an unauthorized discussion he had off the record with BBC journalist Andrew Gilligan about the government's dossier on weapons of mass destruction in Iraq was cited by Gilligan. Kelly's name became known to the media as Gilligan's source and he was called to appear on 15 July 2003 before the parliamentary foreign affairs select committee, where he was aggressively questioned. He was found dead two days later, presumably by suicide.

The Anatomy Lesson of Dr Nicolaes Tulp, 1632[66]
Tiffany Atkinson (2006)

Hanged for thieving a coat in the raw new year
Adriaenszoon lies on the slab for Dr Tulp.
The doctor takes the stage in sweeping gallows black
as the good guildsmen of Amsterdam flock round
in a quackery. This Tulp has a feeling for light
and shade. Behold how he unpicks the knot
of the offender's left hand, the insinuating scalpel
paring back skin like the peplum of a tulip. Such
immaculate work: the smooth-cheeked spectators
press in, anaesthetised by high, white ruffs, purveyors
of tendon and carpal. With watchmaker's nicety,
Tulp applies forceps to the *flexorum digitorum*,
and the dead man's hand becomes fist. All is decorum
as the deadpan Doctor makes a case of Adriaenszoon.
The gentlemen, for the most part, keep their corruption
at arm's length. Tulp's in up to the neck. Between them
they'll have two coats off the poor man's back.

The Vaccination Queue
Kelvin Corcoran (2010)

I queued at the surgery for the flu vaccination. I was with the old, saw our ageing
and I got it. We trailed out of the building and accepted our parts as extras in a
British comedy. A queue is an opportunity to be orderly, anxious and complain in
the service of humour.

- Look it says here, if you are breast feeding or trying to become pregnant, tell
  the nurse.
- Well, I think you're safe then Edie.
- This is like the army. They didn't keep the needles sharp, just jabbed 'em in
  you and off you go to Timbuktu.

Most of the women shouted at most of the men.

- He can't hear me. Stand there, just wait. You're a bit deaf aren't you.

Many were the respectable poor, who no longer exist in any political discourse.
They wear cheap clothes; the men in pressed grey trousers and thin brown slip-ons;
the women in sensible three quarter length coats and shapeless slacks. You queue up
because it's free – and they have paid all their lives. So they act sniffy, like a posh hat
on humility. I'm at home with them and try to be helpful.

---

[66] The poem's title refers to a famous 1632 Rembrandt painting of the dissection of Adriaan Adriaanszoon
(alias Aris Kindt). See Linda Bierds' poem of the same name.

I remembered my mother talked about the doctor visiting. He arrived on a horse.
– He was so tall up there, he'd shout down at you all of your personal business,
   everybody heard. He was a kind old soul though.
   A doctor making house visits on a horse? Have I made this up or read it in the sort
   of novel I don't read?'

One winter my dad came off his bike, cracked his head, staggered home delirious
and collapsed through the door. She tried to lift him up, saw the blood, shrieked
and dropped him smack down on the flagstones. Later, the doctor, discretely
dismounted, asked if she'd tried to kill him – I'd understand Mrs Corcoran but all
the same, best not.

I suppose the accident of him not dying on this occasion, and the succession of
generations, drops me in this queue. It helps me stand here and shuffle forward.
I imagine every one of us standing here must be informed by such events – like a
bright axis of personal identity intersecting the queue unseen and unheard. Our
queue, snaking back through history via Beveridge, the Empire and beyond, is of
course the English class system as vernacular drama. You know your place and
how to behave, thank you. Nobody waiting for the vaccination pushed; one man
faking confusion, cheated. The general disapproval unspoken hung in the air we
all breathed.

A & E
Robin Robertson (2013)

> It was like wetting the bed
> waking up that night, soaked through:
> my sutures open again
> and the chest wound haemorrhaging.
> Pulling on jeans and an overcoat
> I called a car to Camberwell, and
> in through the shivering rubber doors
> presented myself
> at that Saturday-night abattoir
> of Casualty at King's on Denmark Hill.
>
> At this front-line, behind her desk
> and barred window, the triage nurse
> was already waving me away –
> till I parted the tweed to show her
> what I had going on underneath.
> Unfashionable, but striking nonetheless:
> my chest undone like some rare waistcoat,
> with that lace-up front – a black *échelle* –
> its red, wet-look leatherette,
> those fancy, flapping lapels.

Nimzo-Indian[67]
Philip Gross (2014)

Now that all other bearings have led him, astray,
to the last but one ward, now
that even the en-suite bathroom keeps eluding him
like socks or what he started out for from his chair
or family faces, which of us might come in
wearing whose, from when,
now what can I do but... here: the foursquare
board, the rattling-out of chessmen. He looks up.
I set him out white that's gone amber with touch
and he's playing a stout Nimzo-Indian, six
moves or more ahead, away
from this new-scrubbed room with fragments of him
on one shelf. His lips moving. Under his breath,
the cut-glass combinations on a waiter's silver tray
of poise and tremor, upheld,
tinkling, nothing spilled yet but angles of light...
When he slips – yes, his fingertips dither then
go to my knight, not his own – it's the highest mistake
such as God might have made: to reach so deep
into world that (maybe this
is what He longed for) He forgot Himself in it.

The Hospital Punch
Sally Flint (2015)

'*I am sure the air in heaven must be this wonder working gas of delight.*'

Robert Southey

Henry, the anaesthetist, who swayed
like he'd sniffed nitrous oxide all his life,
un-wrapped one of the biggest sterile bowls
used to collect swabs in theatre.
He carried it like a ceremonial platter
to the staff room, leered over his spectacles
and said: 'What we need is alcohol.'
Big Marlon, the porter, brought glasses
out of store, tipped in a hip-flask of rum,
whispered, 'It'll warm the cockles.'
Sister Jacks added Merlot, a gift

---

[67]The Nimzo-Indian Defence is a modern, defensive opening move in the game of chess.

donated by a patient. Spike and Susie X
from the mortuary chilled the mix
as Mr Nash dissected an orange
using a scalpel the same way he cut flesh.
Slices bobbed like harvest moons.
Nancy, now as swollen-eyed
as the grey-faced parents she'd consoled
shook as if she had the palsy. Wrapped
in a cellular blanket, we let her taste first.
She blinked hard, confirmed it was a choker.

The room filled with slurred words
and the funniest jokes ever heard.
Marlene from pharmacy crushed
the contents of her pocket
and, when she thought no-one was looking,
stirred in the powder. Some half dozed,
agreed something smelt lush, almost tropical.
Stella removed her overalls,
put away her bucket and cleaning fluid,
produced cigarettes from a pocket.
But the question of bringing
the dead back to life wouldn't sink.
It was nobody's fault, we chorused.
Life wasn't ours to give or take,
except for the exceptions –
when we'd fought and won.
Slowly, Henry began feeling
dents in the locker doors
when the junior doctor said he couldn't stand
the heat. As the sun slipped
behind the hospital chimney
he swung at the window, made his fist bleed.

Forensic Pathology, The Gordon Museum at Guy's Hospital[68]
Corinna Wagner (2015)

A girl's puckered mouth,
grotesque with its moustache of red hair
forever blows a kiss from its transparent urn.

---

[68]The Gordon Museum of Pathology, part of King's College, London, is the largest medical museum in the UK, containing rare and unique artefacts and specimens. Unlike other medical museums, it is not open to the public, as its primary function remains the training of medical students.

And testifies:
an ode to immortality,
which says nothing about beauty
and only something of truth.

An eternal ode to a drunken impotent boy from the base,
who found brief respite
in a puddle of lardy skin and
the sound of lungs exploding underwater.

Under him,
her pursed lips forced brutally to give way,
forever arrested in a stunned 'O'.

MEDICAL WRITING:

Treatise of the Hypochondriack and Hysterick Diseases
Bernard Mandeville (1730 ed.)

A young gentleman, that understands *Latin,* takes his pleasure at some university, or other, for six or seven years, in which having at his leisure hours gone through the usual stages of logick, natural philosophy, anatomy, botany, and perhaps chemistry, he learns by heart all the distempers incident to human bodies, from head to foot, a few signs by which they are known and distinguished from one another, and what prognostication is commonly made upon every one of them, with the method of cure, and such remedies as the author he reads is pleased to insert and recommend: the gentleman thus instructed being honoured with his degree, which cannot be denied him, is consulted in the most difficult cases, is ready to defend his opinion in mode and figure against all opposers, and thinks himself qualified to be physician to the greatest monarch in the universe; and yet it is certain, that such a one is no more capable of discharging the weighty office of a physician, than a man that should study opticks, proportions, and read of painting and mixing of colours for as many years, would, without having ever touched a pencil, be able to perform the part of a good history-painter.

I own that the studies I have named are necessary for all young Beginners; but they only make up for the easy, the pleasant, the speculative, the prepatory part of physic: the tedious, the difficult, but the only useful part in regard of others, I mean the practical, which is not attempted by many, is only attained by an almost everlasting attendance on the sick, unwearied patience, and judicious as well as diligent observation.

...

As the world grows wiser, physicians of later times have found out more compendious ways to renown and riches; by applying themselves particularly to anatomy, chemistry, etc. and by writing of, or performing something with accuracy in any one only of the shallow auxiliary arts, that all together compose the theory of physic, they know how to insinuate themselves into the favour of the public; and

A B S T R A C T

OF THE

O R D E R S

OF

St. THOMAS's Hospital,

Relating to the

Sifters, Nurfes and Poor Patients, therein.

I. THAT no poor Perfon, at their Entrance, pay any Money or Gratuity, for Garnifh or Footing, on pain of Expulfion of the Perfon that demands or receives it.

II. That no Patients be kept in the Houfe after prefented out, on pain of Expulfion of the Sifter of that Ward where fuch Patient fhall be kept, without Leave from the Treafurer, or Two Governours Takers in.

III. That no Patient be kept in the Houfe, to whom Phyfick or Chyrurgery is not adminiftred within a Week after Admittance, on pain of Expulfion of the Sifter that fo keeps them, without giving Notice to the Treafurer, or the Governours Takers-in.

IV. That the Sifters keep their Wards conftantly neat and clean, and that the Duft and Stools be carried out of their Wards by Six of the Clock in the Morning, to the appointed Places.

V. That no Perfon fetch or carry Fire from one Place to another, in Wooden Veffels, or any other thing that may be dangerous for Fire.

VI. That all the able Men and Women Patients, fhall help the Sifters to cleanfe the Wards, without Money or Reward, upon pain of Expulfion: And that the Sifters fhall wafh, or caufe to be wafh'd, all weak Peoples Clouts, without taking Money or Reward for the fame.

VII. That no Sifter deliver the Patients Fewel, for any other Ufe than the Poor of the Ward to which they belong, upon pain of Five Shillings to be paid by the Sifter.

VIII. That the Patients do conftantly attend the Worfhip of God in the Chappel, at the ufual Times, on the Sabbath Days, and other Days, upon pain of Forfeiture of one Days Allowance for the firft Offence (without reafonable Excufe) and after offending to be punifh'd at the Difcretion of the Treafurer, or Two Governours Takers-in.

IX. That the Sifters be careful there be no playing at Cards, Dice, or other Games in this Houfe, and give Notice to the Treafurer or Committee if any offend therein.

X. That neither Officer nor Poor fhall Swear, or take God's Name in vain.

Nor revile or mifcal one another.

Nor fteal Meat, Drink, Apparel, or other thing from one another.

Nor abufe themfelves by inordinate Drinking, or incontinent Living.

Nor talk or act immodeftly, upon pain of Expulfion.

And that when they go to, or return from their Meals, or Beds, they crave God's Bleffing, and return due Thanks to God.

XI. That none of the Poor contract Matrimony with each other within the Houfe, and that none of the Men go into the Womens Wards, nor the Women into the Mens Wards, without Licenfe, upon pain of Expulfion.

XII. That no Patients fit up in their Wards, or ftay out of the Houfe, after Eight of the Clock at Night, in Winter, and Nine in the Summer, without Licence from the Steward, on pain of Expulfion.

XIII. That no Patient fhall lie out of the Houfe, without fpecial Licenfe from the Steward, on pain of Expulfion.

XIV. That no Patient eat any Meat, or drink any Wine, Brandy, ftrong Ale, or ftrong Beer, or other Drink, but what fhall be directed or allow'd by the Phyfician or Chyrurgeon, under whofe Care fuch Patients fhall be.

XV. That if hereafter any happen to be admitted into this Houfe, that have the Foul Difeafe, they fhall not go into any of the Clean Wards, nor come into the Officers Houfes, nor within the Chappel, nor walk upon the Seats, nor walk about in the Court-Yards, on pain of Expulfion. And if any Perfon having the Foul Difeafe fhall refufe, or neglect to difcover the fame, at the Time of Taking in, every fuch Patient, when difcover'd, fhall be immediately difcharged the Houfe, without Cure. And that no Perfon be admitted twice for the faid Diftemper.

The HOUSE-DIET.

Sunday.	Monday.	Tuefday.	Wednefday.	Thurfday.	Friday.		Saturday.
12 Ounces of Bread. 3 Pints of Beer, Wine Meafure. 8 Ounces of boil'd Beef, without Bones. 1 Quart or 3 Pints of Broth.	12 Ounces of Bread. 3 Pints of Beer. 8 Ounces of boil'd Beef without Bones. 1 Quart or 3 Pints of Broth.	12 Ounces of Bread. 3 Pints of Beer. 8 Ounces of Mutton. 1 Quart or 3 Pints of Mutton-Broth.	12 Ounces of Bread. 3 Pints of Beer. 4 Ounces of Cheefe. 1 Ounce of Butter. 1 Pint of Milk-Pottage, at Night.	12 Ounces of Bread. 3 Pints of Beer. 8 Ounces of boil'd Beef, without Bones. 1 Quart or 3 Pints of Broth.	12 Ounces of Bread. 3 Pints of Beer. 8 Ounces of Mutton. 1 Quart or 3 Pints of Mutton-Broth.	Or inftead of the Mutton and Broth, if the Committee and Treafurer think fit, 1 Quart of Milk-Pottage, and a late Money.	12 Ounces of Bread. 3 Pints of Beer. 4 Ounces of Cheefe. 2 Ounces of Butter. 1 Pint of Rice-Milk, at Night.

FIGURE 4: *Abstract of the Orders of St Thomas's Hospital*, London, c. 1705.

from their giving proofs of their understanding well one inconsiderable branch of their art, are stupidly believed to be equally skilled in the whole. The great anatomist that artfully dissects the dead body of a malefactor, shall therefore be trusted with the live one of the judge, till he has fitted that too for his purpose. The witty philosopher, who can so exactly tell you which way the world was made, that one would think he must have had a hand in it, in his talk cures all diseases by hypothesis, and frightens away the gout with a fine simile, but when he comes to practise oftener reasons a trifling distemper into a consumption.

...

I would have public professors, that should not only instruct others, but spend most of their time in making new experiments, and if possible further discoveries in every one of those useful arts [physic, anatomy, chemistry, etc.]; but I would not have people ridiculously pretend, that because they have more particularly studied and taken pains in any one of them, they therefore understand the practice of physic: such as are designed for the practical part might content themselves with learning as much of the theory as is commonly taught in one, or at most two courses on each branch, and after that presently apply themselves to steady observation, which to come to perfection in, they want above twenty lives.

...

Where shall you find a physician now-a-days that makes that stay with his patients, which it is plain the ancients must have done, to make the noble prognosticks we have from them? But this would not only be too laborious, but a tedious way of getting money; self-interest now gives better lessons to young physicians. If you are not extraordinary in any of the branches I have named, rather than that you should spend your time before the squalid beds of poor patients, and bear with the unsavoury smells of a crowded hospital, show yourself a scholar, write a poem, either a good one, or a long one; compose a Latin oration, or do but translate something out of that language with your name to it. If you can do none of all these, marry into a good family, and your relations will help you into practice: or else cringe and make your court to half a dozen noted apothecaries, promise 'em to prescribe loads of physic.

Petitions to the London Foundling Hospital (1747–57)[69]

Girl (F.H. no. 340) Received 17 July 1747

This Child was born the 24 of May about Eleven o'Clock in the Evening, and was Christened the first of June by the name Elizabeth Green, if it should have the Good

---

[69]These are a small sample of many such petitions that came with foundling children, in the hopes that families could identify them later, or with the idea that the authorities would be more favourably disposed to taking the child. Other parents, some of them illiterate, left a piece of cloth or some small object as identifiers (there are approximately 5,000 small pieces of cloth in the archives). However, only six of the 1384 London children taken in during the early phase, and only 146 of the 14,934 taken in during the General Reception, when the Hospital also received babies from the provinces, were claimed. These three petitions are: A/FH/A/9/1/4; A/FH/A/9/1/6; A/FH/A9/1/55 in the London Metropolitan Archives.

fortune to get into this House, the Parents desire this paper may be preserv'd with the Cloths, as they are in Great Hopes some part of their lives, they may be in such Circumstances as to enable them to own it.

Boy (Foundling Hospital number 497) Received 31 March 1749

Gentleman I do most Humbly request you to preserve this writing, as a Mark that my Child may be known, having a most dear and Tender regard for it. For wch reason I have trusted it to a Charity establish'd upon so good a Foundation as knowing my circumstance will not permit me to take so great a Care of it, as my Duty requireth.

Boy (F.H. No.4478) Received 14 May 1757

To the Honourable Governors and Gentleman of the Foundling Hospital

We present unto Your Care and Protection a Poor Destitute Infant Void of any hopes of being Preserved from the Calamities of want and Money unless provided for by the most compassionate of all the Charity the Donors of this Hospital the Child's Not Baptized but we humbly Beg of you to name it by the name of Jo Isac Walker Being the Same Name of the parents and they expect to see it again if fortune should turn to them once More as they Expect.

And Your Petitioners Shall in Duty Bound for Ever Pray

May 14 1757

P. S. ... the Child has a King Charles Penny, Bearing Date 1688 about his Neck. [St. Luke's, Old Street].

Hygeia
Thomas Beddoes (1802)

'A National Plan for Medical Boards'

The outlines of an effectual system for the ascertainment of the state of the public health, and for its preservation, will readily occur to every person, acquainted with the established forms conducting the great affairs of mankind. Particular regulations will present themselves as soon as the execution of the scheme shall be set about in earnest.

In the first place, it is obvious that a board must be established in the metropolis, and that there must be other boards in cities, towns, and country districts, with which the first is regularly to communicate. The conduct of the business must be entrusted to select individuals, but admission to the place of meeting should be free, at stated times, to members of the medical profession without exception; and all should be invited to give information in writing, when they could not attend. A digest of the whole ought annually to be published. Should a particular emergency demand an extraordinary report, the materials would be at hand. By such an arrangement, the execution, the success, and the comparative merit of the different means of suppressing contagion and chronic disorders would come before the public; and undeniable improvements would pass with expedition from place to place. At present, the rate at which they travel is woefully slow, and thousands perish in the meantime. For if the plan for a fever-house hardly reached Liverpool from Manchester in six years, how long will it be in getting to Bristol, whither the roads for useful public designs have, in all ages, been said to be heavy?

It should be among the principal cares of a national system of medical boards, to extract, from charitable institutions for the relief of the indigent sick, a quantity of medical knowledge, and by consequence, of public benefit, which hitherto they have never yielded.

Currents and Cross-Currents in Medical Science
Oliver Wendell Holmes (1860)

The truth is, that medicine, professedly founded on observation, is as sensitive to outside influences, political, religious, philosophical, imaginative, as is the barometer to the changes of atmospheric density. Theoretically it ought to go on its own straightforward inductive path, without regard to changes of government or to fluctuations of public opinion. But look a moment while I dash a few facts together, and see if some sparks do not reveal by their light a closer relation between the Medical Sciences and the conditions of Society and the general thought of the time, than would at first be suspected.

Observe the coincidences between certain great political and intellectual periods and the appearance of illustrious medical reformers and teachers. It was in the age of Pericles, of Socrates, of Plato, of Phidias, that Hippocrates gave to medical knowledge the form which it retained for twenty centuries. With the world-conquering Alexander, the world-embracing Aristotle,[70] appropriating anatomy and physiology, among his manifold spoils of study, marched abreast of his royal pupil to wider conquests.

...

Look at Vesalius,[71] the contemporary of Luther.[72] Who can fail to see one common spirit in the radical ecclesiastic and the reforming court-physician? Both still to some extent under the dominion of the letter: Luther holding to the real presence; Vesalius actually causing to be drawn and engraved two muscles which he knew were not found in the human subject, because they had been described by Galen,[73] from dissections of the lower animals. Both breaking through old traditions in the search of truth; one, knife in hand, at the risk of life and reputation, the other at the risk of fire and fagot, with that mightier weapon which all the devils could not silence, though they had been thicker than the tiles on the house-tops.

...

And is it to be looked at as a mere accidental coincidence, that while Napoleon was modernizing the political world, Bichat[74] was revolutionizing the science of life

---

[70]All are ancient Greek philosophers, and the founders of the Western philosophical tradition, except Alexander the Great, the famous Greek king, who was tutored by Aristotle.

[71]Andreas Vesalius (1514–64) was an anatomist, physician and author of one of the most influential books on human anatomy, *De humani corporis fabrica (On the Fabric of the Human Body)*.

[72]Martin Luther (1483–1546) was a theologian and the canonical figure of the Protestant Reformation.

[73]Galen (129–c.216 AD) and his theories remained largely unchallenged in Western medicine until the time of Vesalius. Hippocrates (c.460–370 BC) was a Greek physician and founder of the Hippocratic school of medicine.

[74]Marie François Xavier Bichat (1771–1802) was a French anatomist and physiologist, known as the founder of modern histology.

and the art that is based upon it; that while the young general was scaling the Alps, the young surgeon was climbing the steeper summits of unexplored nature.

...

If we come to our own country, who can fail to recognize that Benjamin Rush,[75] the most conspicuous of American physicians, was the intellectual offspring of the movement which produced the Revolution? 'The same hand,' says one of his biographers, 'which subscribed the declaration of the political independence of these States, accomplished their emancipation from medical systems formed in foreign countries, and wholly unsuitable to the state of diseases in America.'

Following this general course of remark, I propose to indicate in a few words the direction of the main intellectual current of the time, and to point out more particularly some of the eddies which tend to keep the science and art of medicine from moving with it, or even to carry them backwards.

The two dominant words of our time are *law* and *average*, both pointing to the uniformity of the order of being in which we live. Statistics have tabulated everything – population, growth, wealth, crime, disease. We have shaded maps showing the geographical distribution of larceny and suicide. Analysis and classification have been at work upon all tangible and visible objects. The Positive Philosophy of Comte[76] has only given expression to the observing and computing mind of the nineteenth century.

In the mean time, the great stronghold of intellectual conservatism, traditional belief, has been assailed by facts which would have been indicted as blasphemy but a few generations ago. Those new tables of the law, placed in the hands of the geologist by the same living God who spoke from Sinai to the Israelites of old, have remodelled the beliefs of half the civilized world. The solemn scepticism of science has replaced the sneering doubts of witty philosophers. The more positive knowledge we gain, the more we incline to question all that has been received without absolute proof.

Border Lines of Knowledge in Some Provinces of Medical Science
Oliver Wendell Holmes (1861)

Science is the topography of ignorance. From a few elevated points we triangulate vast spaces, inclosing infinite unknown details. We cast the lead, and draw up a little sand from abysses we may never reach with our dredges.

The best part of our knowledge is that which teaches us where knowledge leaves off and ignorance begins. Nothing more clearly separates a vulgar from a superior

---

[75]Benjamin Rush (1746–1813) was a physician, politician and social reformer. Rush had a major impact on the emerging medical profession, in his promotion of public health and in his studies of the function of the brain and mental disorders.
[76]Auguste Comte (1798–1857) was a French philosopher and a founder of the discipline of sociology and is regarded as the first modern philosopher of science.

mind, than the confusion in the first between the little that it truly knows, on the one hand, and what it half knows and what it thinks it knows on the other.

That which is true of every subject is especially true of the branch of knowledge which deals with living beings. Their existence is a perpetual death and reanimation. Their identity is only an idea, for we put off our bodies many times during our lives, and dress in new suits of bones and muscles.

...

If it is true that we understand ourselves but imperfectly in health, this truth is more signally manifested in disease, where natural actions imperfectly understood, disturbed in an obscure way by half-seen causes, are creeping and winding along in the dark toward that destined issue, sometimes using our remedies as safe stepping stones, occasionally, it may be, stumbling over them as obstacles.

...

Let us turn to a branch of knowledge which deals with certainties up to the limit of the senses, and is involved in no speculations beyond them. In certain points of view, Human Anatomy may be considered an almost exhausted science. From time to time some small organ which had escaped earlier observers has been pointed out – such parts as the *tensor tarsi*, the otic ganglion, or the Pacinian bodies; but some of our best anatomical works are those which have been classic for many generations. The plates of the bones in Vesalius, three centuries old, are still masterpieces of accuracy, as of art. The magnificent work of Albinus[77] on the muscles, published in 1747, is still supreme in its department, as the constant references of the most thorough recent treatise on the subject, that of Theile,[78] sufficiently show. More has been done in unravelling the mysteries of the fasciae, but there has been a tendency to overdo this kind of material analysis. Alexander Thomson split them up into cobwebs, as you may see in the plates to Velpeau's Surgical Anatomy.[79] I well remember how he used to shake his head over the coarse work of Scarpa and Astley Cooper[80] – as if Denner, who painted the separate hairs of the beard and pores of the skin in his portraits, had spoken lightly of the pictures of Rubens and Vandyk.[81]

...

The great triumph of the microscope as applied to anatomy has been in the resolution of the organs and tissues into their simple constituent anatomical

---

[77]Vesalius's majesterial work *De humani corporus fabrica* (1543) has been referred to often in this anthology. Bernhard Siegfried Albinus (1697–1770) was a German-born Dutch anatomist, best known for his monumental *Tabulae sceleti et musculorum corporis humani* (Leiden, 1747).

[78]Friedrich W. Theile (1801–79) was a German anatomist.

[79]Alfred-Armand-Louis-Marie Velpeau (1795–1867) was an accomplished French anatomist and surgeon.

[80]Antonio Scarpa (1752–1832) was an Italian anatomist and professor. Sir Astley Paston Cooper, 1st Baronet (1768–1841) was an English surgeon and anatomist, who made significant contributions to vascular surgery.

[81]Balthasar Denner (1685–1749) was a German painter, highly regarded as a portraitist. Sir Peter Paul Rubens (1577–1640) was a Flemish painter and proponent of the Baroque style. Sir Anthony van Dyck (1599–1641) was a Flemish Baroque painter who became the leading court painter in England.

elements. It has taken up general anatomy where Bichat left it. He had succeeded in reducing the structural language of nature to syllables, if you will permit me to use so bold an image. The microscopic observers who have come after him have analyzed these *letters*, as we may call them – the simple elements by the combination of which Nature spells out successively tissues, which are her syllables, organs which are her words, systems which are her chapters, and so goes on from the simple to the complex, until she binds up in one living whole that wondrous volume of power and wisdom which we call the human body.

...

Let us turn to Physiology. The microscope, which has made a new science of the intimate structure of the organs, has at the same time cleared up many uncertainties concerning the mechanism of the special functions. Up to the time of the living generation of observers, Nature had kept over all her inner workshops the forbidding inscription, *No Admittance*! If any prying observer ventured to spy through his magnifying tubes into the mysteries of her glands and canals and fluids, she covered up her work in blinding mists and bewildering halos, as the deities of old concealed their favored heroes in the moment of danger. Science has at length sifted the turbid light of her lenses, and blanched their delusive rainbows.

Anatomy studies the organism in space. Physiology studies in also in time. After the study of form and composition follows close that of action, and this leads us along back to the first moment of the germ, and forward to the resolution of the living frame into its lifeless elements. In this way Anatomy, or rather that branch of it which we call Histology, has become inseperably blended with the study of function.

Notes on Nursing
Florence Nightingale (1860)

It appears that scarcely any improvement in the faculty of observing is being made. Vast has been the increase of knowledge in pathology – that science which teaches us the final change produced by disease on the human frame – scarce any in the art of observing the signs of the change while in progress. Or, rather, is it not to be feared that observation, as an essential part of medicine, has been declining?

...

A want of the habit of observing conditions and an inveterate habit of taking averages are each of them often equally misleading.

Men whose profession like that of medical men leads them to observe only, or chiefly, palpable and permanent organic changes are often just as wrong in their opinion of the result as those who do not observe at all. For instance, there is a broken leg; the surgeon has only to look at it once to know; it will not be different if he sees it in the morning to what it would have been had he seen it in the evening. And in whatever conditions the patient is, or is likely to be, there will still be the broken leg, until it is set. The same with many organic diseases. An experienced physician has but to feel the pulse once, and he knows that there is aneurism which will kill some time or other.

But with the great majority of cases, there is nothing of the kind; and the power of forming any correct opinion as to the result must entirely depend upon an enquiry into all the conditions in which the patient lives. In a complicated state of society in large towns, death, as every one of great experience knows, is far less often produced by any one organic disease than by some illness, after many other diseases, producing just the sum of exhaustion necessary for death. There is nothing so absurd, nothing so misleading as the verdict one so often hears: So-and-so has no organic disease – there is no reason why he should not live to extreme old age; sometimes the clause is added, sometimes not: Provided he has quiet, good food, good air, etc., etc., etc.: the verdict is repeated by ignorant people *without* the latter clause; or there is no possibility of the conditions of the latter clause being obtained; and this, the *only* essential part of the whole, is made of no effect. I have heard a physician, deservedly eminent, assure the friends of a patient of his recovery. Why? Because he had now prescribed a course, every detail of which the patient had followed for years. And because he had forbidden a course which the patient could not by any possibility alter.

...

In Life Insurance and such like societies, were they instead of having the person examined by the medical man, to have the houses, conditions, ways of life, of these persons examined, at how much truer results would they arrive! W. Smith appears a fine hale man, but it might be known that the next cholera epidemic he runs a bad chance. Mr and Mrs J. are a strong healthy couple, but it might be known that they live in such a house, in such a part of London, so near the river that they will kill four-fifths of their children; which of the children will be the ones to survive might also be known.

Averages again seduce us away from minute observation. 'Average mortalities' merely tell that so many per cent die in this town and so many in that, per annum. But whether A or B will be among these, the 'average rate' of course does not tell. We know, say, that from 22 to 24 per 1,000 will die in London next year. But minute enquiries into conditions enable us to know that in such a district, nay, in such a street – or even on one side of that street, in such a particular house, or even on one floor of that particular house, will be the excess of mortality, that is, the person will die who ought not to have died before old age.

Now, would it not very materially alter the opinion of whoever were endeavouring to form one, if he knew that from that floor, of that house, of that street the man came.

Much more precise might be our observations even than this, and much more correct our conclusions.

It is well known that the same names may be seen constantly recurring on workhouse books for generations. That is, the persons were born and brought up, and will be born and brought up, generation after generation, in the conditions which make paupers. Death and disease are like the workhouse, they take from the same family, the same house, or in other words, the same conditions.

Why will we not observe what they are?

The close observer may safely predict that such a family, whether its members marry or not, will become extinct; that such another will degenerate morally and physically. But who learns the lesson? On the contrary, it may be well known that the children die in such a house at the rate of 8 out of 10; one would think that nothing more need be said; for how could Providence speak more distinctly? Yet nobody listens, the family goes on living there till it dies out, and then some other family takes it. Neither would they listen 'if one rose from the dead.'

In dwelling upon the vital importance of *sound* observation, it must never be lost sight of what observation is for. It is not for the sake of piling up miscellaneous information or curious facts, but for the sake of saving life and increasing health and comfort. The caution may seem useless, but it is quite surprising how many men (some women do it too), practically behave as if the scientific end were the only one in view, or as if the sick body were but a reservoir for stowing medicines into, and the surgical disease only a curious case the sufferer has made for the attendant's special information. This is really no exaggeration. You think, if you suspected your patient was being poisoned, say, by a copper kettle, you would instantly, as you ought, cut off all possible connection between him and the suspected source of injury, without regard to the fact that a curious mine of observation is thereby lost. But it is not everybody who does so, and it has actually been made a question of medical ethics, what should the medical man do if he suspected poisoning? The answer seems a very simple one – insist on a confidential nurse being placed with the patient, or give up the case.

Hospital Sketches
Louisa May Alcott (1863)

The first thing I met was a regiment of the vilest odors that ever assaulted the human nose, and took it by storm. Cologne, with its seven and seventy evil savors, was a posy-bed to it; and the worst of this affliction was, every one had assured me that it was a chronic weakness of all hospitals, and I must bear it. I did, armed with lavender water, with which I so besprinkled myself and premises, that, like my friend Sairy, I was soon known among my patients as 'the nurse with the bottle'. Having been run over by three excited surgeons, bumped against by migratory coal-hods, water-pails, and small boys, nearly scalded by an avalanche of newly-filled tea-pots, and hopelessly entangled in a knot of colored sisters coming to wash, I progressed by slow stages up stairs and down, till the main hall was reached, and I paused to take breath and a survey. There they were! 'our brave boys,' as the papers justly call them, for cowards could hardly have been so riddled with shot and shell, so torn and shattered, nor have borne suffering for which we have no name, with an uncomplaining fortitude, which made one glad to cherish each as a brother. In they came, some on stretchers, some in men's arms, some feebly staggering along propped on rude crutches, and one lay stark and still with covered face, as a comrade gave his name to be recorded before they carried him away to the dead house. All was hurry and confusion; the hall was full of these wrecks of humanity, for the most exhausted could not reach a bed till duly ticketed and registered; the walls were lined with rows of such as could sit, the floor covered with the more disabled, the steps and doorways filled with helpers and lookers on; the sound of many feet and voices made that usually quiet hour as noisy as noon; and, in the midst of it all, the matron's motherly face brought more comfort to many a poor soul, than the cordial draughts she administered, or the cheery words that welcomed all, making of the hospital a home.

The sight of several stretchers, each with its legless, armless, or desperately wounded occupant, entering my ward, admonished me that I was there to work, not to wonder or weep; so I corked up my feelings, and returned to the path of duty, which was rather 'a hard road to travel' just then. The house had been a hotel before hospitals were needed, and many of the doors still bore their old names; some not so inappropriate as might be imagined, for my ward was in truth a *ball-room*, if gun-shot wounds could christen it. Forty beds were prepared, many already tenanted by tired men who fell down anywhere, and drowsed till the smell of food roused them. Round the great stove was gathered the dreariest group I ever saw – ragged, gaunt and pale, mud to the knees, with bloody bandages untouched since put on days before; many bundled up in blankets, coats being lost or useless; and all wearing that disheartened look which proclaimed defeat, more plainly than any telegram of the Burnside blunder.[82] I pitied them so much, I dared not speak to them, though, remembering all they had been through since the route at Fredericksburg, I yearned to serve the dreariest of them all.

...

'I say, Mrs!' called a voice behind me; and, turning, I saw a rough Michigander, with an arm blown off at the shoulder, and two or three bullets still in him – as he afterwards mentioned, as carelessly as if gentlemen were in the habit of carrying such trifles about with them. I went to him, and, while administering a dose of soap and water, he whispered, irefully:

'That red-headed devil, over yonder, is a reb, damn him! You'll agree to that, I'll bet? He's got shet of a foot, or he'd a cut like the rest of the lot. Don't you wash him, nor feed him, but jest let him holler till he's tired. It's a blasted shame to fetch them fellers in here, along side of us; and so I'll tell the chap that bosses this concern; cuss me if I don't.'

I regret to say that I did not deliver a moral sermon upon the duty of forgiving our enemies, and the sin of profanity, then and there; but, being a red-hot Abolitionist, stared fixedly at the tall rebel, who was a copperhead, in every sense of the word, and privately resolved to put soap in his eyes, rub his nose the wrong way, and excoriate his cuticle generally, if I had the washing of him.

My amiable intentions, however, were frustrated; for, when I approached, with as Christian an expression as my principles would allow, and asked the question – 'Shall I try to make you more comfortable, sir?' all I got for my pains was a gruff – 'No; I'll do it myself.'

---

[82]The Battle of Fredericksburg was fought between 11 and 15 December 1862, in and around Fredericksburg, Virginia, between General Robert E. Lee's Confederate Army of Northern Virginia and the Union Army of the Potomac, commanded by Major General Ambrose Burnside. Burnside ordered multiple frontal assaults against enemy positions on Marye's Heights, all of which were repulsed with heavy losses. On 15 December, Burnside withdrew his army, ending another failed Union campaign.

'Here's your Southern chivalry, with a witness,' thought I, dumping the basin down before him, thereby quenching a strong desire to give him a summary baptism, in return for his ungraciousness; for my angry passions rose, at this rebuff, in a way that would have scandalized good Dr Watts. He was a disappointment in all respects, (the rebel, not the blessed Doctor), for he was neither fiendish, romantic, pathetic, or anything interesting; but a long, fat man, with a head like a burning bush, and a perfectly expressionless face: so I could dislike him without the slightest drawback, and ignored his existence from that day forth. One redeeming trait he certainly did possess, as the floor speedily testified; for his ablutions were so vigorously performed, that his bed soon stood like an isolated island, in a sea of soap-suds, and he resembled a dripping merman, suffering from the loss of a fin. If cleanliness is a near neighbor to godliness, then was the big rebel the godliest man in my ward that day.

...

All having eaten, drank, and rested, the surgeons began their rounds; and I took my first lesson in the art of dressing wounds. It wasn't a festive scene, by any means; for Dr P., whose Aid I constituted myself, fell to work with a vigor which soon convinced me that I was a weaker vessel, though nothing would have induced me to confess it then. He had served in the Crimea, and seemed to regard a dilapidated body very much as I should have regarded a damaged garment; and, turning up his cuffs, whipped out a very unpleasant looking housewife,[83] cutting, sawing, patching and piecing, with the enthusiasm of an accomplished surgical seamstress; explaining the process, in scientific terms, to the patient, meantime; which, of course, was immensely cheering and comfortable. There was an uncanny sort of fascination in watching him, as he peered and probed into the mechanism of those wonderful bodies, whose mysteries he understood so well. The more intricate the wound, the better he liked it. A poor private, with both legs off, and shot through the lungs, possessed more attractions for him than a dozen generals, slightly scratched in some 'masterly retreat;' and had any one appeared in small pieces, requesting to be put together again, he would have considered it a special dispensation.

The amputations were reserved till the morrow, and the merciful magic of ether was not thought necessary that day, so the poor souls had to bear their pains as best they might. It is all very well to talk of the patience of woman; and far be it from me to pluck that feather from her cap, for, heaven knows, she isn't allowed to wear many; but the patient endurance of these men, under trials of the flesh, was truly wonderful. Their fortitude seemed contagious, and scarcely a cry escaped them, though I often longed to groan for them, when pride kept their white lips shut, while great drops stood upon their foreheads, and the bed shook with the irrepressible tremor of their tortured bodies. One or two Irishmen anathematized the doctors with the frankness of their nation, and ordered the Virgin to stand by them, as if she had been the wedded Biddy to whom they could administer the poker, if she didn't; but, as a general thing, the work went on in silence, broken only by some quiet request for roller, instruments, or plaster, a sigh from the patient, or a sympathizing murmur from the nurse.

---

[83]Housewife: a small sewing kit.

It was long past noon before these repairs were even partially made; and, having got the bodies of my boys into something like order, the next task was to minister to their minds, by writing letters to the anxious souls at home; answering questions, reading papers, taking possession of money and valuables; for the eighth commandment was reduced to a very fragmentary condition, both by the blacks and whites, who ornamented our hospital with their presence. Pocket books, purses, miniatures, and watches, were sealed up, labelled, and handed over to the matron, till such times as the owners thereof were ready to depart homeward or campward again. The letters dictated to me, and revised by me, that afternoon, would have made an excellent chapter for some future history of the war; for, like that which Thackeray's 'Ensign Spooney'[84] wrote his mother just before Waterloo, they were 'full of affection, pluck, and bad spelling;' nearly all giving lively accounts of the battle, and ending with a somewhat sudden plunge from patriotism to provender, desiring 'Marm,' 'Mary Ann,' or 'Aunt Peters,' to send along some pies, pickles, sweet stuff, and apples, 'to yourn in haste,' Joe, Sam, or Ned, as the case might be.

The Old Humanities and the New Science[85]
William Osler (1919)

Though small in number, your group [the British Classical Association] has an enormous kinetic value, like our endocrine organs. For man's body, too, is a humming hive of working cells, each with its specific function, all under central control of the brain and heart, and all dependent on materials called hormones (secreted by small, even insignificant-looking structures) which lubricate the wheels of life. For example, remove the thyroid gland just below the Adam's apple, and you deprive man of the lubricants which enable his thought-engines to work – it is as if you cut off the oil-supply of a motor – and gradually the stored acquisitions of his mind cease to be available, and within a year he sinks into dementia. The normal processes of the skin cease, the hair falls, the features bloat, and the paragon of animals is transformed into a shapeless caricature of humanity. These essential lubricators, of which a number are now known, are called hormones – you will recognize from its derivation how appropriate is the term.[86]

...

One of the marvels, so commonplace that it has ceased to be marvellous, is the deep rooting of our civilization in the soil of Greece and Rome – much of our dogmatic religion, practically all the philosophies, the models of our literature, the ideals of our democratic freedom, the fine and the technical arts, the fundamentals of science, and the basis of our law. The Humanities bring the student into contact with the master minds who gave us these things – with the dead who never die, with those immortal lives 'not of now nor of yesterday, but which always were'.

...

---

[84]Ensign Spooney is a character in William Makepeace Thackeray's satirical mid-Victorian novel *Vanity Fair*.
[85]This was Osler's Presidential Address to the Classical Association.
[86]'Hormone' is derived from the Greek *hormon*, meaning 'that which sets in motion'.

The so-called Humanists have not enough Science, and Science sadly lacks the Humanities. This unhappy divorce, which should never have taken place, has been officially recognized in the two reports edited by Sir Frederic Kenyon,[87] which have stirred the pool, and cannot but be helpful. To have got constructive, anabolic action from representatives of interests so diverse is most encouraging. While all agree that neither in the public schools nor in the older universities are the conditions at present in keeping with the urgent scientific needs of the nation, the specific is not to be sought in endowments alone, but in the leaven which may work a much needed change in both branches of knowledge.

...

In Gulliver's voyage to Laputa he paid a visit to the little island of Glubbdubdrib, whose Governor, you remember, had an Endorian command over the spirits, such as Sir Oliver Lodge or Sir Arthur Conan Doyle might envy.[88] When Aristotle and his commentators were summoned, to Gulliver's surprise they were strangers, for the reason that having so horribly misrepresented Aristotle's meaning to posterity, a consciousness of guilt and shame kept them far away from him in the lower world. Such shame, I fear, will make the shades of many classical dons of this university seek shelter with the commentators when they realize their neglect of one of the most fruitful of all the activities of the Master. In biology Aristotle speaks for the first time the language of modern science, and indeed he seems to have been first and foremost a biologist, and his natural history studies influenced profoundly his sociology, his psychology, and his philosophy in general... He must be indeed a dull and muddy-mettled rascal whose imagination is not fired by the enthusiastic – yet true – picture of the founder of modern biology, whose language is our language, whose methods and problems are our own, the man who knew a thousand varied forms of life, – of plant, of bird, and animal, – their outward structure, their metamorphosis, their early development; who studied the problems of heredity, of sex, of nutrition, of growth, of adaptation, and of the struggle for existence'.

...

It is important to recognize that there is nothing mysterious in the method of science or apart from the ordinary routine of life. Science has been defined as the habit or faculty of observation. By such the child grows in knowledge, and in its daily exercise an adult lives and moves. Only a quantitative difference makes observation scientific – accuracy; in that way alone do we discover things as they really are. This is the essence of Plato's definition of science as 'the discovery of things as they really are,' whether in the heavens above, in the earth beneath, or in the observer himself. As a mental operation, the scientific method is equally applicable to deciphering

---

[87]Sir Frederic George Kenyon, GBE, KCB, TD, FBA, FSA (1863–1952), was a British palaeographer and Biblical and classical scholar.
[88]Jonathan Swift's satirical *Gulliver's Travels* (1726) includes a voyage to Laputa, a place where science is pursued for no practical or beneficial purpose. The physicist Sir Oliver Lodge and the writer Sir Arthur Conan Doyle were both spiritualists who viewed spirit communication as similar to work on electricity and radio waves.

a bit of Beneventan script,[89] to the analysis of the evidence of the Commission on Coal-Mines, a study of the mechanism of the nose-dive, or of the colour-scheme in tiger-beetles. To observation and reasoned thought, the Greek added experiment, but never fully used it in biology, an instrument which has made science productive, and to which the modern world owes its civilization.

...

The extraordinary development of modern science may be her undoing. Specialism, now a necessity, has fragmented the specialities themselves in a way that makes the outlook hazardous. The workers lose all sense of proportion in a maze of minutiae. Everywhere men are in small coteries intensely absorbed in subjects of deep interest, but of very limited scope. Chemistry, a century ago an appanage[90] of the Chair of Medicine or even of Divinity, has now a dozen departments, each with its laboratory and literature, sometimes its own society. Applying themselves early to research, young men get into backwaters far from the main stream. They quickly lose the sense of proportion, become hypercritical, and the smaller the field, the greater the tendency to megalocephaly.[91] The study for fourteen years of the variations in the colour scheme of the thirteen hundred species of tiger-beetles scattered over the earth may sterilize a man into a sticker of pins and a paster of labels; on the other hand, he may be a modern biologist whose interest is in the experimental modification of types, and in the mysterious insulation of hereditary characters from the environment. Only in one direction does the modern specialist acknowledge his debt to the dead languages. Men of science pay homage, as do no others, to the god of words whose magic power is nowhere so manifest as in the plastic language of Greece. The only visit many students pay to Parnassus is to get an intelligible label for a fact or form newly discovered.

---

[89]The medieval Beneventan script has typography that is almost indecipherable to modern readers.
[90]Appanage: adjunct.
[91]Megalocephaly: a condition in which the head is abnormally large.

CHAPTER SEVEN

Sex, Evolution, Genetics and Reproduction

Upon the Sight of my Abortive Birth the 31st December 1657
Mary Carey (1658)

What birth is this; a poore despissed creature?
    A little Embrio; voyd of life, and feature:

Seven tymes I went my tyme; when mercy giving
    deliverance unto me; & mine all living:

Stronge, right-proportioned, lovely Girles, & boyes
    There fathers; Mother's present hope't for Joyes:

That was great wisedome, goodnesse, power love praise
    to my deare lord; lovely in all his wayes:

This is no lesse; ye same God hath it donne;
    submits my hart, thats better than a sonne:

In giveing; taking; stroking; striking still;
    his Glorie & my good; is. his. my will:

In that then; this now; both good God most mild,
    his will's more deare to me; then any Child:

I also joy, that God hath gain'd one more;
    To Praise him in the heavens; then was before:

And that this babe (as well as all the rest,)
    since 't had a soule, shal be for ever blest:

That I'm made Instrumentall; to both thes;
    God's praise, babes blesse; it highly doth me please;

May be the Lord lookes for more thankfulnesse,
    and highe esteeme for [of] those I doe posesse:

As limners drawe dead shadds for to sett forth;
    ther lively coullers, & theyr picturs worth;

So doth my God; in this, as all things; wise;
    by my dead formlesse babe; teach me to prise:

My living prety payre; Nat: & Bethia;
    the Childrene deare, (God yett lends to Maria:)

Praisd be his name; thes tow's full Compensation:
    For all thats gone; & yt in Expectation:

And if heere in God hath fulfill'd his Will,
    his hand-maides pleassed, Compleately happy still:

I only now desire of my sweet God
    the reason why he tooke in hand his rodd?

What he doth spy; what is the thinge amisse
    I faine would learne, whilst I ye rod do kisse:

Methinkes I heare Gods voyce, this is thy [the] sinne;
    And Conscience justified ye same within:

Thou often dost present me wth dead frute;
    Why should not my returns, thy presents sute:

Dead dutys; prayers; praises thou dost bring,
    affections dead; dead hart in every thinge;

In hearing; reading; Conference; Meditation;
    in acting graces & in Conversation:

Whose taught or better'd by ye no Relation;
    thou'rt Cause of Mourning, not of Immitation:

Thou doest not answere that great meanes I give;
    my word, and ordinances do teache to live:

Lively: o do't, thy mercyes are most sweet;
    Chastisements sharpe; & all ye meanes that's meet:

Mend now my Child, & lively frute bring me;
    so thou advantag'd much by this wilt be;

My dearest Lord; thy Charge, & more is true;
    I see't; am humbled, and for pardon sue;

In Christ forgive; & henceforth I will be
    what, Nothing Lord; but what thou makest mee;

I am nought, have nought, can doe nought but sinne;
    as my Experience saith, for I'ave ben in:

Several Condissions, tryalls great and many;
  in all I find my nothingness; not any

Thing doe I owne but sinne; Christ is my all;
  that I doe want, can crave; or ever shall:

That good that suteth all my whole desires;
  and for me unto God, all he requires;

It is in Christ; he's mine, and I am his;
  this union is my only happynesse:

But lord since I'm a Child by mercy free;
  Let me by filiall frutes much honnor thee;

I'm a branch of the vine; purge me therefore;
  father, more frute to bring, then heertofore;

A plant in God's house; O that I may be;
  more flourishing in age; a grouing tree:

Let not my hart, (as doth my wombe) miscarrie;
  but precious meanes received, lett it tarie;

Till it be form'd; of Gosplc shape, & sute;
  my meanes, my mercyes, & be pleasant frute:

In my whole Life, lively doe thou make me:
  for thy praise. And name's sake, O quicken mee[1];

Lord I begg quikning grace; that grace aford;
  quicken mee lord according to thy word:

It is a lovely bonne I make to thee.
  after thy loving Kindness quicken mee:

Thy quickning Spirit unto me convey;
  and therby Quicken me; in thine owne way:

And let the Presence of thy spirit deare,
  be wittnessd by his fruts; lett them appeare;

To, & for the; Love; Joy; peace; Gentlenesse;
  longsuffering; goodnesse; faith & meeknesse,

And lett my walking in the Spirit say,
  I live in't & desire it to Obey:

And since my hart thou'st lifted up to the;
  amend it Lord; & keepe it still with thee.

---

[1]Quickening referred to the moment in pregnancy when the woman became aware of the fetus.

from *Dildoides*
Samuel Butler (att.) (1706)

> *Occasioned by a burning of a hogshead of those commodities at Stocks Market,*
> *in the year 1672, pursuant to an Act of Parliament then made for the prohibiting*
> *of French goods.*

Such a sad Tale prepare to hear,
As claims from either Sex a Tear.
Twelve Dildoes (means for the Support
Of aged Lechers of the Court)
Were lately burnt by impious Hand
Of trading Rascals of the Land,
Who envying their curious Frame,
Exposed these *Priapuses* to the flame.
Oh! barbarous Times! where Deities
Are made themselves a Sacrifice.
Some were compos'd of shining Horns,
More precious than ten Unicorns.
Some were of Wax, where every Vein,
And every Fibre, were made plain.
Some were for tender Virgins fit,
Some for the wide salacious slit
Of a rank Lady, tho' so torn,
She hardly feels when Child is born.

Dildoe has Nose, but cannot smell,
No Stink can his great Courage quell;
At sight of Plaister he'd ne'er fail,
Nor faintly ask, What do you ail?
Women must have both Youth and Beauty,
E're – the damn'd Rogue will do his Duty,
And then sometimes he will not stand to
Do what Gallant or Mistress can do.

But I too long have left my Heroes,
Who fell into worse hands than *Nero's*;
Twelve of them shut up in a Box,
Martyrs as true as are in *Fox*,[2]
Were seiz'd upon as Goods forbidden,
Deep under lawful Traffick, hidden,
When Counsel grave, of deepest Beard,
Were call'd from out the City Herd:

---

[2]The *Actes and Monuments*, popularly known as *Foxe's Book of Martyrs*, is a work of Protestant history and martyrology by John Foxe, first published in English in 1563 by John Day. It includes a polemic on the sufferings of Protestants under the Catholic Church, with particular emphasis on England and Scotland.

But see the Fate of cruel Treachery,
Those Goats in Head, but not in Lechery,
Forgetting each his Wife and Daughter,
Condemn'd these *Dildoes* to the Slaughter:
Cuckolds with Rage were blinded so,
They did not their Preservers know.
One less Fanatic than the rest,
Stood up, and thus himself address'd:

These *Dildoes* may do Harm, I know,
But pray what is it may not so?
Plenty has often made Men proud,
And above Law advanc'd the Crowd:
Religion's Self has ruin'd Nations,
And causéd vast Depopulations,
Yet no wise People have refus'd it,
Because Fools sometimes abus'd it:
Unless you fear some merry Grigs
Will wear false P----s as Perriwigs,
And being but to small Ones born,
Will great Ones have of Wax and Horn.
Since even that promotes our Gain,
Methinks unjustly we complain,
If Ladies rather chuse to handle
Our wax in *Dildoe,* than in Candle,
Much good may't do 'em, for they pay for't,
And that the Merchant never stay for't:
For, Neighbours, is't not all one whether
In P----s or Shoes they wear our Leather?
Whether of Horn they make a Comb,
Or Instrument to chafe the Womb.
Like you, I Monsieur *Dildoe* hate,
But the Invention let's translate.
You treat 'em may like *Turks* and *Jews*,
But I'll have two for my own Use.
Priapus[3] was a *Roman* Deity,
And such has been the World's Variety;
I am resolv'd I'll none provoke,
From the humble Garlick to the Oak.
He paus'd, another strait stept in,
With limber – P----k and grisly Chin,
And thus did his harangue begin:

---

[3]In Greek mythology, Priapus was a fertility god, and the protector of livestock, fruit plants, gardens and male genitalia. Priapus is marked by his oversized, permanent erection, which gave rise to the medical term 'priapism', signifying painful and permanent erection.

For Soldiers maim'd by Chance of War,
We artificial Limbs prepare:
Why then should we bear such a Spite
To Lechers maim'd in amorous Fight?
That what the *French* send for Relief,
We thus condemn as witch or thief?
By *Dildoes*, Monsieur sure intends
For his *French*-Pox to make amends;
For such, without the least Disgrace
May well supply the lover's place,
And make our elder Girls ne'er care for't,
Tho' 'twere their Fortune to dance bare-foot.
Lechers, whom Clap or Drink disable,
Might here have *Dildoes* to their Navel.
And with False Heat and Member too,
Rich Widow for Convenience woo.
Did not a Lady of great Honour
Marry a Footman waiting on her?
When one of these timely apply'd,
Had eas'd her Lust, and sav'd her Pride,
Safely her Ladyship might have spent,
While such Gallants in Pocket went.
Honour itself might use the Trade,
While – *Pego* goes in masquerade.[4]
Which of us able to prevent is
His Girl from lying with his 'Prentice,
Unless we other Means provide
For Nature to be satisfy'd?
And what more proper than this Engine,
Which would out-do 'em, should three Men join.
I therefore hold it very foolish,
Things so convenient to abolish;
Which if you burn, we safely may
To that one Act the Ruin lay,
Of all that cast themselves away.

from *Callipaedia, or the Art of Getting Beautiful Children*
Claude Quillet (1710 ed.)[5]

Through strange Meanders and a wandering Maze,
The sprightly Seed, that forms all human Race,
Spreads the warm Flood, whose mingl'd Streams contain

---

[4]Pego: penis.
[5]Trans. William Oldisworth.

What e'er Infections in the Body reign,
Conveying all the noxious Humours down,
From the weak Father, to the sickly Son;
Oft have I seen a poor distemper'd Heir,
Condemn'd his Parents, Sins and Sores to wear,
Load with thick Curses the degenerate Name,
And on the undeserving Gods exclaim;
Let then the well-match'd Pair be fitly join'd,
A healthful Body and an equal Mind,
No happy Progeny shall crown the Bed
Curst with Decay, or with Diseases spread;
The Hind that hopes a Crop from *Ceres*'[6] Hand,
To chear his Household, and to crown his Land,
Chuses the fairest and the brightest Seeds,
And these along the fruitful Furrows spreads;
With the same Care the Harvest of Mankind,
Would yield a Race more noble and refin'd;
Sure, well thou knowest, that Man was form'd to bear
The God like Image of the Thunderer,
To search the Stars, and Heav'nly Secrets know,
And reign sole Monarch in the World below.
Ye Pow'rs, that Guard the genial Bed, and bless
The teeming Earth with Beauty and Increase,
Drive from your Rites and from your Altars far,
The impotent, the Weak, unhealthy Pair,
Left in their Pains their wretched Offspring share,
And by Descent made sickly and unsound,
Their Parents Ghosts with impious Curses wound;
And thou, dread Sire of Gods and Men, support
The sinking World, and from thy awful Court
Send a new Genius o'er the Globe, to raise
The grovelling Kind, and Nature's last Decays:
Then, future Ages shall the Art improve,
And a fair Offspring crown the Joys of Love.
...
How base is he, a Foe to Venus' Pow'r,
Who Riches courts, and doats upon a Dow'r;
On him these Rules are lost, whose lustful Eyes
Seek, for a loving Bride, a golden Prize:
The Churl that Boasts his Bags and spacious Lands,
When bent on Marriage, every Heart commands,

---

[6]In ancient Roman religion, Ceres was a goddess of agriculture, grain crops, fertility and motherly relationships.

The Parents sue, the Virgin trembling stands
And weds a sordid Lump of lifeless Clay,
Curst with Old-Age, and impotent Decay,
Condemn'd perhaps to Sickness, Sores and Pains,
Or to Ill-Nature and eternal Chains.
She hates, but must consent: The nobler Part
Is lost, she gives her Hand, and keeps her Heart.
At Rites like these, no kindly Pow'r appears,
But Discontent, and Grief, and flowing Tears
Wait round the nuptial Bed, the tedious Nights
Pass in imperfect Joys, and vain Delights:
In Beauty she, as he in Strength decays,
Despairing to renew a wretched Race:
The sighing Bride her fading Charms bemoans,
And all the Dotards pall'd Endearments shuns:
But if Revenge and Love by turns inspire,
And prompt an injur'd Wife to loose Desire,
(For Vows and nuptial Ties can never long,
Unite the fair and foul, the old and young)
Then the Town Sparks and gay Gallants repair,
To give her nobler Joys, and him an Heir;
Hence a mixt Offspring, and a motly Race,
With each a diff'rent Sire, and diff'rent Face,
Whose every Look the Mother's Guilt betrays:
This Child a Martial Air and Boldness shows,
And has the *Captain's* Forehead, and his Nose:
Another's like the Merchant and the Citt:
The Footman this resembles, that the Knight:
Thus the dull Dotard's Wealth and numerous Stores,
Laid up by wise and careful Ancestors,
Must now be heap'd upon another's Son,
And all descend to Children not his own.

These Ills, which private Families bewail,
Oft reach to Kings, and o'er the Throne prevail,
From a distemper'd Monarch's lazy Loves,
And sickly Arms, the wanton Queen removes,
And with impatient Hopes of Issue led,
Mounts a less noble and more vigorous Bed:
Hence doubtful Princes rise, pernicious Brood,
In vain the Laws legitimate their Blood,
No Virtues in the Bastard Monarch shine,
Nor is his Person, or his Right Divine:
Beneath his Yoke the luckless Nation mourns,
Who, since not born a King, a Tyrant turns.

The stale decaying Dame, whose aged Brows
Time in a thousand furrow'd Wrinkles plows,
Whose swimming Eyes distil eternal Brine,
Whose *Indian* Teeth the burnish'd Jett outshine,
Rich in the Spoils of some departed Spouse,
Draws a whole Train of Lovers to her House:
And when Catarrhs the amorous Heat excite,
And Love and *Hymen* both their Pow'rs unite,
The Youths all sigh, and flatter, and adore,
Smit with the Charms and Beauties of her Dow'r:
A sprightly Spark, more happy than the rest,
With strong *Ideas* of her Wealth possest,
Finds the short Passage to her aged Breast:
Him to her Arms and Fortune she receives,
And round her mouldring Trunk the Lover cleaves,
And when possest of all, the Passion o'er,
The Wealth and Woman both within his Pow'r
With Age, and Love, and Matrimony cloy'd,
The Dow'r too little, Wife so much enjoy'd,
He rambles through the Sex, the young and fair
Usurp her Pleasures, and her Husband share.
To these with lavish Hands the Rover grants,
The Wealth she gave him, and the Joys she wants;
On the cold Bed lies the forsaken Dame,
Dissolv'd in Tears: The once soft am'rous Flame
Turns to a jealous Rage, whose Transports rouse
And injur'd Bride to punish slighted Vows,
And wreak just Vengeance on a hateful Spouse;
The Fury that so haunts and gnaws her Soul,
Soon guides her Hand to the envenom'd Bowel,
That quickly rids her of the fell Disease,
And kills the Heart she can no more possess.

from *The Economy of Love*
John Armstrong (1745 ed.)

If to progeny thy views extend
Paternal, and the name of Sire invites,
Wouldst thou behold a thriving Race surround
Thy spacious Table, shun the soft Embrace
Emasculent, till twice ten years and more
Have steel'd thy Nerves, and let the holy Rite
License the Bliss. Nor would I urge, precise,
A total Abstinence; this might unman
The genial Organs, unemploy'd so long,

And quite extinguish the prolific Flame,
Refrigerant. But riot oft unblam'd,
On Kisses, sweet repast! ambrosial joy!
Now press with gentle hand the gentle hand,
And, sighing, now the Breasts, that to the touch
Heave amorous. Nor thou, fair Maid, refuse
Indulgence, while thy Paramour discreet
Aspires no farther. Thus thou mayst expect
Treasure hereafter, when the Bridegroom, warm,
Trembling with keen Desire, profusely pours
The rich Collection of enamour'd years;
Exhaustless, blessing all thy nuptial Nights.

But O my Son, whether the generous care
Of Propagation and domestic Charge,
Or soft Encounter more attract, renounce
The Vice of Monks recluse, the early Bane
Of rising Manhood. Banish from thy Shades
Th'ungenerous, selfish, solitary Joy.
Hold, Parricide, thy hand! For thee alone
Did Nature form thee? for thy narrow self
Grant thee the means of Pleasure? Dream'st thou so?
...
A train
Of ills of tedious count and horrid name.
Such as of old distress'd the Man else squar'd
To God's own heart, but that he wide debauch'd
Jersualem fair Daughters to his Flames
Unquench'd; nor from the holy Marriage bed
Refrain'd his loose Embraces, when the Wife
Of wrong'd *Urias*[7] he seduc'd; nor stopt
Till Murder crown'd his Lust. Hence him the Wrath
Of righteous Heaven, awaking, long pursu'd
With sore Disease, and fill'd his Loins with Pain.
All Day he roar'd, and all the tedious Night
Bedew'd his Couch with Tears; and still his Groans
Breathe musical in sacred Song. What Woes!
What Pains he try'd! But now this Plague attacks
With double rancour, and severely marks
Modern Offenders: undermines at once

---

[7]In the Bible, Urias (Uriah) was an officer in the Israelite army and the husband of Bathsheba. He was sent to die in battle so that David could marry his wife.

The Fame and Nose, that by unseemly Lapse,
Awkward deforms the human Face divine
With ghastly Ruins. Tho' this Breach, they say,
Nice *Taliacotius*'[8] Art, with substitute
From Porters borrow'd, or the callous Breech
Of sedentary Weaver, oft repair'd,
Precarious; for no sooner Fate demands
The parent Stock, than (pious Sympathy!)
Revolts th'adopted Nose – Such Ills attend
Th'obscene Embrace of Harlots.

...

But in these vicious Days great *Nature*'s Laws
Are spurn'd; eternal *Virtue*, which no Time
Nor Place can change, nor Custom changing all,
Is mock'd to scorn; and *lewd Abuse* instead,
Daughter of Night, her shameless Revels holds
O'er half the Globe, while the chaste Face of Day
Eclipses at her Rites. For Man with Man,
And Man with Woman, (monstrous to relate!)
Leaving the natural Road, themselves debase
With Deeds unseemly and Dishonour foul.
Britons, for shame! be Male and Female still.
Banish this foreign Vice; it grows not here;
It dies neglected; and in Clime so chaste
Cannot but by forc'd Cultivation thrive.
So cultivated swells the more our Shame,
The more our Guilt. And shall not greater Guilt
Meet greater Punishment and heavier Doom?
Not lighter for Delay. Did Justice spare
The Men of *Sodom*[9] erst? Like us they sinn'd,
Like us they sought the Paths of monstrous Joy;
Till, urg'd to Wrath at last, all-patient Heaven
Descending, wrapt them in sulphureous Storm;
And where proud Palaces appear'd, the Haunts
Of Luxury, now sleeps a sullen Pool:
Vengeful Memorial of almighty Ire,
Against the Sons of Lewdness exercis'd!

---

[8]Gaspar Taliacotius (1546–99) was professor of medicine and anatomy in the university of Bologna. He practised the art of restoring lost body parts, particularly the nose.

[9]In Genesis, the Hebrew Bible, the New Testament and the Qur'an, Sodom and Gomorrah were two of the five 'cities of the plain', situated on the plain of the River Jordan in the southern region of Canaan. God passed judgment on the sinning cities, and they were consumed by fire and brimstone.

Poems from Aristotle's Masterpiece
Pseudo-Aristotle (1784 ed.)[10]

'The parts of Generation in men and women'

And thus man's nobler parts we see,
For such the parts of generation be;
And they that carefully survey will find
Each part is fitted for the use design'd.
The purest blood, we find, if well we heed,
is in the testicles turn'd into seed.
Which by most proper channels is transmitted
Into the place by Nature for it fitted;
With highest sense of pleasure to excite
In amorous combatants the more delight.
For Nature does in this work design
Profit and pleasure in one act to join.

Thus the woman's secrets I have survey'd
And let them see how curiously they're made.
And that, though they of different sexes be,
Yet in the whole they are the same as we.
For those that have the strictest searchers been,
Find women are but men turn'd outside in:
And men, if they but cast their eyes about,
May find they're women with their inside out.

Thus Nature nothing does in vain produce,
But fits each part for what's its proper use;
And though of different sexes formed we be,
Yet betwixt these there is that unity,
That we in nothing can a greater find,
Unless the soul that's to the body joined:
And sure in this Dame Nature's in the right,
The strictest union yields the most delight.

'Carnal Copulation'

Who to forbidden pleasures are inclin'd
Will find at last they leave a sting behind.

---

[10]We have chosen the 1784 edition here, but the poems were composed and circulated earlier. Many versions and editions of this text were published from the late seventeenth century, and various authors contributed at certain times. This popular book is likely the most widely reprinted text on a medical subject in the eighteenth and early nineteenth century. For more on the various forms of *Aristotle's Masterpiece* and *The Works of Aristotle*, see Mary E. Fissell (2007), 'Hairy Women and Naked Truths: Gender and the Politics of Knowledge in Aristotle's Masterpiece', *The William and Mary Quarterly* 60(1), 43–74.

'Of Monsters and Monstrous Births'

Heaven in our first formation did provide
Two arms and legs: but what we have beside
Renders us monstrous and misshapen too,
Nor have we any work for them to do,
Two arms, two legs, are all that we can use,
And to have more there's no wise man will chuse.

Nature does to us sometimes Monsters show,
That we by them may our own Mercies know;
And thereby Sin's Deformity may see,
Than which there's nothing can more monstrous be.

from *Infancy, or the Management of Children*
Hugh Downman (1790)

'The lacteal springs; or, apostrophe to tender affection'

O luckless Babe, born in an evil hour!
Who shall thy numerous wants attend? explore
The latent cause of ill? thy slumbers guard?
And when awake, with nice sedulity
Thy every glance observe? A parent might;
A Hireling cannot; tho of blameless mind,
Tho conscious duty prompt her to the task,
She feels not in her breast th' impulsive goad
Of instinct, all the fond, the fearful thoughts
Awakening: Say, at length that habit's power
Can something like maternal kindness give,
Yet, ere that time, may the poor nursling die.
Besides, who can assure the lacteal springs
Clear, and untained? Oft disorder lurks
Beneath the vivid bloom, and cheerful eye,
Promising health; and poisonous juice secrete,
Slow undermining life, stains what should be
The purest nutriment. Hence, worse than death,
Long years of misery to thy blasted child.
A burthen to himself, by others shunn'd,
He wishes for the grave, and wastes his days
In solitary woe; or haply weds,
And propagates the hereditary plague;
Entailing on his name the bitter curse
Of generations yet unborn, a race
Pithless, and weak, of faded texture, wan;
Like some declining plant, with mildew'd leaves,

Whose root a treacherous insect gnaws unseen.

'Nature to be satisfied'

These truths regard;
By Nature heeded, when with care She form'd
The lacteal fluid; a peculiar Mixt,
Skilfully blended; by digestion due,
Or in it's winding passage thro the glands
Animalized, and render'd fit to tame
The ferment of acidity, to which
Childhood is prone. Whence we conclude, that now
When from the breast exiled, as far as Art
Her nicer laws can imitate, 'tis right
T' adapt it's food, and mingle aliment
Of alkalescent quality, with that
Which might t' incorrigible acid turn.

'The Confinement of Daughters'

Call'd by society to tread the paths
Of busy life, from it's hard slavery soon
The stronger Sex was freed; and ere too late,
Haply by Nature's potent air restored,
Could boast a frame of vigour unimpair'd,
And undeformed. But to long sufferings doom'd,
The female Race, so will'd perverted taste,
For many a year pined underneath the force
Of this domestic torture. For as erst
The Mother strove t' assist their infant nerves,
And give to weakness strength: She now assay'd
Her progeny t' embellish, and their shape
To mould, as fancied beauty in her eye
Deceptive shone. Heaven! that the human Mind
Warp'd by imagination, should believe,
Or e'en suggest it possible, the form,
Whose archetype the Deity Himself
Created in his image, could be changed
From it's divine proportion, and receive
By alteration, comeliness and grace!
That round the Zone which awkwardly reduced
E'en to an insect ligament the waist,
The blooming loves should sport, enticing charms,
And young attractions! Heaven! that e'er a Bard,
(The genuine Bard is Nature's sacred Priest)
Forgetful of his charge, should deck with praise
As fair and lovely, what would strike the soul

Unwarp'd by custom, as a subject fit
For scorn, indignant spleen, or ridicule.
Yet Prior![11] tho nor taste nor reason blend
Their essence with the verse, while lasts the tongue
Thy numbers help'd to polish, while the powers
Of melody bear sway, the verse shall live,
Beauteous description of a Gothic Shape.

Oh! may the manners of thy nut-brown Maid,
Her artless truth, simplicity of soul,
Her fondness, and intrepid constancy,
Long in the bosoms of the British Fair,
Tho banisht every other region, dwell,
Delighted inmates! May their eyes still beam
With all her speaking rays, their cheeks endue
Her modest crimson! But may never more
'The Boddice aptly laced' their panting hearts
Confine, or mutilate that symmetry
Of limb and figure, whence a Zeuxis' hand[12]
His all-accomplisht Helen might have form'd,
Or a Praxiteles with happiest art
Sculptured a Venus.[13] Tho Meridian day
Behold them drest as potent fashion bids,
Girt with exterior ornaments uncouth,
Trappings disgustful; yet at morn, or eve,
Or when they to the genial bed repair,
Still may they charm the melting eye of love
With elegance and grace, the fabled Dames
Of classic soil transcending, native grace,
And elegance unveil'd, which mocks attire.

'Exercise, Curiosity, the formation of Body and Mind'

Much hath Anatomy distinguish'd, much
Remains unknown; the rudiments of life
Who ever shall explore? Where dwells the Power
Inherent, or acquired, which first expands
The comprehensive germ? Which moulds, propells,
And inorganic fluid can convert
To animated fibre? In the Brain

---

[11] Matthew Prior (1664–1721) was an English poet, who wrote a poem based on the ballad 'The Nut-Brown Maid', which was included in Thomas Percy's *Reliques of Ancient English Poetry*.
[12] Zeuxis of Heraclea (5th century BC) was a Greek painter and pioneer of the ideal nude; allegedly, he could not find a woman beautiful enough to pose as Helen of Troy, so he painted a composite of various models.
[13] Praxiteles of Athens (4th century BC) was the most renowned of the Attic sculptors. He was the first to sculpt the nude female form in a life-size statue.

Does it reside? Or in the central Heart?
Or do they both their energy combine?
Is it subtle, elastic, and derived
From that ethereal Essence which perchance
All space informs, and every substance fills?
Or is it from the blood by wondrous means
Secreted, render'd volatile, sublimed,
A pure, peculiar spirit? From his state
Of vegetable torpor when released,
Whate'er it be, by this the Infant lives,
By this He moves; by this th' absorbents bear
Their nurture from the stomach to the veins,
The wasted blood's supply, whose finer parts
Perpetually exhale; this gives the lungs
To play, which from the circumambient air
It's vital principle inspire, and yield
Th' effete mephitic vapour back again.
This stimulates the heart, and by the heart
And irritated fibres is in turn
Excited, quicken'd, strengthen'd: This extends
The solids, and enlarges, hasting on
The circulating stream. This generates,
Or is of living Heat the copious fount,
Active while it exists, without it's aid
Soon changed to deadly cold. By this, the nerves
Of every various sense with speed convey
Each impulse to the Brain, infixing there
The indelible ideas, there arranged,
Connected, modified, they haply form
Or seem at least to form the Soul Itself,
Immortal, immaterial: Hence the stores
Of wisdom are establish'd; hence the flash
Of wit bursts forth; and hence with keenest glance
Imagination darts her eye throughout
This mundane space, pierces beyond its bounds,
And Worlds creates, and Beings all her own.

from *Temple of Nature*
Erasmus Darwin (1803)

'Non-sexual Reproduction'

Where no new Sex with glands nutritious feeds,
Nurs'd in her womb, the solitary breeds;
No Mother's care their early steps directs,
Warms in her bosom, with her wings protects;
The clime unkind, or noxious food instills

To embryon nerves hereditary ills;
The feeble births acquired diseases chase,
Till Death extinguish the degenerate race.

So grafted trees with shadowy summits rise,
Spread their fair blossoms, and perfume the skies;
Till canker taints the vegetable blood,
Mines round the bark, and feeds upon the wood.
So, years successive, from perennial roots
The wire or bulb with lessen'd vigour shoots;
Till curled leaves, or barren flowers, betray
A waning lineage, verging to decay;
Or till, amended by connubial powers,
Rise seedling progenies from sexual flowers.

'Sexual Selection and Inbreeding in Humans'
E'en where unmix'd the breed, in sexual tribes
Parental taints the nascent babe imbibes;
Eternal war the Gout and Mania wage
With fierce uncheck'd hereditary rage;

Sad Beauty's form foul Scrofula surrounds[14]
With bones distorted, and putrescent wounds;
And, fell Consumption! thy unerring dart[15]
Wets its broad wing in Youth's reluctant heart.

With pausing step, at night's refulgent noon,
Beneath the sparkling stars, and lucid moon,
Plung'd in the shade of some religious tower,
The slow bell counting the departed hour,
O'er gaping tombs where shed umbrageous Yews
On mouldering bones their cold unwholesome dews;
While low aerial voices whisper round,
And moondrawn spectres dance upon the ground;
Poetic Melancholy loves to tread,
And bend in silence o'er the countless Dead;
Marks with loud sobs infantine Sorrows rave,
And wring their pale hands o'er their Mother's grave;

Hears on the new-turn'd sod with gestures wild
The kneeling Beauty call her buried child;
Upbraid with timorous accents Heaven's decrees,
And with sad sighs augment the passing breeze.
'Stern Time,' She cries, 'receives from Nature's womb
Her beauteous births, and bears them to the tomb;

---

[14]Scrofula is the swelling of the cervical lymph nodes, associated with tuberculosis.
[15]Consumption, now called tuberculosis.

Calls all her sons from earth's remotest bourn,
And from the closing portals none return!'

Urania[16] paused – upturn'd her streaming eyes,
And her white bosom heaved with silent sighs;
With her the Muse laments the sum of things,
And hides her sorrows with her meeting wings;
Long o'er the wrecks of lovely Life they weep,
Then pleased reflect, 'to die is but to sleep;'
From Nature's coffins to her cradles turn,
Smile with young joy, with new affection burn.
'Sexual Love: Cupid and Psyche'

Now on broad pinions from the realms above
Descending Cupid seeks the Cyprian grove;
To his wide arms enamour'd Psyche springs,
And clasps her lover with aurelian wings.
A purple sash across His shoulder bends,
And fringed with gold the quiver'd shafts suspends;
The bending bow obeys the silken string,
And, as he steps, the silver arrows ring.
Thin folds of gauze with dim transparence flow
O'er Her fair forehead, and her neck of snow;
The winding woof her graceful limbs surrounds,
Swells in the breeze, and sweeps the velvet grounds;
As hand in hand along the flowery meads
His blushing bride the quiver'd hero leads;
Charm'd round their heads pursuing Zephyrs throng,[17]
And scatter roses, as they move along;
Bright beams of Spring in soft effusion play,
And halcyon Hours invite them on their way.

Delighted Hymen hears their whisper'd vows,
And binds his chaplets round their polish'd brows,
Guides to his altar, ties the flowery bands,
And as they kneel, unites their willing hands.
'Behold, he cries, Earth! Ocean! Air above,
And hail the Deities of Sexual Love!
All forms of Life shall this fond Pair delight,
And sex to sex the willing world unite;

Shed their sweet smiles in Earth's unsocial bowers,
Fan with soft gales, and gild with brighter hours;

---

[16]Darwin casts Urania, the classical muse of astronomy, as his scientific muse.
[17]In Greek mythology, Zephyr was the god of the west wind.

Fill Pleasure's chalice unalloy'd with pain,
And give Society his golden chain.'

Now young Desires, on purple pinions borne,
Mount the warm gales of Manhood's rising morn;
With softer fires through virgin bosoms dart,
Flush the pale cheek, and goad the tender heart.
Ere the weak powers of transient Life decay,
And Heaven's ethereal image melts away;
Love with nice touch renews the organic frame,
Forms a young Ens,[18] another and the same;
Gives from his rosy lips the vital breath,
And parries with his hand the shafts of death;
While Beauty broods with angel wings unfurl'd
O'er nascent life, and saves the sinking world.

To The Siamese Twins
Hannah F. Gould (1832)

Mysterious tie by the Hand above,
Which nothing below must part!
Thou visible image of faithful love,
Firm union of heart and heart;
The mind to her utmost bound may run,
And summon her light in vain
To scan the *twain* that must still be *one*;
The *one* that will still be *twain*!

The beat of this bosom forbears to reach
Where the other distinctly goes;
Yet, the stream that empurples the veins of each
Through the breast of his brother flows!
One grief must be felt by this two-fold mark,
As the points of a double dart;
And the joy lit up by a single spark
Is sunshine in either heart.

O wonder, to baffle poor human skill
In clay of the human mould!
But a greater mystery all must still,
In the union of souls, behold.
Ye are living harps, by your silken strings
In a heavenly concord bound;
And who o'er one but a finger flings

---

[18]Ens: an entity.

Awakens you both to sound.

But, what do you do when your slumbers come,
When ye've sweetly sunken to rest?
Do your spirits, side by side, fly home,
Still linked, to your mother's breast?
Did ye ever dream that your bond was broke;
That ye were asunder thrown?
And how did ye feel at the severing stroke,
When each was forever alone?

No – ye would not think of yourselves apart,
Even in fancy's wildest mood,
For each would seem but a broken heart,
And the world but a solitude!
Dear youths, may your lives be a flowery way,
And, watched by your Maker's eye,
May both, at the close, one call obey
To shine as twin stars on high!

'This is the female form', from I Sing the Body Electric
Walt Whitman (1867)

This is the female form;
A divine nimbus exhales from it from head to foot;
It attracts with fierce undeniable attraction!
I am drawn by its breath as if I were no more than a helpless vapor –
    all falls aside but myself and it;
Books, art, religion, time, the visible and solid earth, the atmosphere and
    the clouds, and what was expected of heaven or fear'd of hell, are now
    consumed;
Mad filaments, ungovernable shoots play out of it, the response likewise
    ungovernable!
Hair, bosom, hips, bend of legs, negligent falling hands, all diffused – mine
    too diffused;
Ebb stung by the flow, and flow stung by the ebb – love-flesh swelling and
    deliciously aching;
Limitless limpid jets of love hot and enormous, quivering jelly of love, white-
    blow and delirious juice;
Bridegroom night of love, working surely and softly into the prostrate dawn;
Undulating into the willing and yielding day,
Lost in the cleave of the clasping and sweet-flesh'd day.

This is the nucleus – after the child is born of woman, the man is born of
    woman;
This is the bath of birth – this is the merge of small and large, and the outlet
    again.

Be not ashamed, women – your privilege encloses the rest, and
    is the exit of the rest,
You are the gates of the body, and you are the gates of the soul.

The female contains all qualities, and tempers them – she is in her place,
    and moves with perfect balance;
She is all things duly veil'd – she is both passive and active;
She is to conceive daughters as well as sons, and sons as well as daughters.

As I see my soul reflected in nature;
As I see through a mist, one with inexpressible completeness and beauty,
See the bent head, and arms folded over the breast – the female I see.

The male is not less the soul, nor more – he too is in his place;
He too is all qualities – he is action and power;
The flush of the known universe is in him;
Scorn becomes him well, and appetite and defiance become him well;
The wildest largest passions, bliss that is utmost, sorrow that is utmost,
    become him well – pride is for him;
The full-spread pride of man is calming and excellent to the soul;
Knowledge becomes him – he likes it always – he brings everything to the
    test of himself;

Whatever the survey, whatever the sea and the sail, he strikes soundings at
    last only here;
Where else does he strike soundings, except here?

A Ballade of Evolution
Grant Allen (1881)

In the mud of the Cambrian main[19]
Did our earliest ancestor dive:
From a shapeless albuminous grain
We mortals our being derive.
He could split himself up into five,
Or roll himself round like a ball;
For the fittest will always survive,
While the weakliest go to the wall.

As an active ascidian again[20]
Fresh forms he began to contrive,
Till he grew to a fish with a brain
And brought forth a mammal alive.

---

[19]The Cambrian (c.541–c.485 m.y.a.) was the first geological period of the Paleozoic Era.
[20]Ascidians, or tunicates (sea squirts), are marine invertebrate filter feeders.

With his rivals he next had to strive,
To woo him a mate and a thrall;
So the handsomest managed to wive,
While the ugliest went to the wall.

At length as an ape he was fain
The nuts of the forest to rive;
Till he took to the low-lying plain,
And proceeded his fellow to knive.
Thus did cannibal men first arrive,
One another to swallow and maul;
And the strongest continued to thrive,
While the weakliest went to the wall.

from *Evolutionary Erotics*
Constance Woodhill Naden (1887)

Natural Selection

I had found out a gift for my fair,
I had found where the cave-men were laid;
Skull, femur, and pelvis were there,
And spears, that of silex they made.

But he ne'er could be true, she averred,
Who would dig up an ancestor's grave –
And I loved her the more when I heard
Such filial regard for the Cave.

My shelves, they are furnished with stones
All sorted and labelled with care,
And a splendid collection of bones,
Each one of them ancient and rare;

One would think she might like to retire
To my study – she calls it a 'hole!'
Not a fossil I heard her admire,
But I begged it, or borrowed, or stole.

But there comes an idealess lad,
With a strut, and a stare, and a smirk;
And I watch, scientific though sad,
The Law of Selection at work.

Of Science he hasn't a trace,
He seeks not the How and the Why,

But he sings with an amateur's grace,
And he dances much better than I.

And we know the more dandified males
By dance and by song win their wives –
'Tis a law that with *Aves* prevails,
And even in *Homo* survives.

Shall I rage as they whirl in the valse?
Shall I sneer as they carol and coo?
Ah no! for since Chloe is false,
I'm certain that Darwin is true!

Solomon Redivivus

What am I? Ah, you know it,
I am the modern Sage,
Seer, savant, merchant, poet –
I am, in brief, the Age.

Look not upon my glory
Of gold and sandal-wood,
But sit and hear a story
From Darwin and from Buddh.[21]

Count not my Indian treasures,
All wrought in curious shapes,
My labours and my pleasures,
My peacocks and my apes;

For when you ask me riddles,
And when I answer each,
Until my fifes and fiddles
Burst in and drown our speech,

Oh then your soul astonished
Must surely faint and fail,
Unless, by me admonished,
You hear our wondrous tale.

We were a soft Amoeba
In ages past and gone,
Ere you were Queen Of Sheba,
And I King Solomon.

---

[21]Darwin and Buddh: Charles Robert Darwin (1809–82), was an English naturalist and geologist, best known for his contributions to evolutionary theory, as outlined in *On the Origin of Species* (1859). Buddh is the shortened form of Buddha.

Unorganed, undivided,
We lived in happy sloth,
And all that you did I did,
One dinner nourished both:

Till you incurred the odium
Of fission and divorce –
A severed pseudopodium
You strayed your lonely course.

When next we met together
Our cycles to fulfil,
Each was a bag of leather,
With stomach and with gill.

But our Ascidian morals[22]
Recalled that old mischance,
And we avoided quarrels
By separate maintenance.

Long ages passed – our wishes
Were fetterless and free,
For we were jolly fishes,
A-swimming in the sea.

We roamed by groves of coral,
We watched the youngsters play –
The memory and the moral
Had vanished quite away.

Next, each became a reptile,
With fangs to sting and slay;
No wiser ever crept, I'll
Assert, deny who may.

But now, disdaining trammels
Of scale and limbless coil,
Through every grade of mammals
We passed with upward toil.

Till, anthropoid and wary
Appeared the parent ape,
And soon we grew less hairy,
And soon began to drape.

So, from that soft Amoeba,
In ages past and gone,

---

[22]Ascidian: of the class of marine animals that include sea squirts.

You've grown the Queen of Sheba,
And I, King Solomon.

Siamese Twins
Eugene Lee-Hamilton (1894)

Know you how died those twins, famed far and near,
Who, tethered hip to hip, with Fate's strong thread,
Were forced to walk through life with equal tread,
And to be friends and share at last one bier?

How one awoke one day, and could not hear
His brother's breath, and felt, and found him dead;
And how, compelled to share a dead man's bed,
He died of an unutterable fear?

Body and Mind have link of like dread kind:
Woe to the Body, blind and helpless clod,
That wakes one day, and hears the Mind no more;

But ten times woe to the surviving Mind,
Born to create, command, and play the god:
Bound to a corpse, it struggles still to soar.

Heredity
Thomas Hardy (1917)

I am the family face;
Flesh perishes, I live on,
Projecting trait and trace
Through time to times anon,
And leaping from place to place
Over oblivion.

The years-heired feature that can
In curve and voice and eye
Despise the human span
Of durance – that is I;
The eternal thing in man,
That heeds no call to die.

Complaint
William Carlos Williams (1921)

They call me and I go.
It is a frozen road
past midnight, a dust
of snow caught

in the rigid wheeltracks.
The door opens.
I smile, enter and
shake off the cold.
Here is a great woman
on her side in the bed.
She is sick,
perhaps vomiting,
perhaps laboring
to give birth to
a tenth child. Joy! Joy!
Night is a room
darkened for lovers,
through the jealousies the sun
has sent one golden needle!
I pick the hair from her eyes
and watch her misery
with compassion.

The Mother
Gwendolyn Brooks (1945)

Abortions will not let you forget.
You remember the children you got that you did not get,
The damp small pulps with a little or with no hair,
The singers and workers that never handled the air.
You will never neglect or beat
Them, or silence or buy with a sweet.
You will never wind up the sucking-thumb
Or scuttle off ghosts that come.
You will never leave them, controlling your luscious sigh,
Return for a snack of them, with gobbling mother-eye.

I have heard in the voices of the wind the voices of my dim killed
          children.
I have contracted. I have eased
My dim dears at the breasts they could never suck.
I have said, Sweets, if I sinned, if I seized
Your luck
And your lives from your unfinished reach,
If I stole your births and your names,
Your straight baby tears and your games,
Your stilted or lovely loves, your tumults, your marriages, aches,
          and your deaths,
If I poisoned the beginnings of your breaths,
Believe that even in my deliberateness I was not deliberate.
Though why should I whine,

Whine that the crime was other than mine? –
Since anyhow you are dead.
Or rather, or instead,
You were never made.
But that too, I am afraid,
Is faulty: oh, what shall I say, how is the truth to be said?
You were born, you had body, you died.
It is just that you never giggled or planned or cried.

Believe me, I loved you all.
Believe me, I knew you, though faintly, and I loved, I loved you
All.

The Human Species
Raymond Queneau (1948)[23]

The human species has given me
the right to be mortal
the duty to be civilised
a conscience
2 eyes that don't always function very well
a nose in the middle of my face
2 feet 2 hands
speech

the human species has given me
my father and mother
some brothers maybe who knows
a whole mess of cousins
and some great-grandfathers
the human species has given me
its 3 faculties
feeling intellect and will
each in moderation
32 teeth 10 fingers a liver
a heart and some other viscera
the human species has given me
what I'm supposed to be satisfied with

To A Baby Born Without Limbs
Kingsley Amis (1966)

This is just to show you whose boss around here.
It'll keep you on your toes, so to speak,

---

[23]Trans. Teo Savory.

Make you put your best foot forward, so to speak,
And give you something to turn your hand to, so to speak.
You can face up to it like a man,
Or snivel and blubber like a baby.
That's up to you. Nothing to do with Me.
If you take it in the right spirit,
You can have a bloody marvelous life,
With the great rewards courage brings,
And the beauty of accepting your LOT.
And think how much good it'll do your Mum and Dad,
And your Grans and Gramps and the rest of the shower,
To be stopped being complacent.
Make sure they baptise you, though,
In case some murdering bastard
Decides to put you away quick,
Which would send you straight to LIMB-O, ha ha ha.
But just a word in your ear, if you've got one.
Mind you DO take this in the right spirit,
And keep a civil tongue in your head about Me.
Because if you DON'T,
I've got plenty of other stuff up My sleeve,
Such as Leukemia and polio,
(Which incidentally you're welcome to any time,
Whatever spirit you take this in.)
I've given you one love-pat, right?
You don't want another.
So watch it, Jack.

Twins
Robert Graves (1968)

Siamese twins: one, maddened by
The other's moral bigotry,
Resolved at length to misbehave
And drink them both into the grave.

Against Coupling
Fleur Adcock (1971)

I write in praise of the solitary act:
of not feeling a trespassing tongue
forced into one's mouth, one's breath
smothered, nipples crushed against the
rib-cage, and that metallic tingling
in the chin set off by a certain odd nerve:

unpleasure. Just to avoid those eyes would help –
such eyes as a young girl draws life from,
listening to the vegetal
rustle within her, as his gaze
stirs polypal fronds in the obscure
sea-bed of her body, and her own eyes blur.

There is much to be said for abandoning
this no longer novel excercise –
for not 'participating in
a total experience' – when
one feels like the lady in Leeds who
had seen *The Sound Of Music* eighty-six times;

or more, perhaps, like the school drama mistress
producing *A Midsummer Night's Dream*
for the seventh year running, with
yet another cast from 5B.
Pyramus and Thisbe[24] are dead, but
the hole in the wall can still be troublesome.

I advise you, then, to embrace it without
encumbrance. No need to set the scene,
dress up (or undress), make speeches.
Five minutes of solitude are
enough – in the bath, or to fill
that gap between the Sunday papers and lunch.

Cadaver
John Stone, 1972

'*The initial lesion of syphilis may result over the years in a gradual weakening and dilatation (aneurysm) of the aorta. This aneurysm may ultimately rupture and lead to death of the patient.*'

Medical Textbook

Fitting the labels
in our books
to our own tense tendons
slipping in their sheaths

we memorized the body
and the word

---

[24]Pyramus and Thisbe were ill-fated lovers, originally from Ovid's *Metamorphoses*. The story is enacted in Shakespeare's *A Midsummer Night's Dream* (V: i).

stripped the toughened skin
from the stringing nerve
the giving muscle.

Ribs sprang like gates.

In the chest
like archaeologists
we found it:
dotted, swollen,
aneurysmal
sign of an old sin –

the silent lust
that had buried itself
in the years
growing
in the hollow of his chest

still rounded by her arms
clinging
belly to belly
years beyond that first seed

to the rigid final fact

of a body.

To a Fourteen-Year-Old Girl in Labor and Delivery
John Stone (1972)

I cannot say it to you, Mother, Child.
Nowhere now is there a trace of the guile
that brought you here. Near the end of exile

I hold you prisoner, jailer, in my cage –
with no easy remedy for your rage
against him and the child. Your coming of age

is a time of first things: a slipping of latches;
of parallels like fire and the smell of matches.
The salmon swims upstream. The egg hatches.

Fetus
Robert Lowell (1977)

The convicted abortion-surgeon
and his Harvard lawyers are Big League,

altruistic, unpopular men lost in the clouds
above the friendly municipal court.
The long severe tiers of windows
are one smear of sunlight multiplied;
the new yellow brick has a cutting edge.

'The law is a sledgehammer,
not a scalpel.'

The court cannot reform the misstep
of the motionless moment...
So many killers are cleared of killing,
yet we are shocked a fetus can be murdered –
its translucence looms to attention
in bilious X-ray
too young to be strengthened
by our old New England hope of heaven
made unsentimental by our certainty in hell.

Our germ –
no number in the debtbook
to say it lived
once unembarrassed by the flesh.

When the black arrow arrives on the silver tray,
the fetus has no past,
not even an immovable wall of paintings –
no room to stir its thoughts,
no breathless servility
overacting the last day,
writhing like a worm
under the contradicting rays of science –
no scared eye on the audience.

Wrap me close, but not too close –
when we wake to our unacceptable age,
will we find our hearts enlarged
and wish all men our brothers –
hypocrites pretending to answer
what we cannot hear?

How much we carry away with us
before dying,
learning we have nothing to take,
like the fetus, the homunculus,
already at four months one pound,
with shifty thumb in mouth –

Our little model...

As I drive on, I lift my eyes;
the focus is spidered
with black winter branches
and blackened concrete stores
bonneted for Easter with billboards...
Boston snow contracting
like a yellow surgical bandage –
the slut of struggle.
The girl high on the billboard
was ten years my senior in life;
she would have teased my father –
unkillable, unlaid,
disused as the adolescent tan on my hand.
She is a model, and cannot lose her looks,
born a decade too soon for any buyer.

Talking Shop
Peter Reading (1984)

The three sterilizations went OK,
except for the advanced C. uterine cervix
(just my damned luck to find that) – anyway,
apart from that it all went normally.
The one in Number 2 was staggered when
I said 'We found your coil, by the way –
worked its way through the womb into the space
between the womb and stomach.' Number 3
(non compos mentis, got eight kids already)
asked me when 'it' would be alright again.
I said 'If you endeavour to avoid
sexual intercourse for about two nights...'
She said 'he won't wait. He *will* have his rights.'

The Moment the Two Worlds Meet
Sharon Olds (1987)

That's the moment I always think of – when the
slick, whole body comes out of me,
when they pull it out, not pull it but steady it
as it pushes forth, not catch it but keep their
hands under it as it pulses out,
they are the first to touch it,
and it shines, it glistens with the thick liquid on it.

That's the moment, while it's sliding, the limbs
compressed close to the body, the arms
bent like a crab's cloud-muscle legs, the
thighs packed plums in heavy syrup, the
legs folded like the wings of a chicken –
that is the center of life, that moment when the
juiced bluish sphere of the baby is
sliding between the two worlds, wet, like sex, it *is* sex,
it is my life opening back and back
as you'd strip the reed from the bud, not strip it but
watch it thrust so it peels itself and the
flower is there, severely folded, and
then it begins to open and dry
but by then the moment is over,
they wipe off the grease and wrap the child in a blanket and
hand it to you entirely in this world.

Sex
Hugo Williams (1990)

'Sex' seems to be a word that most people understand,
so there is a fair chance that the woman will understand
what the man is getting at when he mentions the subject.

Perhaps he is finding difficulty getting into the passage
and it may be necessary to ask why. Perhaps she is dry
because there is no natural lubricant for the penis,

or perhaps she is very tense and unable to accept him.
It may be that the fault lies with the man, if he cannot
complete the sexual act, or his climax comes too soon.

At this point it may be necessary to enquire about orgasm.
As sexual excitement reaches its climax (orgasm), the man
will recognize that the jerking out of his semen (sperm)

is about to start and that it is inevitable. His semen
is said to be 'coming' and if any discussion is needed
the verb 'to come' may be used without causing offence.

For instance, the woman may be asked if she understands
what the word 'coming' means in this context
and whether she has ever experienced such a thing.

Does she feel herself to be on the verge of 'coming',
only to find herself drawing back from it because of some
unspecified mental problem, and if so, what?

Poem to my Uterus
Lucille Clifton (1991)

> you uterus
> you have been patient
> as a sock
> while i have slippered into you
> my dead and living children
> now
> they want to cut you out
> stocking i will not need
> where i am going
> where am i going
> old girl
> without you
> uterus
> my bloody print
> my estrogen kitchen
> my black bag of desire
> where can i go
> barefoot
> without you
> where can you go
> without me

To My Last Period
Lucille Clifton (1991)

> well, girl, goodbye,
> after thirty-eight years.
> thirty-eight years and you
> never arrived
> splendid in your red dress
> without trouble for me
> somewhere, somehow.
>
> now it is done,
> and I feel just like
> the grandmothers who,
> after the hussy has gone,
> sit holding her photograph
> and sighing, *wasn't she*
> *beautiful? wasn't she beautiful?*

Genes, Likenesses
Elizabeth Jennings (1994)

What is this in me called spirit or
Soul or being, self which I call me?
So many qualities I owe to more
Than one ancestor but my self is free
Of them. It knows of law

And duty, choice, responsibility,
Yet it is dressed in clothes much like those of
Some member of my huge past family
And closer ones whom I know best through love,
And then there's liberty

Whose boundaries are often hard to know.
My voice, my eyes, my hair, my shape of head
Are easy likenesses to see although
They are so mingled, but my present need
Moves further, deeper too.

My spirit's part of my imagination
And also part of thought and memory.
Then there are ways of feeling, also passion.
Can spirits look alike? Is soul not free
To be unique and its own revelation?
I say my history's me.

Saint Sex
C. K. Williams (1995)

there are people whose sex
keeps growing even when they're old whose
genitals swell like tumors endlessly
until they are all sex and nothing else nothing
that moves or thinks nothing
but great inward and outward handfuls of gristle

think of them men
who ooze their penises out like snail
feet whose testicles clang in their scrotums women
are like anvils to them the world an
anvil they want to take whole buildings
in their arms they want
to come in the windows to run antennas
through their ducts like ramrods and women
these poor women who dream and dream of
the flower they can't sniff it sends buds

into their brain they feel their neural
river clot with moist fingers the ganglia[25]
hardening like ant eggs the ends
burning off

pity them these people there are no wars
for them there is no news no
summer no reason they are so humble they want
nothing they have no hands or faces
pity them at night whispering I love
you to themselves and during the day how they
walk along smiling and suffering pity;
them love them they are
angels

Vasectomy
Philip Appleman (1996)

After the steaming bodies swept
through the hungry streets of swollen cities;
after the vast pink spawning of family
poisoned the rivers and ravaged the prairies;
after the gamble of latex and
diaphragms and pills;
I invoked the white robes, gleaming blades
ready for blood, and, feeling the scourge
of Increase and Multiply, made
affirmation: *Yes*, deliver us from
complicity.
And after the precision of scalpels,
I woke to a landscape of sunshine where
the catbird mates for life and
maps trace out no alibis—stepped
into a morning of naked truth,
where acts mean what they really are:
the purity of loving
for the sake of love.

A Puppy Called Puberty
Adrian Mitchell (1996)

It was like keeping a puppy in your underpants
A secret puppy you weren't allowed to show to anyone
Not even your best friend or your worst enemy

---

[25]A ganglion (pl. ganglia) is a nerve cell cluster.

You wanted to pat him stroke him cuddle him
All the time but you weren't supposed to touch him

He only slept for five minutes at a time
Then he'd suddenly perk up his head
In the middle of school medical inspection
And always on bus rides
So you had to climb down from the upper deck
All bent double to smuggle the puppy off the bus
Without the buxom conductress spotting
Your wicked and ticketless stowaway.

Jumping up, wet-nosed, eagerly wagging –
He only stopped being a nuisance
When you were alone together
Pretending to be doing your homework
But really gazing at each other
Through hot and hazy daydreams

Of those beautiful schoolgirls on the bus
With kittens bouncing in their sweaters.

A Dog Called Elderly
Adrian Mitchell (1996)

And now I have a dog called Elderly
And all he ever wants to do
Is now and then be let out for a piss
But spend the rest of his lifetime
Sleeping on my lap in front of the fire.

The Man Who is Married to Siamese Twins Joined at the Skull
Lyn Lifshin (1996)

In our huge bed
from a bird's eye view
we look like a three
petaled flower.
I rub my wife's
neck. It's always
sore from leaning
over in chairs, on
trains, walking thru
the aisles of the
A & P.[26] We're happy,

---

[26]A&P refers to an American supermarket chain.

the three of us. Her
sister shuts us out
when I get to
rutting loud in her.
Then we all sing
oh where oh where
has my little
dog gone in the
shower and I
bring them both
hot chocolate.
We can lie on our
backs with the
tv swinging
from the ceiling
and laugh at the
news. Her sister
threatens to
run off and I kiss
her soundly. They
think the same
jokes are funny.
Sometimes when my
wife is asleep I talk
to her sister. She
can't imagine
what it would be
like to be separated,
have half of her
sliced away

Abortion
Haki R. Madhubuti (1997)

she,
walla (queen) anderson
miss booker t. washington jr. high of 1957,
miss chicago bar maid of 1961
had her first abortion at 32
after giving birth to
john (pee wee) jackson at 14,
mary smith at 15 and a half,
janice wilson at 17,
dion jones at 19,
sara jones at 21,

and
richard (cream) johnson at 27.

on a sun-filled day
during her 32nd year
after
as many years of aborting
weak men who would not stand
behind their own creations
she
walla (queen) anderson
by herself alone without consultation
went under the western butchers
to get her insides
out.

Monogamous Orgasms
Nin Andrews (2000)

Every day when Joe goes to work in the morning, he puts my orgasms in a medicine bottle, securing them with a cotton plug before capping the bottle. Sometimes they attempt to fly out but to no avail. When Joe gets lonely, he takes them out. He is soothed by their sweet voices.

Out of the Bag
Seamus Heaney (2001)

1.
All of us came in Doctor Kerlin's bag.
He'd arrive with it, disappear to the room
And by the time he'd reappear to wash

Those nosy, rosy, big soft hands of his
In the scullery basin, its lined insides
(The colour of a spaniel's inside lug)

Were empty for all to see, the trap-sprung mouth
Unsnibbed and gaping wide. Then like a hypnotist
Unwinding us, he'd wind the instruments

Back into their lining, tie the cloth
Like an apron round itself,
Darken the door and leave

With the bag in his hand, a plump ark by the keel...
Until the next time came and in he'd come
In his fur-lined leather collar which was also spaniel-coloured

And go stooping up to the room again, a whiff
Of disinfectant, a Dutch interior gleam
Of waistcoat satin and highlights on the forceps.

Getting the water ready, that was next –
Not plumping hot, and not lukewarm, but soft,
Sud-luscious, saved for him from the rain-butt

And savoured by him afterwards, all thanks
Denied as he towelled hard and fast,
Then held his arms out suddenly behind him

To be squired and silk-lined into the camel coat.
At which point once he turned his eyes upon me,
Hyperborean, beyond-the-north wind blue,

Two peepholes to the locked room I saw into
Every time his name was mentioned, skimmed
Milk and ice, swabbed porcelain, the white

And chill of tiles, steel hooks, chrome surgery tools
And blood dreeps in the sawdust where it thickened
At the foot of each cold wall. And overhead

The little, pendent, teat-hued infant parts
Strung neatly from a line up near the ceiling –
A toe, a foot and shin, an arm, a cock

A bit like the rosebud in his buttonhole.

2.
Poeta doctus[27] Peter Levi says
Sanctuaries of Asclepius (called asclepions)
Were the equivalent of hospitals

In ancient Greece, or of shrines like Lourdes,
Says poeta doctus Graves. Or of the cure
By poetry that cannot be coerced,

Say I, who realized at Epidaurus[28]
That the whole place was a sanatorium
With theatre and gymnasium and baths,

A site of incubation, where 'incubation'
Was technical and ritual, meaning sleep
When epiphany occurred and you met the god...

---

[27]Poeta doctus, from Latin, meaning 'learned poet'.
[28]Epidaurus was the birth place of Asclepius, the Greek god of medicine.

Hatless, groggy, shadowing myself
As the thurifer[29] I was in an open-air procession
In Lourdes in '56

When I nearly fainted from the heat and fumes,
Again I nearly fainted as I bent
To pull a bunch of grass and hallucinated

Doctor Kerlin at the steamed-up glass
Of the scullery window, starting in to draw
With his large pink index finger dot-faced men

With button-spots in a straight line down their fronts
And women with dot breasts, giving them all
A set of droopy sausage-arms and legs

That soon began to run. And then as he dipped and laved
In the generous suds again, *miraculum*:
The baby bits all came together swimming

Into his soapy big hygienic hands
And I myself came to, blinded with sweat,
Blinking and shaky in the windless light.

3.
Bits of the grass I pulled I posted off
To one going in to chemotherapy
And one who had come through. I didn't want

To leave the place or link up with the others.
It was midday, mid-May, pre-tourist sunlight
In the precincts of the god,

The very site of the temple of Asclepius.
I wanted nothing more than to lie down
Under hogweed, under seeded grass

And to be visited in the very eye of the day
By Hygeia, his daughter, her name still clarifying
The haven of light she was, the undarkening door.

4.
The room I came from and the rest of us all came from
Stays pure reality where I stand alone,
Standing the passage of time, and she's asleep

---

[29]Thurifer: an acolyte who carries incense in a religious ceremony.

In sheets put on for the doctor, wedding presents
That showed up again and again, bridal
And usual and useful at births and at deaths.

Me at the bedside, incubating for real,
Peering, appearing to her as she closes
And opens her eyes, then lapses back

Into a faraway smile whose precinct of vision
I would enter every time, to assist and be asked
In that hoarsened whisper of triumph,

'And what do you think
Of the new wee baby the doctor brought for us all
When I was asleep?'

Double Helix
Peter Carpenter (2002)

It's a shape cut in time,
a tracer line from the year dot

moving on from its first form: a pulse,
a curl in fluid, continuous creation

lightning sketched, a steady course
that cannot be charted or rolled

in fire then beaten out of us.
We follow its orders with a smile,

a double-take, something in the eyes.
It ripples like the bars of a mackerel sky,

turns sun to ice, shore to tide.
We cannot break the code, however hard we try.

IVF
Kona Macphee (2002)

I come home early, feel the pale house close
around me as the pressure of my blood
knocks at my temples, feel it clench me in
its cramping grasp, the fierceness of its quiet
sanctioning the small and listless hope
that I might find it mercifully empty.

Dazed, I turn the taps to fill the empty
tub, and draw the bathroom door to close
behind me. I lie unmoving, feel all hope

leaching from between my legs as blood
tinges the water, staining it the quiet
shade of a winter evening drifting in

on sunset. Again, no shoot of life sprouts in
this crumbling womb that wrings itself to empty
out the painfully-planted seeds. The quiet
doctors, tomorrow, will check their notes and close
the file, wait for the hormones in my blood
to augur further chances, more false hope.

My husband holds to patience, I to hope,
and yet our clockworks are unwinding. In
the stillness of the house, we hear our blood
pumped by our hearts that gall themselves, grow empty:
once, this silence, shared, could draw us close
that now forebodes us with a desperate quiet.

I hear him at the door, but I lay quiet,
as if, by saying nothing, I may hope
that somehow his unknowingness may close
a door on all the darkness we've let in:
the nursery that's seven years too empty;
the old, unyielding stains of menstrual blood.

Perhaps I wish the petitioning of my blood
for motherhood might falter and fall quiet,
perhaps I wish that we might choose to empty
our lives of disappointment, and of hope,
but wishes founder – we go on living in
the shadow of the cliffs now looming close:

the blood that's thick with traitorous clots of hope;
the quiet knack we've lost, of giving in;
the empty room whose door we cannot close.

Mapping the Genome
Michael Symmons-Roberts (2004)

Geneticist as driver, down the gene
codes in, let's say, a topless coupé
and you keep expecting bends,

real tyre-testers on tight
mountain passes, but instead it's dead
straight, highway as runway,

helix unravelled as vista,
as vanishing point. Keep your foot
down. This is a finite desert.

You move too fast to read it,
the order of the rocks, the cacti,
roadside weeds, a blur to you.

Every hour or so, you glimpse a shack
which passes for a motel here:
tidy faded rooms with TVs on

for company, the owner pacing out
his empty parking lot. And after
each motel you hit a sandstorm

thick as fog, but agony.
Somewhere out there are remnants
of our evolution, genes for how

to fly south, sense a storm,
hunt at night, how to harden
your flesh into hide or scales.

These are the miles of dead code.
Every desert has them.
You are on a mission to discover

why the human heart still slows
when divers break the surface,
why mermaids still swim in our dreams.

Crick, Watson and the Double Helix
Christopher Southgate (2006)

A single insight made the Book of Life cohere,
Sent two men shouting into a Cambridge bar.
More slowly there steals upon us the power, the fear.

The X-ray from King's, and Chargaff's pairs,[30]
Not one helix, but two, fugues on a common air;
A single insight made the Book of Life cohere.

An amazing future, suddenly laid bare –
New drugs, cheap insulin, strawberries all the year.
More slowly there steals upon us the power, the fear.

---

[30]An X-ray image, 'Photo 51', which showed the structure of DNA, was taken at King's College London. Erwin Chargaff (1905–2002) was an Austrian professor of biochemistry at Columbia University medical school, whose discoveries contributed to the discovery of the double helix structure of DNA.

They were to find the grammar of genes trickier
Than expected, the syntax harder by far.
But a single insight had made the Book of Life cohere.

They could see the Nobel, and the patenting wars,
The complex hunger for profit, healing, honour.
More slowly there steals upon us the power, the fear.

It was all there, in the thin Cambridge beer,
The Text of Texts, laid ready for the sequencer,
A single insight made the Book of Life cohere.

Harder to take in the tears at the screening centre,
The many deaths of unborn others,
But slowly there steals upon us the power, the fear.

Now we face the uninsurable cancer,
Anticipate the repertoire of the baby-tweaker.
A single insight made the Book of Life cohere,
And slowly there steals upon us the power, the fear.

The Dirty Thirties – A manual of theory and practice
Alexis Lykiard (2007)

'We consider certain precautions and even treatment useful as a means of reducing this necessary evil to a minimum' (Drs. A. Costler, A. Willy et al., *Encyclopaedia of Sexual Knowledge*, 1934).

'I read those two guides to "sexual knowledge" which Mr Arthur Koestler wrote in the guise of Professor Costler. They are most excellent works... It is hard to imagine how the topic could be elucidated better' (Robert Aickman, *The Attempted Rescue*, 1966).

'*The Encyclopaedia of Sexual Knowledge*... argues that an open and honest approach to sex has been submerged by hypocrisy... taking a very relaxed line towards masturbatio' (David Cesarani and Arthur Koestler, *The Homeless Mind*, 1998).

1.
The treatment of onanism[31] must be carried out
as follows: Absolute cleanliness of the whole body.
A bath, at first in tepid (30° C.) and later in cool (25° C.) water
is to be taken in the morning on rising. The sexual organs
are to be washed with mild soap or with pure cool water.
If any irritants, dirt, or hardened smegma are found

---

[31]Onanism, or masturbation.

under the foreskin, they must be removed,
for irritation makes the cure of onanism
very difficult if not impossible.

The presence of worms is one
of the contributing causes of onanism,
especially in girls, and their elimination
is an urgent necessity.
Constipation should be relieved by an enema
at 30° C. A well-chosen diet with a daily ration
of sour milk will also be helpful.
All stimulants are also to be rigidly avoided.

Wine, beer, liqueurs, and even fermented fruit-wine
are equally harmful to the onanist, as are also
coffee and China or Russian tea.
Meat should be eaten only sparingly,
and pork, smoked meat, ripe cheese and caviar
should never be taken. Spices
such as cinnamon, pepper, and cayenne pepper
are also to be avoided.

Rice, maize, oats, barley, green vegetables
and carrots (but not celery), green salads, fruit
stewed and in every form may be recommended
as most suitable and sufficiently nourishing.
Water is the best drink, and even when a palate
is spoilt, an apple, a pear, or a few strawberries
will satisfy thirst much better than a cool glass of beer.

2.

Daily exercises and games in the open air
played to the point of fatigue,
occasional sawing or wood-chopping,
rowing, gymnastics, swimming, running,
hard and tiring house-work
are splendid diversions. The onanist
should go to bed thoroughly tired,
and rise as soon as he wakens.
The patient (for so we must call him)
should not be allowed to lie in bed awake.

Before retiring it is desirable
that the bowels should be emptied;
in any case the bladder should
be emptied. The hands should be placed
outside the blankets before sleep begins.

The bed should contain no soft lower portion.
The mattress is quite sufficient
in winter as in summer. Feather-beds
should be replaced by horse-hair cushions
and quilts or woollen blankets lined with linen.

The patient should lie, if possible, on his side;
he should avoid lying on his back,
as this posture produces pressure
on the seminal vesicles, due
to the filling of the bladder,
and brings about an erection.
The bedroom should be cool, and at least
one upper window may be left half open.
Tight clothes are forbidden.
Woollen underclothes should not be worn,
as they irritate the skin. The trouser pockets
should be at the back above the waist
and not at the sides or in front.

Girls should never wear corsets as they
produce congestion in the lower abdomen
and favour onanism or hinder its cure.
For obvious reasons they should not use
a sewing machine during adolescence.
On the other hand, daily gymnastic exercises are
essential if onanism is to be
successfully combated.

3.
All reading matter should be carefully chosen.
Humorous articles, sea stories, adventures
which awaken enthusiasm, are not only
strong incentives to activity, but also indispensable
as a source of recreation and diversion...
Obscene thoughts are most difficult to combat...
In difficult cases of onanism hypnotic suggestion
may be employed in conjunction with the precepts
given above and will be found to be
a sovereign remedy... As for drugs,
the doctor may sometimes recommend
bromide and other sedatives. In recent times,
certain practitioners have resorted
to puncturing the skin in order to reduce
the sensitiveness of the body.

> At all events, the last thing
> a doctor should do when faced
> with a young masturbater
> is to frighten him, or to threaten
> castration or other
> similar punishments.

MEDICAL WRITING:

Onania
John Marten (1723)[32]

The afflictions which may, and often do fall upon those who are or have been guilty of the sinful practice of self-pollution, belong either to the soul or the body: I shall begin with those of the least concern. In the first place, it manifestly hinders the growth, both in boys and girls, and few of either sex, that in their youth commit this sin to excess for any considerable time, come ever to that robustness or strength, which they would have arrived to without it. In men as well as boys, the very first attempt of it has often occasioned a *phymosis* in some, and a *paraphymosis*[33] in others; I shall not explain these terms further, let it suffice that they are accidents which are very painful and troublesome, and may continue to be tormenting for some time, if not bring on ulcers and other worse symptoms; especially if managed by raw unskilful people, whom to employ, it is most commonly the fate of young men, who being conscious of their guilt, have not the assurance to address themselves to men of worth and experience. Whoever wants to know the signification of those words, any surgeon will inform him.

The frequent use of this pollution; likewise causes stranguries,[34] priapisms,[35] and other disorders of the penis and testes, but especially gonorrheas, more difficult to be cured than those contracted from women actually labouring under foul diseases. When the seminal vessels are first strained, and afterwards relaxed, the ferment in the testes is destroyed and the seed grown thin and waterish, comes away unelaborated, without any provocation; this distemper often proves fatal, even under the hands of the most skilful.

...

In some it has been the cause of fainting fits and epilepsies; in others of consumptions; and many young men, who were strong and lusty before they gave themselves over to this vice, have been worn out by it, and by robbing the body of its balmy and vital moisture, without cough or spitting, dry and emaciated, sent to their graves. In others again, whom it has not killed, it has produced nightly and

---

[32]Onania (onanism), or masturbation. The first edition was likely 1717 or 1718, and it was republished throughout the century.
[33]Phymosis and paraphymosis refer to the inability to retract the foreskin, or the inability of a retracted foreskin, which has become trapped behind the glans of the penis, to return to a flaccid state.
[34]Strangeries refers to painful slow urination.
[35]Priaprism is the condition of persistent erection.

excessive seminal emissions; a weakness in the penis, and loss of erection, as if they had been castrated.

…

In some men of very strong constitutions, the mischiefs may not be so visible, and themselves perhaps capable of marrying; and yet the blood and spirits impaired, and the seed rendered infertile, so as to make them unfit for procreation, by its changing the crasis[36] of the spermatick parts, making them become barren, as land becomes poor by being overtilled; and few of those that have been much accustomed to this vice in their youth, have ever much reason to boast of the fruits of their marriage-bed; for if by nature's extraordinary helps, they should get any children, which happens not often, they are commonly weakly little ones, that either die soon, or become tender, sickly people, always ailing and complaining; a misery to themselves, a dishonour to humane race and a scandal to their parents.

…

In women self-pollution if frequently practised, relaxes and spoils the retentive faculty, occasions the *fluor albus*,[37] an obnoxious as well as perplexing illness attending that sex, which upon account of the womb, may draw on a whole legion of diseases; among other disorders, it makes them look pale, and those who are not of a good complexion, swarthy and hagged. It frequently is the cause of histerick fits, and sometimes, by draining away all the radical moisture, consumptions. But what is more often produced than either is barrenness, and at length a total ineptitude to the act of generation itself, misfortunes very afflicting to them, because seldom to be redressed.

The Compleat Midwife's Companion
Jane Sharp (1725)[38]

'What things are required for the Procreation of Children'

I have in the former part made a short explanation of the parts of both sexes, that are needful for this use; but yet some think there is no need of describing the parts of them both, because some have written that the generative parts in men, differ not from those in women, but in respect of place and situation in the body, and that a woman may become a man; and that one *Tyesias* was a man for many years, and after that was strangely metamorphosed into a woman, and again from a woman to a man; and that in regard he had been of both sexes, he was chosen as the most fit judge to determine that great question, which of the two, male or female find most pleasure in time of copulation?[39] Some again hold, that man may be changed into a woman, but a woman can never become a man. But let every man abound in his own opinion;

---

[36]Crasis is the mixture of physical qualities that gives rise to a certain state of health.
[37]*Fluor albus* is vaginal discharge, indicating infection.
[38]The original version of this was *The Midwives Book*; or, *The Whole Art of Midwifery Discovered*, published in 1671.
[39]In this story, Juno blinded Tiresias (who was born male and bore children while living as female) for stating that women experienced more sexual pleasure then men.

certain it is, that neither of these opinions is true: for the parts in men and women are different in number and likeness, substance and proportion: the cod of a man[40] turned inside outward, is like the womb, yet the difference is so great, that they can never be the same: for the cod is a thin wrinkled skin, but the womb at the bottom is a thick membrane, all fleshy within and woven with many small fibres, and the seed vessels are implanted so that they can never change their place; and moreover their stones are for shape, magnitude and composition, too different to suffer a change of the sex; so that of necessity there must be a conjunction of male and female for the begetting of children. Insects and imperfect creatures are bred sundry ways, without conjunction; but it is not so with mankind, but both sexes must concur, by mutual embracements, and there must be a perfect mixture of seed issuing from them both, which virtually contain the infant that must be formed from them. God made all things of nothing, but man must have some matter to work upon, or he can produce nothing.

A New Description of Merryland
Thomas Stretzer (1741)[41]

Merryland is well watered by a River, which takes its Rise from a large Reservoir or Lake in the Neighbourhood called VSCA, and discharges itself with a most impetuous Current and fearful Cataract towards the *Terra Firma* near the Entry of the Great Gulph; of this River I shall treat more particularly in another Chapter.

There is a spacious CANAL runs through the midst of this Country, from one End almost to the other; it is so deep that Authors affirm it has no Bottom. I have often sounded it in many Parts, and though I don't doubt but it has a Bottom, I must own I never could reach it; perhaps, had my Sounding-line been a few Fathoms longer, it might have reached the Bottom.

We are told of Solomon's Wells or Cisterns at a Place the Turks call Roselayne, which, like this Canal, are reputed to be unfathomable; and the current Tradition is, that they are filled from a subterraneous River, which when flesh becomes word that wise King, by his great Sagacity, knew to run under-ground in that Place. Vide De Bruyn. Voyag. au Levant. Whether this might not as properly be called Solomon's Canal, I leave to the Reader's Judgment; it is certain, that wise King was no Stranger to this Country, but spent a great deal in Improvements he made in several Provinces of it.

All the superfluous Moisture of the Country is drained off through this Canal, and it is likewise the Conveyance of all Provisions to the up per Part of MERRYLAND; all the Seed sowed in that Country is conveyed this Way to the Great Storehouse at the upper End of it; and in short, there is no Commodity imported into MERRYLAND, but by this Road; so that you may easily conceive it to be a Place of great Traffic. We may say of this Canal, as the learned Doctor Cheyne says of the alimentary Tube, 'that it is, as it were, a Common-Sewer, which may be fouled or cleaned in various Manners, and with great Facility; it is wide, open, and reasonably strong.'

---

[40]Cod: scrotum; stones: testicles.
[41]The author identified in the editor's preface in other editions as Roger Pheuquewell, i.e. Thomas Stretser. The imprint is false, as are the publication details (it was published in London by Edmund Curll).

The Country is generally fertile enough, where duly manured; and some Parts are so exceedingly fruitful as to bear two or three Crops at a time; a Dutch Traveller tells us, there was once known to be as many Crops as Days in the Year; but this I look upon as apocryphal. Other Provinces are so utterly barren, that though a Man should leave no Stone unturned but labour and toil for ever, no Seed will take Root in them; yet so whimsical are many of the Inhabitants, that they would choose one of these barren Spots, rather than the more fertile ones; and indeed there is some Reason for it, People having found by Experience several great Inconveniencies by too fruitful a Crop. 'Tis a lamentable Thing for a Man to have a large Crop, when his Circumstances can't afford Houses to keep it in, or Thatch to cover it; to let it perish would be infamous, and what can a poor Man do? For he can't dispose of it immediately, it must be kept several Years at great Expence to him, before it is fit for the Market, or capable of making the least Return for his Labour and Expence. These are melancholy Circumstances for the poor Farmers:

Quæque ipse miserrima vidi, Et Quorum pars magna fui.[42]

This Peculiarity has put some People on inventing Means to prevent the Seed taking Root, or to destroy it before it comes to Maturity; but such Practices are only used by Stealth, and not openly approved of; it is looked on as a bad Practice, and we are told it was formerly punished with Death.

It sounds odd, but it is no less true than strange, that many have been ruined and forced to run away, by the Greatness of their Crops; and on the other hand, many are in a manner miserable and never satisfied, because their Spots prove barren – Strange Contradiction in People's Tempers! that what would be one Man's Delight, should be another Man's Torment!

An Essay upon Nursing and the Management of Children
William Cadogan (1749)

When a man takes upon him to contradict received opinions and prejudices sanctified by time, it is expected he should bring valid proof of what he advances. The truth of what I say, that the treatment of children in general is wrong, unreasonable and unnatural, will in great measure appear, if we but consider what a puny valetudinary race most of our people of condition are; chiefly owing to bad nursing, and bad habits contracted early. But let any one, who would be fully convinced of this matter, look over the bills of mortality; there he may observe, that almost half of the number of those, that fill up that black list, die under five years of age: so that half the people that come into the world, go out of it again before they become of the least use to it, or themselves. To me, this seems to deserve serious consideration; and yet I cannot find, that any one man of sense, and publick spirit, has ever attended to it at all; notwithstanding the maxim in

---

[42]*'Which I, alas! have seen, and deeply felt'.*

every one's mouth, that a multitude of inhabitants is the greatest strength and best support of a commonwealth.

...

When a child sucks its own mother, which, with a very few exceptions, would be best for every child, and every mother, nature has provided it with such wholesome and suitable nourishment; supposing her a temperate woman, that makes some use of her limbs; it can hardly do amiss.

The mother would likewise, in most hysterical, nervous cases, establish her own health by it, though she were weak and sickly before, as well as that of her offspring, for these reasons I could wish, that every woman that is able, whose fountains are not greatly disturbed or tainted, would give suck to her child. I am very sure that forcing back the milk, which most young women must have in great abundance, may be of fatal consequence: sometimes it endangers life, and often lays the foundation of many incurable diseases. The reasons that are given for this practice are very frivolous, and drawn from false premises; that some women are too weak to bear such a drain, which would rob them of their own nourishment. This is a very mistaken notion; for the first general cause of most people's diseases is, not want of nourishment, as is here imagined, but too great a fullness and redundancy of humours; good at first, but being more than the body can employ or consume, the whole mass becomes corrupt, and produces many diseases. This is confirmed by the general practice of physicians, who make holes in the skin, perpetual blisters, issues, *etc.* to let out the superfluity.

...

It is not so common for children to inherit the diseases of their parents, as is generally imagined; there is much vulgar error in this opinion; for people that are very unhealthy seldom have children, especially if the bad health be of the female side; and it is generally late in life when chronic diseases take place in most men, when the business of love is pretty well over: certainly children can have no title to those infirmities, which their parents have acquired by indolence and intemperance long after their birth. It is not common for people to complain of ails they think hereditary, until they are grown up; that is, until they have contributed to them by their own irregularities and excesses, and then are glad to throw their own faults back upon their parents; and lament a bad constitution, when they have spoiled a very good one.

...

The plain natural plan I have laid down, is never followed; because most mothers, of any condition, either cannot, or will not undertake the troublesome task of suckling their own children; which is troublesome only for want of proper method; were it rightly managed, there would be much pleasure in it, to every woman that can prevail upon herself to give up a little of the beauty of her breast to feed her offspring. There would be no fear of offending the husband's ears with the noise of the squalling brat. The child, was it nursed in this way, would be always quiet, in good humour, ever playing, laughing, or sleeping. In my opinion, a man of sense cannot have a prettier rattle (for rattles he must have of one kind or other) than such a young child.

'Of Monstrous Births', from *A Collection of Preternatural Cases*
William Smellie (1765)

Collection XXXVIII: Case 1

The history below, is of two children adhering to one another at the side of the breasts and bellies: they have both hairlips, and but one navel-string; the vessels separate as they enter the skin of their bellies, and each child has its own. Both were sent to me by the same gentleman, and are amongst my collection of foetuses, together with other useful preparations collected from time to time for the information and improvement of students; and now in the hands of Dr Harvie, my successor in the teaching of midwifery.

Sir,
Agreeable to my promise I have sent the preparation, which I hope will fully answer your expectation. The mother, who before had seven or eight children, miscarried with these at the end of twenty weeks, from her great uneasiness, she imagines in longing for a chop of bacon. She was taken at first with a considerable flooding, which was moderated by blooding and anodyne medicines. The next day finding some strong pains, her midwife was sent for, who delivered her in a few hours; notwithstanding their smallness, and one of them presenting with the feet, she found great difficulty in extracting them, as you will see by the laceration of one of them which is stitched up again. They had no signs of life. The mother has since had two fine children. This happened in the year 1735.

It is remarkable of the father of these children, that he had no teeth before the age of one or two and twenty; but has now as good a set as ever I saw, and can lift up very great weights with them, etc. From Henry North, surgeon in Stirminster Newton, in the county of Dorset, 4th July 1747.

Case 2

A child born, in which part of the skull was wanting, 1747, from Mr Pierce of St. Thomas's Hospital, apothecary.

It was a male child of an uncommon size in his body and limbs, with very broad shoulders, and a thick brawny neck. The head was smaller than those of most infants that come in due season, as this did. The nose was broad and flat, the eyes full, large, and very prominent, so that the lids could not cover them, the ears were remarkably large and thick. There was no skull to cover the brain, and the edges of the bones of the loser part of the head were as straight and smooth as if they had been sawn asunder immediately above the orbits of the eyes. There was wanting the *Os Frontis* on the fore-part, and on the back-part almost the whole of the *Occipitis*. The *Ossa Bregmatis* were entirely wanting, and as there was no scalp, the brain was covered by nothing but the *pia* and *dura mater*,[43] which looked of a dark livid colour, and was pushed out in diverse places by the brain, so that it made an unequal surface

---

[43]Smellie describes how the cranial bones are missing, leaving only the membranes (*pia* and *dura mater*).

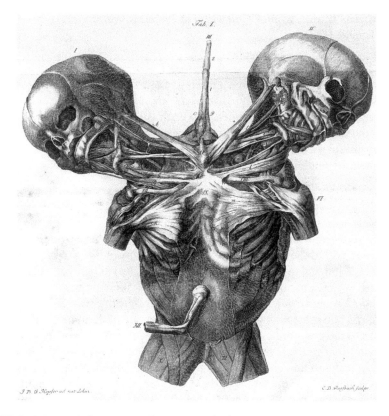

FIGURE 5: J. F. Meckel, 'Conjoined twins,' *De duplicitate monstrosa commentarius*, 1815.
Courtesy Wellcome Library, London.

for want of bones to confine it. This inequality and softness, together with the edge
of the bones, was what surprised the midwife, and made her expect a more difficult
delivery. The account then given by the mother, as the probable occasion of this
disaster, is as follows:

Upon the ninth of April 1747, when she was near two months gone with child,
she was grievously frightened with thinking on Lord Lovat, who was that day to
be beheaded.[44] Her husband was gone to see the execution among the crowd on
Tower-Hill, and when the news came to her hearing, that a scaffold was fallen down, by
which accident many people were hurt, and some killed on the spot, she immediately
feared that her husband might be of the number, and was greatly affected. While she
was under this dread and apprehension, an officious idle woman came to her and said,
that a friend of hers, for whom she had a great regard, was killed on the spot, and
that she saw his brains on the ground; upon this the poor woman put both her hands
on her head in great agony, and immediately fainted away.

---

[44]Simon Fraser, 11th Lord Lovat (1667–1747) was convicted of treason (for his part in the Battle of
Culloden) and became the last man to be beheaded in Britain.

Nymphomania
M. D. T. de Bienville (1775)

By the *Nymphomania* is understood an irregular, and disturbed motion of the fibres, in the organical parts of woman. This disorder is different from most others which are sudden in their attack, and declare, nearly at once, by evident symptoms, all their malignity; the *Nymphomania* on the contrary, lurks, almost without exception, under the imposing outside of an apparent calm, and frequently hath acquired a dangerous nature, when not only its progress, but its beginnings elude our perception. Sometimes the fair one, who is attacked by it, stands with one foot upon the precipice, without suspecting that she is in peril. It is a serpent which hath insensibly glided into her heart; and fortunate must she be, if before it can have mortally wounded her, she should exert a powerful resolution, and flee with speed, from this cruel and destructive foe.

...

Debauched girls who, during a long time, have lived amidst the disorders of a voluptuous life, are on a sudden, attacked by this malady. This is frequently the case, when an involuntary retreat drives them far off from the opportunities of indulging their fatal inclinations. Married women are not exempted from this distemper, particularly, when they are united either to a husband of so feeble a temperament, as to exact continence in his pleasures, or to a cold mate, but little sensible of the delights of enjoyment.

To this disorder, young widows are frequently liable, especially if death hath deprived them of a strong, and vigorous man, during a commerce with whom, by acts briskly repeated, they had acquired an habitude in pleasures, the dangerous remembrance of which too often affects them with that bitter regret, which produces uneasinesses, agitations, and motions at the first involuntary, but which, in the end, soon throw the mind into the most alarming situation.

In a word, all, when once they yield themselves a prey to this disorder, are uninterruptedly busied with equal perseverance and eagerness in the search of such objects as may kindle their passions at the infernal firebrand of lubricity; and if they engage with particular ardour in the pursuit, it is because they are impelled to it, by the natural vehemence of their constitution.

This natural vehemence must be simulated, and increased, when they read such luxurious novels as begin by preparing the heart for the impression of every tender sentiment, and end by leading it to the knowledge of all the grosser passions, and causing it to glow with each lascivious sensation. They also add fuel to the flames which devour them, by learning the most amorous songs: their impassioned voices incessantly accompany the tunes, and words of these which breathe into their souls the poison destined to destroy them.

In particular conversations with their companions, they are so far from using any efforts to banish the most seducing subjects from their imaginations, that they are assiduous in making them the leading topics. If, in spite of all their art, they cannot prevent the discourse from taking a turn quite opposite to their passions, they sink into languor, and pine under an incurable disquiet, which they have not the power to conceal.

They perpetually dishonour themselves in secret by habitual pollutions, of which they are themselves the unfortunate agents, until they have openly passed the bounds of modesty; but when impudence enlists itself on their side, they are no longer fearful of procuring this dreadful, and detestable pleasure from the assisting hand of a stranger.

Always disposed to listen to the flattering and seducing compliments of the men who surround them, they shudder at the most trifling employments whensoever they prove capable of turning them, for one moment aside from those lascivious subjects, which are the favourite pleasures of their imagination.

From the walks, where the most innocent sports of nature are, in their pre-occupied minds, the lively attractions of voluptuousness, they proceed to luxurious tables, at which the sharp, stimulating, and poisoned meats give the finishing stroke to that horrible disorder, into which the blood had previously been thrown.

Strong wines with which they are incessantly drenched, spirituous liquors which they swallow, as if they were water, the abused, and excessive use of chocolate; all these articles, (a single one of which is capable of corrupting the animal harmony) when united, impart additional fury to the flames which burn for their destruction; all these throw such sparks amongst the passions, as set fire to the most shameful and unbridled lust.

I grant that all these alarming accidents, of which it is impossible to draw a picture sufficiently hideous, are, at the first, supportable; but the dismal events which they produce, soon become of the highest concern, unless the most prudent means to repress their course, be instantly and earnestly embraced. On the contrary, the women who have neither the resolution, nor the power to turn back, after having taken their first step in this labyrinth of horrors, fall insensibly, and almost without any perception of their conduct, into those excesses which, having wounded their reputation, conclude by depriving them of life.

...

One of the principal points to which a physician ought to attach himself, is the study of the effects of the imagination, in the disorders which occur to him, in the course of his practice. A neglect of this important business must either involve us in mistakes, or plunge us into a total ignorance of the real causes of particular complaints.

...

The knowledge of interior and exterior physical symptoms, so absolutely necessary on all occasions, is, unfortunately, too limited, and the most learned physician may, in this respect, prove likely to be embarrassed, and even err daily in giving his opinion, and prescribing the conduct to be pursued.

...

There are cases which will admit of a cure from a simple attention to the imagination; but there are no cases (or, at least, scarcely any) in which physical remedies can alone effect a radical cure. There is no constitution without a germ of this natural and generative fire, unless some vice, or some accident contrary to the order of nature, should have excluded it; and this cannot be a case in any manner relative to the *Nymphomania*.

**Pseudo-Aristotle, 'Of Abortion and Untimely Birth', from *Aristotle's Masterpiece*
Anonymous (1777 ed.)**[45]

Why do women that eat unwholesome meats easily miscarry?

Because it breeds putrefied seed in them, which the mind abhorring doth cast it out
of the womb, as unfit for the most noble shape which is adapted to receive the soul.

Why doth wrestling or leaping cause the casting of the child as some subtile women
used to do on purpose?

The vapour is burning and doth easily hurt the tender substance of the child,
entering in at the pores of the matrix. Albertus says, if the child be near delivery,
lightning and thunder will kill it.

Why doth thunder and lightning rather cause young women than old to miscarry?

Because the bodies of young women are fuller of pores, and more slender and
therefore the lightning sooner enters into their body; but old ones have a thick skin,
well compacted, therefore the vapours cannot enter.

Why do much joy cause a woman to miscarry?

Because in the time of joy a woman is destitute of heat, and so the miscarriage
doth follow.

Why do women easily miscarry when they are first with child, viz., the first, second,
or third month?

As apples and pears easily fall at first, because the knots and ligaments are weak,
so it is of a child in the womb.

Why is it hard to miscarry when they are come to the midst of their times, as three,
four, five, or six months?

Because then the ligaments are stronger and well fortified.

**'Of the Sexual Intercourse', from *Lectures on Diet and Regimen*
A. F. M. Willich (1800)**

There are a variety of circumstances, by which either the utility or the insalubrity of
the sexual intercourse is, in general, to be determined. It is conducive to the well-
being of the individual, if Nature (not an extravagant or disordered imagination)
induces us to satisfy this inclination, especially under the following conditions:

1 In young persons, that is, adults, or those of a middle age; as, from the
   flexibility of their vessels, the strength of their muscles, and the abundance
   of their vital spirits, they can the better sustain the loss occasioned by this
   indulgence.

---

[45]Many versions and editions of this text were published from the late seventeenth century, and various authors
contributed at certain times. This popular book is likely the most widely reprinted text on a medical subject
in the eighteenth and early nineteenth century. For more on the various forms of *Aristotle's Masterpiece* and
The Works of Aristotle, see Mary E. Fissell (2007). 'Hairy Women and Naked Truths: Gender and the Politics
of Knowledge in Aristotle's Masterpiece'. *The William and Mary Quarterly* 60 (1): 43–74.

2 In robust persons, who lose no more than is almost immediately replaced.

3 In sprightly individuals, and such as are particularly addicted to pleasure; for, the stronger the natural desire, the safer is its gratification.

4 In persons who are accustomed to it – for Nature pursues a different path, accordingly as she is habituated to the re-absorption, or to the evacuation of this fluid.

5 With a beloved object; as the power animating the nerves and muscular fibres is in proportion to the pleasure received.

6 After a sound sleep; because then the body is more energetic; is provided with a new stock of vital spirits; and the fluids are duly prepared: hence the early morning appears to be designed by Nature for the exercise of this function; as the body is then most vigorous; and, being unemployed in any other pursuit, its natural propensity to this is the greater: besides, at this time, a few hours sleep can be readily obtained, by which the expended powers are, in a great measure, renovated.

7 With an empty stomach; for the office of digestion, so material to the restoration of bodily strength, is then uninterrupted. Lastly,

8 In the vernal months; as Nature, at this season in particular, incites all the lower animals to sexual intercourse; as we are then most vigorous and sprightly; and as the spring is not only the safest, but likewise the best time, with respect to the consequences resulting from that intercourse. It is well ascertained by experience, that children begotten in spring are of more solid fibres, and consequently more vigorous and robust, than those generated in the heat of summer, or cold of winter.

It may be collected from the following circumstances, whether or not the gratification of the sexual impulse has been conducive to the well-being of the body; namely, if it be not succeeded by a peculiar lassitude; if the body do not feel heavy, and the mind averse to reflection: all which are favourable symptoms, indicating that the various powers have sustained no essential loss, and that superfluous matter only has been evacuated.

Farther, the healthy appearance of the urine, in this case, as well as cheerfulness and vivacity of mind, also prove a proper coction of the fluids, and sufficiently evince an unimpaired slate of the animal functions, a due perspiration, and a free circulation of the blood.

There are, however, many cases in which this gratification is the more detrimental to health, when it has been immoderate, and without the impulse of Nature, but particularly in the following situations:

1 In all debilitated persons; as they do not possess sufficient vital spirits; and their vigour, after this enervating emission, is consequently much exhausted. Their digestion necessarily suffers, perspiration is checked, and the body becomes languid and heavy.

2 In the aged, whole vital heat is diminished, whose frame is enfeebled by the moderate enjoyment, and whole strength, already reduced, suffers a

still greater diminution, from every loss, that is accompanied with a violent convulsion of the whole body.

3 In persons not arrived at the age of maturity: by an early intercourse with the other sex, they become enervated and emaciated, and inevitably shorten their lives.

4 In dry, choleric, and thin persons: these, even at a mature age, should seldom indulge in this passion, as their bodies are already in want of moisture and pliability, both of which are much diminished by the sexual intercourse, while the bile is violently agitated, to the great injury of the whole animal frame. Lean persons generally are of a hot temperament; and the more heat there is in the body, the greater will be the subsequent dryness. Hence, likewise, to persons in a state of intoxication, this intercourse is extremely pernicious; because in such a state the increased circulation of the blood towards the head, may be attended with dangerous consequences, such as burning of blood vessels, apoplexy, etc. – the plethoric[46] are particularly exposed to these dangers.

5 Immediately after meals; as the powers requisite to the digestion of food are thus diverted, consequently the aliment remains too long unassimilated, and becomes burdensome to the stomach.

6 After violent exercise; in which case it is still more hurtful than in the preceding, where muscular strength was not consumed, but only required to the aid of another function. After bodily fatigue, on the contrary, the necessary energy is in a manner exhausted, so that every additional exertion of the body must be peculiarly injurious.

7 In the heat of summer, it is less to be indulged in than in spring and autumn; because the process of concoction and assimilation is effected less vigorously in summer than in the other seasons, and consequently the losses sustained are not so easily recovered. For a similar reason, the sexual commerce is more debilitating, and the capacity for it sooner extinguished, in hot than in temperate climates. The same remark is applicable to every warm temperature combined with moisture, which is extremely apt to debilitate the solid parts. Hence hatters, dyers, bakers, brewers, and all those exposed to steam, generally have relaxed fibres.

8 In a posture of body, which requires great muscular exertion, it is comparatively more enfeebling; as, in this cafe, various powers are exhausted at once.

On The Origin of Species
Charles Darwin (1859)

Sexual Selection – Inasmuch as peculiarities often appear under domestication in one sex and become hereditarily attached to that sex, the same fact probably occurs under

---

[46]Plethoric or sanguine: characterized by overabundant blood.

nature, and if so, natural selection will be able to modify one sex in its functional relations to the other sex, or in relation to wholly different habits of life in the two sexes, as is sometimes the case with insects. And this leads me to say a few words on what I call Sexual Selection. This depends, not on a struggle for existence, but on a struggle between the males for possession of the females; the result is not death to the unsuccessful competitor, but few or no offspring. Sexual selection is, therefore, less rigorous than natural selection. Generally, the most vigorous males, those which are best fitted for their places in nature, will leave most progeny. But in many cases, victory will depend not on general vigour, but on having special weapons, confined to the male sex. A hornless stag or spurless cock would have a poor chance of leaving offspring. Sexual selection by always allowing the victor to breed might surely give indomitable courage, length to the spur, and strength to the wing to strike in the spurred leg, as well as the brutal cock-fighter, who knows well that he can improve his breed by careful selection of the best cocks. How low in the scale of nature this law of battle descends, I know not; male alligators have been described as fighting, bellowing, and whirling round, like Indians in a war-dance, for the possession of the females; male salmons have been seen fighting all day long; male stag-beetles often bear wounds from the huge mandibles of other males. The war is, perhaps, severest between the males of polygamous animals, and these seem oftenest provided with special weapons. The males of carnivorous animals are already well armed; though to them and to others, special means of defence may be given through means of sexual selection, as the mane to the lion, the shoulder-pad to the boar, and the hooked jaw to the male salmon; for the shield may be as important for victory, as the sword or spear.

Amongst birds, the contest is often of a more peaceful character. All those who have attended to the subject, believe that there is the severest rivalry between the males of many species to attract by singing the females. The rock-thrush of Guiana, birds of Paradise, and some others, congregate; and successive males display their gorgeous plumage and perform strange antics before the females, which standing by as spectators, at last choose the most attractive partner. Those who have closely attended to birds in confinement well know that they often take individual preferences and dislikes: thus Sir R. Heron has described how one pied peacock was eminently attractive to all his hen birds. It may appear childish to attribute any effect to such apparently weak means: I cannot here enter on the details necessary to support this view; but if man can in a short time give elegant carriage and beauty to his bantams, according to his standard of beauty, I can see no good reason to doubt that female birds, by selecting, during thousands of generations, the most melodious or beautiful males, according to their standard of beauty, might produce a marked effect. I strongly suspect that some well-known laws with respect to the plumage of male and female birds, in comparison with the plumage of the young, can be explained on the view of plumage having been chiefly modified by sexual selection, acting when the birds have come to the breeding age or during the breeding season; the modifications thus produced being inherited at corresponding ages or seasons, either by the males alone, or by the males and females; but I have not space here to enter on this subject.

Thus it is, as I believe, that when the males and females of any animal have the same general habits of life, but differ in structure, colour, or ornament, such differences have been mainly caused by sexual selection; that is, individual males have had, in successive generations, some slight advantage over other males, in their weapons, means of defence, or charms; and have transmitted these advantages to their male offspring. Yet, I would not wish to attribute all such sexual differences to this agency: for we see peculiarities arising and becoming attached to the male sex in our domestic animals (as the wattle in male carriers, horn-like protuberances in the cocks of certain fowls, etc.), which we cannot believe to be either useful to the males in battle, or attractive to the females. We see analogous cases under nature, for instance, the tuft of hair on the breast of the turkey-cock, which can hardly be either useful or ornamental to this bird; – indeed, had the tuft appeared under domestication, it would have been called a monstrosity.

The Functions and Disorders of the Reproductive Organs
William Acton (1867 ed.)

'Marital Excesses'

Any warning against sexual dangers would be very incomplete if it did not extend to the excesses too often committed by married persons in ignorance of their ill-effects. Too frequent emission of the life-giving fluid, and too frequent sexual excitement of the nervous system, is as we have seen, in itself most destructive. Whether it occurs in married or unmarried people has little, if anything, to do with the result. The married man who thinks that, because he is a married man, he can commit no excess, however often the act of sexual congress is repeated, will suffer as certainly and as seriously as the debauchee who acts on the same principle in his indulgences – perhaps more certainly, from his very ignorance and from his not taking those precautions and following those rules which a career of vice is apt to teach a man.

Many a man has, until his marriage, lived a most continent life – so has his wife. But as soon as they are wedded, intercourse is indulged in night after night, neither party having any idea that this is an excess which the system of neither can bear, and which to the man, at least is simple ruin. The practice is continued till health is impaired, sometimes permanently, and when a patient is at last obliged to seek medical advice he is thunderstruck at learning that his sufferings arise from such a cause as this. People often appear to think that connection may be repeated just as regularly and almost as often as meals may. Till they are told, the idea never enters their heads that they have been guilty of great and almost criminal excess; nor is this to be wondered at, as such a cause of disease is seldom hinted at by the medical man they consult.

Some years ago a young man called on me, complaining that he was unequal to sexual congress, and was suffering from spermatorrhoea,[47] the result, he said, of self-abuse.[48] He was cauterized, and I lost sight of him until March, 1856, when he

---

[47]Spermatorrhoea is excessive, involuntary ejaculation.
[48]Self-abuse refers to masturbation.

returned complaining that he was scarcely able to move alone. His mind had become enfeebled, there was great pain in the back, and he wished me to repeat the operation.

On cross-examining the patient, I found that he had recovered his powers after the previous cauterization, and, strange to say had been in the habit of indulging in connection (ever since I had seen him, two years ago) three times a week, without any idea that he was committing an excess, or that his present weakness could depend upon this cause. This is far from being an isolated instance of men who, having been reduced by former excesses, still imagine themselves equal to any excitement, and when their powers are recovered, to any expenditure of vital force. Some go so far as to believe that indulgence may increase these powers, just as gymnastic exercise does the muscles. This is a popular error, and requires correction. Such patients should be told that the shock on the system, each time connection is indulged in, is very powerful, and that the expenditure of seminal fluid must be particularly injurious to organs already debilitated. It is thus that premature old age and complaints of the generative organs are brought on. A few months later I again saw this young man, and all his symptoms had improved under abstinence, care, and tonics.

...

I will give one more instance. A medical man called on me, saying he found himself suffering from spermatorrhoea. There was general debility, inaptitude to work, disinclination for sexual intercourse, in fact, he thought he was losing his senses. The sight of one eye was affected. The only way in which he lost semen was, as he thought, by a slight occasional oozing from the penis. I asked him at once if he had ever committed excesses. As a boy, he acknowledged having abused himself, but he married seven years ago, being then a hearty, healthy man, and it was only lately that he had been complaining. In answer to my further inquiry, he stated that since his marriage he had had connection two or three times a week, and often more than once a night! This one fact, I was obliged to tell him, sufficiently accounted for all his troubles. The symptoms he complained of were similar to those we find in boys who abuse themselves. It is true that it may take years to reduce some strong, healthy men, just as it may be a long time before some boys are prejudicially influenced, but the ill effects of excesses are sooner or later sure to follow.

...

'Indisposition for Connection among Single Men'

This condition may arise from a variety of causes. We find, for instance, that some men reach adult age without having experienced any sexual desire at all. That complete sexual quiescence, which we have noticed as being the proper condition of childhood continues, in these cases, during the period of youth, and even into adult age.

So unusual a phenomenon as the entire non-development of the sexual desire must always be rather an alarming and suspicious circumstance; unfortunately, in the majority of cases the medical man is not consulted, as neither the patient nor his friends are aware that there is anything unusual in his condition until it is accidentally discovered. When the surgeon is consulted, however, he will usually find that the individual is fat, without hair on his face; or even down on the pubes; the testes and penis are small, almost rudimentary, like those of a young child, no sexual desire ever troubles him, and his voice is often weak and almost falsetto in quality; in fact, the condition is much the same as that of the castrated individual or eunuch.

In such a case it is clear that the non-development of the testes has produced this state of eunuchism,[49] as well as most of the peculiar changes which, both in animals and in human beings, attend the condition of castration.

The undeveloped state of the reproductive system, whether permanent or temporary, usually indicates itself by, among other signs, a marked indifference to manly sports and exercise, and a visible deficiency in virile attributes generally.

...

It should be recollected that other causes produce indifference to the opposite sex and deficiency in manly vigor. The most common of such causes is the wretched habit of masturbation... A youth who masturbates himself and continues the practice as he grows up to manhood, generally evinces, even after he has arrived at the marriageable age, no disposition towards the other sex. Only his own solitary pleasure can give him any gratification; as far as women are concerned, he is virtually impotent. Lallemand[50] gives the following perhaps rather too graphic account of such a person's state of feeling towards the opposite sex: 'Their solitary vice has a tendency to separate those practicing it from women. At first, of course, it is on the sex that their thoughts dwell, and they embellish an ideal being with all the charms of imaginary perfection; the habit, however, which enslaves them little by little, changes and depraves the nature of their ideas, and at last leaves nothing but indifference for the very reality of which the image has been so constantly evoked to aid their criminal indulgence. At a later period, when erection is only temporary and is too incomplete for them to think of sexual intercourse, they abandon themselves with fury to their fatal habit, notwithstanding the almost complete flaccidity in which the erectile tissues are left. At this period the handsomest women only inspire these patients with repugnance and disgust; and they ultimately acquire an instinctive aversion, a real hatred for the sex.'

...

'Want of Sexual Feeling in the Female a Cause of Impotence'

I should say that the majority of women (happily for them) are not very much troubled with sexual feeling of any kind. What men are habitually, women are only exceptionally. It is too true, I admit, as the divorce courts show, that there are some few women who have sexual desires so strong that they surpass those of men, and shock public feeling by their exhibition. I admit, of course, the existence of sexual excitement terminating even in nymphomania, a form of insanity that those accustomed to visit lunatic asylums must be fully conversant with; but, with these sad exceptions, there can be no doubt that sexual feeling in the female is in the majority of cases in abeyance, and that it requires positive and considerable excitement to be roused at all; and even if roused (which in many instances it never can be) is very moderate compared with that of the male. Many men, and particularly young men,

---

[49]Eunuchism: having non-functioning, or castrated testes.
[50]Claude François Lallemand (1790–1854) was a French physician, who was instrumental in establishing spermatorrhea as a disease (peculiar to the nineteenth century) brought on by masturbation.

form their ideas of women's feelings from what they notice early in life among loose or, at least, low and vulgar women. There is always a certain number of females who, though not ostensibly in the rank of prostitutes, make a kind of trade of a pretty face. They are fond of admiration, they like to attract the attention of those immediately above them. Any susceptible boy is easily led to believe, whether he is altogether overcome by the syren or not, that she, and therefore all women, must have at least as strong passions as himself. Such women however give a very false idea of the condition of female sexual feeling in general. Association with the loose women of London streets, in casinos, and other immoral haunts (who, if they have not sexual feeling, counterfeit it so well that the novice does not suspect but that it is genuine), all seem to corroborate such an impression, and as I have stated above, it is from these erroneous notions that so many young men think that the marital duties they will have to undertake are beyond their exhausted strength, and from this reason dread and avoid marriage.

Married men – medical men – or married women themselves, would, if appealed to, tell a very different tale, and vindicate female nature from the vile aspersions cast on it by the abandoned conduct and ungoverned lusts of a few of its worst examples.

There are many females who never feel any sexual excitement whatever. Others, again, immediately after each period, do become, to a limited degree, capable of experiencing it; but this capacity is often temporary, and will cease entirely till the next menstrual period. The best mothers, wives, and managers of households, know little or nothing of sexual indulgences. Love of home, children, and domestic duties, are the only passions they feel.[51]

As a general rule, a modest woman seldom desires any sexual gratification for herself. She submits to her husband, but only to please him; and, but for the desire of maternity, would far rather be relieved from his attentions. No nervous or feeble young man need, therefore, be deterred from marriage by any exaggerated notion of the duties required from him. The married woman has no wish to be treated on the footing of a mistress.

One instance may better illustrate the real state of the case than much description.

In —, 186 – , a barrister, about thirty years of age, came to me on account of sexual debility. On cross-examination, I found he had been married a twelvemonth, and that connection had taken place but once since the commencement of the year, and that there was some doubt as to the completion of the act then. He brought his wife with him, as she was, he said, desirous of having some conversation with me.

I found the lady a refined but highly sensitive person. Speaking with a freedom equally removed from assurance, or *mauvaise honte*, she told me she thought it

---

[51]Author's note: 'The physiologist will not be surprised that the human female should in these respects differ but little from the female among animals. We well know it, as a fact, that the dog or stallion is not allowed approach to the female except at particular seasons. In the human female, indeed, I believe, it is rather from the wish of pleasing or gratifying the husband than from any strong sexual feeling, that cohabitation is so habitually allowed. Certainly, it is so during the months of gestation. I have known instances where the female has during gestation evinced positive loathing for any marital familiarity whatever. In some of these instances, indeed, feeling has been sacrificed to duty, and the wife has endured, with all the self-martyrdom of womanhood, what was almost worse than death.'

her duty to consult me. She neither blushed nor faltered in telling her story, and I regret that my words must fail to convey the delicacy with which her avowal was made.

Her husband and herself, she said, had been acquainted since childhood, had grown up together, became mutually attached, and married. She believed him debilitated, but – as she was fully convinced – from no indiscreet acts on his part. She believed it was his natural condition. She was dotingly attached to him, and would not have determined to consult me but that she wished, for his sake, to have a family, as it would, she hoped, conduce to their mutual happiness. She assured me that she felt no sexual passions whatever; that if she was capable of them, they were dormant. Her passion for her husband was of a Platonic kind, and far from wishing to stimulate his frigid feelings, she doubted whether it would be right or not. She loved him as he was and would not desire him to be otherwise except for the hope of having a child.

I believe this lady is a perfect ideal of an English wife and mother, kind, considerate, self-sacrificing, and sensible, so pure-hearted as to be utterly ignorant of and averse to any sexual indulgence, but so unselfishly attached to the man she loves, as to be willing to give up her own wishes and feelings for his sake.

A great contrast to the unselfish sacrifices such married women make of their feelings in allowing cohabitation is offered by others, who, either from ignorance or utter want of sympathy, although they are model wives in every other respect, not only evince no sexual feeling, but, on the contrary, scruple not to declare their aversion to the least manifestation of it. Doubtless this may, and often does, depend upon disease, and if so, the sooner the suffering female is treated the better. Much more frequently, however, it depends upon apathy, selfish indifference to please, or unwillingness to overcome the natural repugnance which such females feel for cohabitation.

Sexual Selection in Man
Havelock Ellis (1905)

In his famous *Descent of Man*, wherein he first set forth the doctrine of sexual selection, Darwin injured an essentially sound principle by introducing into it a psychological confusion whereby the physiological sensory stimuli through which sexual selection operates were regarded as equivalent to aesthetic preferences. This confusion misled many, and it is only within recent years... that the investigations and criticisms of numerous workers have placed the doctrine of sexual selection on a firm basis by eliminating its hazardous aesthetic element. Love springs up as a response to a number of stimuli to tumescence, the object that most adequately arouses tumescence being that which evokes love; the question of aesthetic beauty, although it develops on this basis, is not itself fundamental and need not even be consciously present at all. When we look at these phenomena in their broadest biological aspects, love is only to a limited extent a response to beauty; to a greater extent beauty is simply a name for the complexus of stimuli which most adequately arouses love. If we analyze these stimuli to tumescence as they proceed from a person of the opposite sex we find that they are all appeals which must come through the channels of four senses: touch, smell, hearing, and, above all, vision.

When a man or a woman experiences sexual love for one particular person from among the multitude by which he or she is surrounded, this is due to the influences of a group of stimuli coming through the channels of one or more of these senses. There has been a sexual selection conditioned by sensory stimuli. This is true even of the finer and more spiritual influences that proceed from one person to another, although, in order to grasp the phenomena adequately, it is best to insist on the more fundamental and less complex forms which they assume. In this sense sexual selection is no longer a hypothesis concerning the truth of which it is possible to dispute; it is a self-evident fact. The difficulty is not as to its existence, but as to the methods by which it may be most precisely measured. It is fundamentally a psychological process, and should be approached from the psychological side. This is the reason for dealing with it here. Obscure as the psychological aspects of sexual selection still remain, they are full of fascination, for they reveal to us the more intimate sides of human evolution, of the process whereby man is molded into the shapes we know.

...

'Vision' is the main channel by which man receives his impressions. To a large extent it has slowly superseded all the other senses. Its range is practically infinite; it brings before us remote worlds, it enables us to understand the minute details of our own structure. While apt for the most abstract or the most intimate uses, its intermediate range is of universal service. It furnishes the basis on which a number of arts make their appeal to us, and, while thus the most aesthetic of the senses, it is the sense on which we chiefly rely in exercising the animal function of nutrition. It is not surprising, therefore, that from the point of view of sexual selection vision should be the supreme sense, and that the love-thoughts of men have always been a perpetual meditation of beauty.

...

There is [a] reason why the sexual organs should be discarded as objects of sexual allurement, a reason which always proves finally decisive as a people advances in culture. They are not aesthetically beautiful. It is fundamentally necessary that the intromittent organ of the male and the receptive canal of the female should retain their primitive characteristics; they cannot, therefore, be greatly modified by sexual or natural selection, and the exceedingly primitive character they are thus compelled to retain, however sexually desirable and attractive they may become to the opposite sex under the influence of emotion, can rarely be regarded as beautiful from the point of view of aesthetic contemplation. Under the influence of art there is a tendency for the sexual organs to be diminished in size, and in no civilized country has the artist ever chosen to give an erect organ to his representations of ideal masculine beauty. It is mainly because the unaesthetic character of a woman's sexual region is almost imperceptible in any ordinary and normal position of the nude body that the feminine form is a more aesthetically beautiful object of contemplation than the masculine. Apart from this character we are probably bound, from a strictly aesthetic point of view, to regard the male form as more aesthetically beautiful. The female form, moreover, usually overpasses very swiftly the period of the climax of its beauty, often only retaining it during a few weeks.

The following communication from a correspondent well brings out the divergences of feeling in this matter:

> You write that the sex organs, in an excited condition, cannot be called aesthetic. But I believe that they are a source, not only of curiosity and wonder to many persons, but also objects of admiration. I happen to know of one man, extremely intellectual and refined, who delights in lying between his mistress's thighs and gazing long at the dilated vagina. Also another man, married, and not intellectual, who always tenderly gazes at his wife's organs, in a strong light, before intercourse, and kisses her there and upon the abdomen. The wife, though amative, confessed to another woman that she could not understand the attraction. On the other hand, two married men have told me that the sight of their wives' genital parts would disgust them, and that they have never seen them.
>
> If the sexual parts cannot be called aesthetic, they have still a strong charm for many passionate lovers, of both sexes, though not often, I believe, among the unimaginative and the uneducated, who are apt to ridicule the organs or to be repelled by them. Many women confess that they are revolted by the sight of even a husband's complete nudity, though they have no indifference for sexual embraces. I think that the stupid bungle of Nature in making the generative organs serve as means of relieving the bladder has much to do with this revulsion. But some women of erotic temperament find pleasure in looking at the penis of a husband or lover, in handling it, and in kissing it. Prostitutes do this in the way of business; some chaste, passionate wives act thus voluntarily. This is scarcely morbid, as the mammalia of most species smell and lick each others' genitals. Probably primitive man did the same.

'The Sexual Aberrations', from *Three Contributions to the Sexual Theory* Sigmund Freud (1910)

The fact of sexual need in man and animal is expressed in biology by the assumption of a 'sexual impulse.' This impulse is made analogous to the impulse of taking nourishment, and to hunger. The sexual expression corresponding to hunger not being found colloquially, science uses the expression 'libido.'

Popular conception assumes very different ideas concerning the nature and qualities of this sexual impulse. It is supposed to be absent during childhood and to commence about the time of and in connection with the maturing process of puberty; it is supposed that it manifests itself in irresistible attractions exerted by one sex upon the other, and that its aim is sexual union or at least such actions as would lead to union.

But we have every reason to see in these assumptions a very untrustworthy picture of reality. On closer examination they are found to abound in errors, inaccuracies and hasty conclusions.

If we introduce two terms and call the person from whom the sexual attraction emanates the sexual object, and the action towards which the impulse strives the sexual aim, then the scientifically examined experience shows us many deviations in reference to both sexual object and sexual aim, the relations of which to the accepted standard require thorough investigation.

1. 'Deviation in Reference to the Sexual Object'

The popular theory of the sexual impulse corresponds closely to the poetic fable of dividing the person into two halves – man and woman – who strive to become reunited through love. It is therefore very surprising to hear that there are men for whom the sexual object is not woman but man, and that there are women for whom it is not man but woman. Such persons are called contrary sexuals, or better, inverts; that is, these form the actualities of inversion. They exist in very considerable numbers, although their definite ascertainment is subject to difficulties.

...

I. Inversion

Conception of Inversion.

The first attention bestowed upon inversion gave rise to the conception that it was a congenital sign of nervous degeneration. This harmonized with the fact that doctors first met it among the nervous, or among persons giving such an impression. There are two elements which should be considered independently in this conception: the congenitality, and the degeneration.

Degeneration.

This term *degeneration* is open to the objections which may be urged against the promiscuous use of this word in general. It has in fact become customary to designate all morbid manifestations not of traumatic or infectious origin as degenerative... Under the circumstances it is a question what use and what new content the meaning of 'degeneration' still possesses. It would seem more appropriate not to speak of degeneration: Where there are not many marked deviations from the normal; where the capabilities and the capacity to exist do not in general appear markedly impaired.

That the inverted are not degenerates in this qualified sense can be seen from the following facts:

1 The inversion is found among persons who otherwise show no marked deviation from the normal.

2 It is found also among persons whose capabilities are not disturbed, who on the contrary are distinguished by especially high intellectual development and ethical culture.

3 If one disregards the patients of one's own practice and strives to comprehend a wider field of experience, he will in two directions encounter facts which will prevent him from assuming inversions as a degenerative sign.

...

The Sexual Object of Inverts.

The theory of psychic hermaphroditism presupposed that the sexual object of the inverted is the reverse of the normal. The inverted man, like the woman, succumbs to the charms emanating from manly qualities of body and mind; he feels himself like a woman and seeks a man.

But however true this may be for a great number of inverts it by no means indicates the general character of inversion. There is no doubt that a great part of the male inverted have retained the psychic character of virility, that proportionately they show but little the secondary characters of the other sex, and that they really look for real feminine psychic features in their sexual object. If that were not so it would be incomprehensible why masculine prostitution, in offering itself to inverts, copies in all its exterior, today as in antiquity, the dress and attitudes of woman. This imitation would otherwise be an insult to the ideal of the inverts.

...

2. 'Deviation in Reference to the Sexual Aim'

The union of the genitals in the characteristic act of copulation is taken as the normal sexual aim. It serves to loosen the sexual tension and temporarily to quench the sexual desire (gratification analogous to satiation of hunger). Yet even in the most normal sexual process those additions are distinguishable, the development of which leads to the aberrations described as perversions. Thus certain intermediary relations to the sexual object connected with copulation, such as touching and looking, are recognized as preliminary to the sexual aim. These activities are on the one hand themselves connected with pleasure and on the other hand they enhance the excitement which persists until the definite sexual aim is reached.

One definite kind of contiguity, consisting of mutual approximation of the mucous membranes of the lips in the form of a kiss, has among the most civilized nations received a sexual value, though the parts of the body concerned do not belong to the sexual apparatus but form the entrance to the digestive tract. This therefore supplies the factors which allow us to bring the perversions into relation with the normal sexual life, and which are available also for their classification. The perversions are either (a) anatomical transgressions of the bodily regions destined for the sexual union, or (b) a lingering at the intermediary relations to the sexual object which should normally be rapidly passed on the way to the definite sexual aim.

(a) Anatomical Transgression

Overestimation of the Sexual Object – The psychic estimation in which the sexual object as a wish-aim of the sexual impulse participates, is only in the rarest cases limited to the genitals; generally it embraces the whole body and tends to include all sensations emanating from the sexual object. The same over-estimation spreads over the psychic sphere and manifests itself as a logical blinding (diminished judgment) in the face of the psychic attainments and perfections of the sexual object, as well as a blind obedience to the judgments issuing from the latter. The full faith of love thus becomes an important, if not the most primordial source of authority.

...

Sexual Utilization of the Mucous Membrane of the Lips and Mouth – The significance of the factor of sexual over-estimation can be best studied in the man, in whom alone the sexual life is accessible to investigation, whereas in the woman it is veiled in impenetrable darkness, partly in consequence of cultural stunting and partly on account of the conventional reticence and dishonesty of women.

The employment of the mouth as a sexual organ is considered as a perversion if the lips (tongue) of the one are brought into contact with the genitals of the other, but not when the mucous membrane of the lips of both touch each other. In the latter exception we find the connection with the normal. He who abhors the former as perversions, though these since antiquity have been common practices among mankind, yields to a distinct feeling of loathing which protects him from adopting such sexual aims. The limit of such loathing is frequently purely conventional; he who kisses fervently the lips of a pretty girl will perhaps be able to use her tooth brush only with a sense of loathing, though there is no reason to assume that his own oral cavity for which he entertains no loathing is cleaner than that of the girl. Our attention is here called to the factor of loathing which stands in the way of the libidinous over-estimation of the sexual aim, but which may in turn be vanquished by the libido. In the loathing we may observe one of the forces which have brought about the limitations of the sexual aim. As a rule these forces halt at the genitals; there is, however, no doubt that even the genitals of the other sex themselves may be an object of loathing. Such behavior is characteristic of all hysterics, especially women. The power of the sexual impulse by preference occupies itself with the overcoming of this loathing.

Wise Parenthood
Marie Stopes (1919 ed.)

A few fortunate people who really understand their own physiology, or by happy instinct have chanced upon the right use of their bodies and have been in the habit of practising satisfactory methods [of birth control], may say or think that such simple and direct instruction as follows is not needed. To them the answer is that the personally fortunate are ever the most callous and unaware of the needs of others. I have overwhelming evidence and experience that ignorance is rife even in the very places where knowledge might be expected to hold sway. For some time past, scarcely a day has gone by without my receiving letter after letter from people who have long been married, from people who have consulted physicians, from people who have tried many experiments, and who are yet ignorant of any really *satisfactory* means of achieving what they have been perforce achieving in unsatisfactory ways. I once asked a medical woman who had had a practice for fifteen years what method [of birth control] she would advise: she knew of no method whatever. A well-known doctor in London, who for twenty years had had a general and important family practice, asked me if I could tell him of any method other than the sheath, which was the only one he knew, as his patients were inquiring and he did not know what to tell them. Many married couples who are even told by the doctor that for the wife to have another child would be fatal, are at the same time not told any rational method of prevention. With variations depending on the temperament of the writer, I get appeals one after the other saying: 'We have asked our doctor, but he tells us nothing which is of any use. We have therefore to go on using this, that, or the other method, which we feel to be unsatisfactory, because we do not know what else to do.'

Churchmen recommend (though I wonder if they practise) 'absolute continence.' Where the mated pair are young, normal, and in love, such advice is not only impracticable, it is detrimental. A rigid and enforced abstinence can be as destructive of health as incontinence.

Destructive of the health of both mother and child are the frantic efforts of women 'caught' prematurely after a birth, or too frequently in their lives, by undesired motherhood. The desolating effects of attempted abortion can only be exterminated by a sound knowledge of the control of conception.

...

Women, driven to despair, to madness, by the incessant horror of pregnancies they dread, will by hook or by crook, from the street corner or the gutter, find out how to strangle the life which should never have begun.

...

To those who protest that we have no right to interfere with the course of Nature, one must point out that the whole of civilisation, everything which separates men from animals, is an interference with what such people commonly call Nature.

Nothing in the cosmos could be against Nature, for it all forms part of the great processes of the universe.

Actions differ, however, in their relative positions in the scale of things. Only those actions are worthy which lead the race always to a higher and fuller completion and the perfecting of its powers, which steer the race into the main current of that stream of life and vitality which courses through us and impels us forward.

It is a sacred duty of all who dare to hand on the awe-inspiring gift of life, to hand it on in a vessel as fit and perfect as they can fashion, so that the body may be the strongest and most beautiful instrument possible in the service of the soul they summon to play its part in the mystery of material being.

CHAPTER EIGHT

Aging and Dying

from *The Old, Old, Very Old Man*
John Taylor (1635)[1]

He is a Wonder, worthy Admiration,
He's (in these times filled with Iniquity)
No *Antiquary*, but *Antiquity*;
For his Longevity's of such extent,
That he's a living mortal Monument.
And as high Towers, (that seem the sky to shoulder)
By eating time, consume away, and moulder,
Until at last in piece meal they do fall;
Till they are buried in their Ruins All:
So this Old Man, his limbs their strength have left,
His teeth all gone, (but one) his sight bereft,
His sinews shrunk, his blood most chill and cold,
Small solace, Imperfections manifold:
Yet still his spirits possess his mortal Trunk;
Nor are his senses in his ruins shrunk,
But that his Hearing's quick, his stomach good,
He'll feed well, sleep well, well digest his food.
He will speak heartily, laugh, and be merry;
Drink Ale, and now and then a cup of Sherry;
Loves Company, and Understanding talk,
And (on both sides held up) will sometimes walk.
And though old Age his face with wrinkles fill,
He hath been handsome, and is comely still,
Well fac'd; and though his Beard not oft corrected,
Yet neat it grows, not like a Beard neglected;
From head to heel, his body hath all over,
A Quick-set, Thick-set natural hairy cover.
And thus (as my dull weak Invention can)
I have anatomized this poor Old Man.

---

[1]Originally published in 1635, this poem was consistently republished throughout the eighteenth and nineteenth centuries. The version here is very slightly modernized, reflective of the later editions.

Though Age be incident to most transgressing,
Yet time well spent, make Age to be a blessing.
And if our studies would but deign to look,
And seriously to ponder Nature's Book,
We there may read, that Man, the noblest Creature,
By riot and excess doth murder Nature.
This man never fed on dear compounded dishes,
Of Metamorphosed beasts, fruit, fowls, and fishes,
The earth, the air, the boundless Ocean
Were never raked nor foraged for this Man;
Nor ever did Physician to (his cost)
Send purging Physic through his guts in post;
In all his lifetime he was never known,
That drinking other's health, he lost his own;
The Dutch, the French, the Greek, and Spanish grape,
Upon his reason never made a rape;
For *Ryot*, is for *Troy*, an anagram;
And *Ryot*, wasted *Troy*, with sword and flame:
And surely that which will a kingdom spill,
Hath much more power one silly man to kill,
Whilst sensuality the palate pleases,
The body's filled with surfeits, and diseases;
By riot (more than war) men slaughtered be,
From which confusion this old man is free.
He once was catched in the venereal sin,
And (being punished) did experience win,
That careful fear his Conscience so did strike,
He never would again attempt the like.
Which to our understandings may express
Men's days are shortened through lasciviousness,
And that a competent contenting diet
Makes men live long, and soundly sleep in quiet.
Mistake me not, I speak not to debar
Good fare of all sorts; for all Creatures are
Made for man's use, and may by Man be used,
Not by voracious Gluttony abused.
For he that dares to scandal or deprave
Good house-keeping; Oh hang up such a knave,
Rather commend (what is not to be found)
Than injure that which makes the world renowned.
Bounty hath got a spice of *Lethargy*,
And liberal noble *Hospitality*
Lies in consumption, almost pinned to death,
And Charity benumbed, near out of breath.
May *England's* few good house-keepers be blest
With endless glory, and eternal Rest;

And my their goods, lands, and their happy seed
With heaven's blest blessings multiply and breed.

To a Gentleman that Cut off his Hair… in his Old Age
Thomas Brown (1700)

Thou, that not many months ago
Wast white as Swan, or driven Snow,
Now blacker far than *Aesop's* Crow,
Thanks to thy Wig, set'st up for Beau,
    Faith, *Harry*, thou'rt in the wrong box,
Old Age these vain endeavours mocks,
And time that knows thou'st hoary locks,
Will pluck thy Mask off with a pox.

A Song of a Young Lady to Her Ancient Lover
John Wilmot, Earl of Rochester (1705)

Ancient Person, for whom I
All the flattering Youth defy,
Long be it e'er thou grow Old,
Aking, shaking, crasie cold;
But still continue as thou art,
Ancient Person of my Heart.

On thy wither'd Lips and dry,
Which like barren Furrows lye,
Brooding Kisses I will pour,
Shall they youthful Heart restore,
Such kind Show'rs in autumn fall,
And a second Spring recall;
Nor from thee will ever part,
Ancient Person of my Heart.

Thy Nobler Parts, which but to name
In our Sex would be counted Shame,
By Ages frozen Grasp posses'd,
From their Ice shall be releas'd,
And, sooth'd by my reviving Hand,
In former Warmth and Vigour stand.
All a Lover's Wish can reach,
For thy Joy my Love shall teach;
And for they Pleasure shall improve
All that Art can add to Love.
Yet still I love thee without Art,
Ancient Person of my Heart.

from *A Dialogue Between a Blind-man and Death*
Richard Standfast (c. 1750–90 eds.)[2]

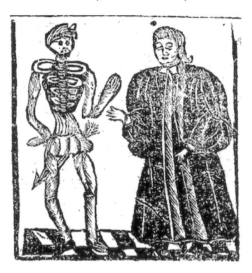

Blind-Man: The more men see, the less they do enquire;
The worse they see, the more they do desire;
Others to grant what Blindness cannot give,
And for intelligence grow inquisitive.
They ask to be inform'd, who cannot see.
I know by sad experience, Woe is me!

The B L I N D - M A N.

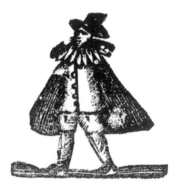

Death: What are you, Sir, thus standing all alone,
I did suppose 'twas you, by that sad moan:

---

[2]This verse dialogue was written in the late seventeenth century, but was reproduced and reprinted throughout the eighteenth century in England, Scotland and America, indicating the perennial popularity of the themes of mortality, religion and the perceived limits of medicine. We have reconciled the later editions here, and have included the woodcut illustrations of the London c.1750 edition, and the frontispiece of the Bristol c.1720 edition.

Coming this way to gather what's my due,
I thought it not amiss, to call on you.

Blind-Man: I do not know that voice; 'tis sure some Stranger;
And by his words, he seems to bode me danger.

Death: You guess aright, and before I go,
I'll make you know me, whether you will or no.

D   E   A   T   H.

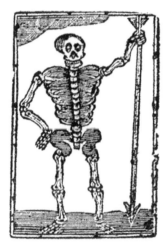

Blind-Man: Why, what are you? Pray tell me what's your name,
And what's your business, and from whence you came?

Death: I will declare what no man can deny,
There's none so great a Traveller as I;
Yet you must know, I am no wandering rover,
For my dominion lies the world all over;
I march through court and country, town and city,
I know not how to fear, nor how to pity.
The highest cedar, and the lowest flower,
Sooner or later do both feel my power.
The mightiest Emperors do submit to me,
Nor is the poorest tatter'd beggar free.
In Peace, I glean here one, and there another;
Sometimes I sweep whole streets together:
In time of War, thus much I can divine,
Whoever gets the day, the triumph's mine.
I am a potent and a high commander,
'Twas I that conquered the Great Alexander,
And after all the victory he had won,
Compell'd him to confess he was a man.

Were you Goliath great, or Sampson strong,
Were you as wise and rich as Solomon,
Were you as Nestor old; as infant young,
Had you the fairest cheek, the sweetest tongue
Yet you must stoop, all this will not avail,
For my arrest does not admit of bail:
And to deal plainly, Sir, my name is Death,
And it's my business to resign your breath.

Blind-Man: My breath and life shall both go out together.

Death: And on that errand 'twas that I came hither.
I'll have both breath and life without delay,
You must and shall dispatch, come, come, away.

Blind-Man: What needs such posting haste? Pray change your mind,
'Tis a poor conquest to surprise the Blind.

Death: You may not call it postings or surprise,
For you had warning when you lost your eyes;
Nor could you hope your house could long be free,
When once Windows were possessed by me.

Blind-Man: But Life is sweet; who would not, if he might
Have a long day before he bids good night?
O spare me yet awhile, slight not my tears.

Death: Hard hearts and hungry bellies have no ears.

Blind-Man: I am not yet quite ready for the table.

Death: All's one to me; I am inexorable.

Blind-Man: Yet, by your favour, I may slip aside?

Death: Be not deceived; it is in vain to hide,
My forces are dispersed through all places,
And act for me without respect of faces:
I have a thousand ways to shorten life,
Besides a rapier, pistol, sword, or knife;
A fly, a hair, a splinter, or a thorn,
A little scratch, the cutting of a corn,
Have sometimes done my business heretofore,
So to the full, that I need wish no more.
Should all these fail, enough of humours lurk
Within your body, Sir, to do my work.

Blind-Man: Well then, let some one run to my physician,
Tell him I want his aid in this condition.

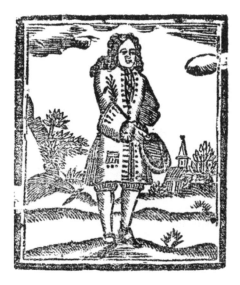

Death: Run boy and fetch him, call the whole college do,
For I intend to have them shortly too.
I value not their portions and their pills,
Nor all the cordials in their doctor's bills.
When my time's come, let them do what they can,
I'll have my due, so vain a thing is man.
Should Galen and Hippocrates join,
And Paracelsus with them combine,[3]
Let them all meet to countermand my strength
Yet they shall be my prisoners at length.
I grant that men of learning, worth and art,
May have the better of me at the start;
But in long running they'll give out and tire,
And quit the field, and leave me my desire.
As for those quacks who threaten to undo me,
They are my friends; and speed some patients to me.

Blind-Man: Well, If I must, I'll yield to you the day,
So its enacted, and I must obey;
Henceforth I count myself among your debtors,
For 'tis, I see, the measure of my betters.
But tell me now, when did your power commence?

---

[3]Galen (129–c.216 AD) was a prominent Greek physician, surgeon and philosopher. Hippocrates (c.460–370 BC) was a Greek physician and canonical figure in the history of medicine. Paracelsus (1493–1541), born Philippus Aureolus Theophrastus Bombastus von Hohenheim, was a Swiss-German Renaissance physician, botanist, alchemist and founder of toxicology.

Death: My Power began from Adam's first offence.

Blind-Man: From Adam's first offence! O base beginning,
Whose very first original was sinning.

Death: My rising did from Adam's fall begin,
And ever since my strength and sting's from sin.

Blind-Man: To know wherein the enemy's strength doth lie,
In my conceit is half a victory;
Have you commission now?

Death: What's that to you?

Blind-Man: Yes very much, for now I understand,
I am not totally at your command;
My life at his who gave you this commission;
To him I'll therefore make with my petition:
I'll seek his love, and on his mercy trust;
And when my sins are pardoned, do your worst.

Death: That you may know how far my power extends,
I will divorce you from your dearest friends;
You shall resign your jewels, money, plate,
Your earthly joys shall all be out of date.
I will deprive you of your dainty fare,
And strip you to the skin, naked and bare.
Linen or woolen you shall have to wind you,
As for the rest, all must be left behind you.
Bound hand and foot, I'll bring you to my den,
Where constant dreadful darkness reigns, and then
Your only dwelling-house shall be a cave;
Your lodging-room, a little narrow grave;
A chest, your closet; and a sheet, your dress;
And your companions, worms and rottenness.

Blind-Man: If this be all the mischief you can do,
Your harbingers deserve more dread than you.
Diseases are your harbingers, I'm sure;
Many of which are grievous to endure;
But when once dead, I shall not then complain
Of cold, or hunger, poverty or pain.

Death: There's one thing more, which here to mind I call,
When once I come, then come I once for all:
And when my stroke doth soul and body sever,
What's left undone, must be undone forever.

On an Infant Dying as Soon as Born
Charles Lamb (1836)

I saw where in the shroud did lurk
A curious frame of Nature's work.
A flow'ret crushed in the bud,
A nameless piece of Babyhood,
Was in a cradle-coffin lying;
Extinct, with scarce the sense of dying;
So soon to exchange the imprisoning womb
For darker closets of the tomb!
She did but ope an eye, and put
A clear beam forth, then strait up shut
For the long dark: ne'er more to see
Through glasses of mortality.
Riddle of destiny, who can show
What thy short visit meant, or know
What thy errand here below?
Shall we say, that Nature blind
Check'd her hand, and changed her mind,
Just when she had exactly wrought
A finish'd pattern without fault?
Could she flag, or could she tire,
Or lack'd she the Promethean fire
(With her nine moons' long workings sicken'd)
That should thy little limbs have quicken'd?
Limbs so firm, they seem'd to assure
Life of health, and days mature:
Woman's self in miniature!
Limbs so fair, they might supply
(Themselves now but cold imagery)
The sculptor to make Beauty by.
Or did the stern-eyed Fate descry,
That babe, or mother, one must die;
So in mercy left the stock,
And cut the branch; to save the shock
Of young years widow'd; and the pain,
When Single State comes back again
To the lone man who, 'reft of wife,
Thenceforward drags a maimed life?
The economy of Heaven is dark;
And wisest clerks have miss'd the mark,
Why Human Buds, like this, should fall,
More brief than fly ephemeral,
That has his day; while shrivel'd crones

Stiffen with age to stocks and stones;
And crabbed use the conscience sears
In sinners of an hundred years.
Mother's prattle, mother's kiss,
Baby fond, thou ne'er wilt miss.
Rites, which custom does impose,
Silver bells and baby clothes;
Coral redder than those lips,
Which pale death did late eclipse;
Music framed for infants' glee,
Whistle never tuned for thee;
Though thou want'st not, thou shalt have them,
Loving hearts were they which gave them.
Let not one be missing; nurse,
See them laid upon the hearse
Of infant slain by doom perverse.
Why should kings and nobles have
Pictured trophies to their grave;
And we, churls, to thee deny
Thy pretty toys with thee to lie,
A more harmless vanity?

The Wounded
Sydney Dobell (1855)[4]

'See to my brother, Doctor; I have lain
All day against his heart; it is warm there;
This stiffness is a trance; he lives! I swear –
I swear he lives!' 'Good Doctor, tell my ain
Auld Mother' – but his pale lips moved in vain.
'Doctor, when you were little Master John,
I left the old place; you will see it again.
Tell my poor Father – turn down the wood-lane
Beyond the home-field – cross the stepping stone
To the white cottage, with the garden gate –
O God!' – he died. 'Doctor, when I am gone
Send this to England.' 'Doctor, look upon
A countryman!' 'Devant mon Chef? Ma foi!'
'Oui, il est blessé beaucoup plus que moi'.[5]

---

[4]From a collection of poems written on the Crimean War.
[5]'Before my Chief? My faith!' 'Yes, he's hurt a lot more than me'.

from *To Think of Time*
Walt Whitman (1860)

To think of it! To think of time – of all that retrospection!
To think of to-day, and the ages continued henceforward!

Have you guessed you yourself would not continue?
Have you dreaded those earth-beetles?
Have you feared the future would be nothing to you?

Is to-day nothing? Is the beginningless past nothing?
If the future is nothing, they are just as surely nothing.

To think that the sun rose in the east! that men and women were flexible, real,
    alive! that everything was alive!
To think that you and I did not see, feel, think, nor bear our part!
To think that we are now here, and bear our part!

Not a day passes – not a minute or second, without an accouchement!
Not a day passes – not a minute or second, without a corpse!

The dull nights go over, and the dull days also,
The soreness of lying so much in bed goes over,
The physician, after long putting off, gives the silent and terrible look for an
    answer,
The children come hurried and weeping, and the brothers and sisters are sent for,
Medicines stand unused on the shelf – (the camphor-smell has long pervaded
    the rooms,)
The faithful hand of the living does not desert the hand of the dying,
The twitching lips press lightly on the forehead of the dying,
The breath ceases, and the pulse of the heart ceases,
The corpse stretches on the bed, and the living look upon it,
It is palpable as the living are palpable.

The living look upon the corpse with their eye-sight,
But without eye-sight lingers a different living, and looks curiously on the corpse.

To think that the rivers will flow, and the snow fall, and fruits ripen, and act
    upon others as upon us now – yet not act upon us!
To think of all these wonders of city and country, and others taking great
    interest in them – and we taking no interest in them!

To think how eager we are in building our houses!
To think others shall be just as eager, and we quite indifferent!

I see one building the house that serves him a few years, or seventy or eighty
    years at most,
I see one building the house that serves him longer than that.

Slow-moving and black lines creep over the whole earth – they never cease –
    they are the burial lines,
He that was President was buried, and he that is now President shall surely be
    buried.

Cold dash of waves at the ferry-wharf – posh and ice in the river, half-frozen
    mud in the streets, a gray, discouraged sky overhead, the short, last daylight
    of Twelfth Month,
A hearse and stages – other vehicles give place – the funeral of an old Broadway
    stage-driver, the cortege mostly drivers.

Steady the trot to the cemetery, duly rattles the death-bell, the gate is passed,
    the new-dug grave is halted at, the living alight, the hearse uncloses,
The coffin is passed out, lowered and settled, the whip is laid on the coffin, the
    earth is swiftly shovelled in,
The mound above is flatted with the spades – silence,
A minute – no one moves or speaks – it is done,
He is decently put away – is there anything more?

He was a good fellow, free-mouthed, quick-tempered, not bad-looking, able to
    take his own part, witty, sensitive to a slight, ready with life or death for a
    friend, fond of women, gambled, ate hearty, drank hearty, had known what it
    was to be flush, grew low-spirited toward the last, sicken'd, was help'd by a
    contribution, died, aged forty-one years – and that was his funeral.

Thumb extended, finger uplifted, apron, cape, gloves, strap, wet-weather
    clothes, whip carefully chosen, boss, spotter, starter, hostler, somebody
    loafing on you, you loafing on somebody, headway, man before and man
    behind, good day's work, bad day's work, pet stock, mean stock, first out,
    last out, turning-in at night;
To think that these are so much and so nigh to other drivers – and he there
    takes no interest in them!

Growing Old
Matthew Arnold (1867)

What is it to grow old?
Is it to lose the glory of the form,
The lustre of the eye?
Is it for beauty to forego her wreath?
Yes, but not for this alone.

Is it to feel our strength –
Not our bloom only, but our strength – decay?
Is it to feel each limb
Grow stiffer, every function less exact,

Each nerve more weakly strung?

Yes, this, and more! but not,
Ah, 'tis not what in youth we dreamed 'twould be!
'Tis not to have our life
Mellowed and softened as with sunset-glow,
A golden day's decline!

'Tis not to see the world
As from a height, with rapt prophetic eyes,
And heart profoundly stirred;
And weep, and feel the fulness of the past,
The years that are no more!

It is to spend long days
And not once feel that we were ever young.
It is to add, immured
In the hot prison of the present, month
To month with weary pain.

It is to suffer this,
And feel but half, and feebly, what we feel:
Deep in our hidden heart
Festers the dull remembrance of a change,
But no emotion – none.

It is – last stage of all –
When we are frozen up within, and quite
The phantom of ourselves,
To hear the world applaud the hollow ghost
Which blamed the living man.

A March in the Ranks Hard-prest, and the Road Unknown
Walt Whitman (1881–82)

A march in the ranks hard-prest, and the road unknown,
A route through a heavy wood with muffled steps in the darkness,
Our army foil'd with loss severe, and the sullen remnant retreating,
Till after midnight glimmer upon us the lights of a dim–lighted building,
We come to an open space in the woods, and halt by the dim–lighted building,
'Tis a large old church at the crossing roads, now an impromptu hospital,
Entering but for a minute I see a sight beyond all the pictures and poems ever made,
Shadows of deepest, deepest black, just lit by moving candles and lamps,
And by one great pitchy torch stationary with wild red flame and clouds of smoke,
By these, crowds, groups of forms vaguely I see on the floor, some in the pews
    laid down,

At my feet more distinctly a soldier, a mere lad, in danger of bleeding to death,
    (he is shot in the abdomen,)
I stanch the blood temporarily, (the youngster's face is white as a lily,)
Then before I depart I sweep my eyes o'er the scene fain to absorb it all,
Faces, varieties, postures beyond description, most in obscurity, some of
    them dead,
Surgeons operating, attendants holding lights, the smell of ether, the odor of
    blood,
The crowd, O the crowd of the bloody forms, the yard outside also fill'd,
Some on the bare ground, some on planks or stretchers, some in the death-
    spasm sweating,
An occasional scream or cry, the doctor's shouted orders or calls,
The glisten of the little steel instruments catching the glint of the torches,
These I resume as I chant, I see again the forms, I smell the odor,
Then hear outside the orders given, *Fall in, my men, fall in*;
But first I bend to the dying lad, his eyes open, a half-smile gives he me,
Then the eyes close, calmly close, and I speed forth to the darkness,
Resuming, marching, ever in darkness marching, on in the ranks,
The unknown road still marching.

Corpse-Washing
Rainer Maria Rilke (1908)[6]

They had grown used to him. But when
the kitchen lamp came and burned restlessly
in the dark draft, the one no one knew
grew utterly unknown. They washed his neck,

and since they knew nothing of his fate,
they made up another one out of lies,
all the while washing. The first had to cough,
and put the heavy vinegar-soaked sponge

down on his face. Then there was a pause
while the other rested. From her hard brush
the drops kept falling; while his terrible
cramped hand tried to make the whole house see
that he no longer thirsted.

He got through to them. With a short cough,
as if embarrassed, they took up the task
more urgently, so that on the wallpaper
their hunched shadows writhed and twisted

---

[6]Trans. Edward Snow.

in the mute patterns as though in a net,
until the washings came to an end.
The night in the curtainless window-frame
was pitiless. And one without names
lay there bare and clean and gave decrees.

Anaesthesia
Arthur Stringer (1914)

I caught the smell of ether
From the glass-roofed room
Where the hospital stood.
Suddenly all about me
I felt a mist of anguish
And the old, old hour of dread
When Death had shambled by.

Yellow with time it is,
This letter on which I look;
But up from it comes a perfume
That stabs me still to the heart;
And suddenly, at the odour,
Through a ghost-like mist I know
Rapture and love and wild regret
When Life, and You, went by.

On a Subaltern Killed in Action
Francis Brett Young (1919)

Into that dry and most desolate place
With heavy gait they dragged the stretcher in
And laid him on the bloody ground: the din
Of Maxim fire ceased not. I raised his head,
And looked into his face,
And saw that he was dead.
Saw beneath matted curls the broken skin
That let the bullet in;
And saw the limp, lithe limbs, the smiling mouth...
(Ah, may we smile at death
As bravely...) the curv'd lips that no more drouth
Should blacken, and no sweetly stirring breath
Mildly displace.
So I covered the calm face
And stripped the shirt from his firm breast, and there,

A zinc identity disc, a bracelet of elephant hair
I found... Ah, God, how deep it stings
This unendurable pity of small things!

But more than this I saw,
That dead stranger welcoming, more than the raw
And brutal havoc of war.
England I saw, the mother from whose side
He came hither and died, she at whose hems he had play'd,
In whose quiet womb his body and soul were made.
That pale, estrangèd flesh that we bowed over
Had breathed the scent in summer of white clover;
Dreamed her cool fading nights, her twilights long,
And days as careless as a blackbird's song
Heard in the hush of eve, when midges' wings
Make a thin music, and the night-jar spins.
(For it is summer, I thought, in England now...)
And once those forward gazing eyes had seen
Her lovely living green: that blackened brow
Cool airs, from those blue hills moving, had fann'd –
Breath of that holy land
Whither my soul aspireth without despair:
In the broken brain had many a lovely word
Awakened magical echoes of things heard,
Telling of love and laughter and low voices,
And tales in which the English heart rejoices
In vanishing visions of childhood and its glories:
Old-fashioned nursery rhymes and fairy stories:
Words that only an English tongue could tell.

And the firing died away; and the night fell
On our battle. Only in the sullen sky
A prairie fire, with huge fantastic flame
Leapt, lighting dark clouds charged with thunder.
And my heart was sick with shame
That there, in death, he should lie,
Crying: 'Oh, why am I alive, I wonder?'

In a dream I saw war riding the land:
Stark rode she, with bowed eyes, against the glare
Of sack'd cities smouldering in the dark,
A tired horse, lean, with outreaching head,
And hid her face of dread...
Yet, in my passion would I look on her,
Crying, O hark,
Thou pale one, whom now men say bearest the scythe

Of God, that iron scythe forged by his thunder
For reaping of nations overripened, fashioned
Upon the clanging anvil whose sparks, flying
In a starry night, dying, fall hereunder...
But she, she heeded not my cry impassioned
Nor turned her face of dread,
Urging the tired horse, with outreaching head,
O thou, cried I, who choosest for thy going
These bloomy meadows of youth, these flowery ways
Whereby no influence strays
Ruder than a cold wind blowing,
Or beating needles of rain,
Why must thou ride again
Ruthless among the pastures yet unripened,
Crushing their beauty in thine iron track
Downtrodden, ravish'd in thy following flame,
Parched and black?
But she, she stayed not in her weary haste
Nor turned her face; but fled:
And where she passed the lands lay waste...

And now I cannot tell whither she rideth:
But tired, tired rides she.
Yet know I well why her dread face she hideth:
She is pale and faint to death. Yea, her day faileth,
Nor all her blood, nor all her frenzy burning,
Nor all her hate availeth:
For she passeth out of sight
Into that night
From which none, none returneth
To waste the meadows of youth,
Nor vex thine eyelids, Routhe,
O sorrowful sister, soother of our sorrow.
And a hope within me springs
That fair will be the morrow,
And that charred plain,
Those flowery meadows, shall rejoice at last
In a sweet, clean
Freshness, as when the green
Grass springeth, where the prairie fire hath passed.

A Death-bed
Rudyard Kipling (1919)

'This is the State above the Law.
    The State exists for the State alone.'

(This is a gland at the back of the jaw,
    And an answering lump by the collar-bone.)

Some die shouting in gas or fire;
    Some die silent, by shell and shot.
Some die desperate, caught on the wire;
    Some die suddenly. This will not.

'Regis suprema voluntas Lex'[7]
    (It will follow the regular course of – throats.)
Some die pinned by the broken decks,
    Some die sobbing between the boats.

Some die eloquent, pressed to death
    By the sliding trench as their friends can hear.
Some die wholly in half a breath.
    Some – give trouble for half a year.

'There is neither Evil nor Good in life.
    Except as the needs of the State ordain.'
(Since it is rather too late for the knife,
    All we can do is mask the pain.)

Some die saintly in faith and hope –
    Some die thus in a prison-yard –
Some die broken by rape or the rope;
    Some die easily. This dies hard.

'I will dash to pieces who bar my way.
    Woe to the traitor! Woe to the weak!'
(Let him write what he wishes to say.
    It tires him out if he tries to speak.)

Some die quietly. Some abound
    In loud self-pity. Others spread
Bad morale through the cots around...
    This is a type that is better dead.

'The war was forced on me by my foes.
    All that I sought was the right to live.'
(Don't be afraid of a triple dose;
    The pain will neutralize half we give.)

Here are the needles. See that he dies
    While the effects of the drug endure...
What is the question he asks with his eyes? –
    Yes, All-Highest, to God, be sure.)

---

[7]*King of the supreme Law.*

On the kitchen shelf the dusty medicine bottles
Charles Reznikoff (1919)

> On the kitchen shelf the dusty medicine bottles;
> she in her room heaped under a sheet,
> and men and women coming in with clumsy steps.

Death like his is right and splendid...
W. H. Auden (1936)

> Death like his is right and splendid;
> That is how life should have ended!
> He cannot calculate nor dread
> The mortifying in the bed,
> Powers wasting day by day
> While the courage ebbs away.
> Ever-charming, he will miss
> The insulting paralysis,
> Ruined intellect's confusion,
> Ulcer's patient persecution,
> Sciatica's intolerance
> And the cancer's sly advance;
> Never hear, among the dead,
> The rival's brilliant paper read,
> Colleague's deprecating cough
> And the praises falling off;
> Never know how in the best
> Passion loses interest;
> Beauty sliding from the bone
> leaves the rigid skeleton.

An Aged Woman
Mina Loy (1949)[8]

> The past has come apart
> events are vagueing
> the future is inexplicable
> the present   pain.
>
> Not even pain has that precision
> with which it struck in youth-time.
>
> More like moth
> eroding internal organs

---

[8]As in Loy's manuscripts, this poem was signed off with a future date (1984), though written some decades earlier.

hanging or falling down
in a spoiled closet

Does you mirror Bedevil you
Or is the impossible
possible to senility
enabling the erstwhile agile
narrow silhouette of self
to hold in huge reserve
this excessive incognito
of a Bulbous stranger
only to be exorcised by death

Dilation has entirely dominated
your long reality.
                    Mina Loy
                    July 12
                    1984

Death in Leamington
John Betjeman (1958)

She died in the upstairs bedroom
By the light of the ev'ning star
That shone through the plate glass window
From over Leamington Spa.

Beside her the lonely crochet
Lay patiently and unstirred,
But the fingers that would have work'd it
Were dead as the spoken word.

And Nurse came in with the tea-things
Breast high 'mid the stands and chairs –
But Nurse was alone with her own little soul,
And the things were alone with theirs.

She bolted the big round window,
She let the blinds unroll,
She set a match to the mantle,
She covered the fire with coal.

And 'Tea!' she said in a tiny voice
'Wake up! It's nearly *five*'
Oh! Chintzy, chintzy cheeriness,
Half dead and half alive!

Do you know that the stucco is peeling?
Do you know that the heart will stop?

From those yellow Italianate arches
Do you hear the plaster drop?

Nurse looked at the silent bedstead,
At the gray, decaying face,
As the calm of a Leamington ev'ning
Drifted into the place.

She moved the table of bottles
Away from the bed to the wall;
And tiptoeing gently over the stairs
Turned down the gas in the hall.

Terminal Days at Beverly Farms
Robert Lowell (1959)

At Beverly Farms, a portly, uncomfortable boulder
bulked in the garden's center
an irregular Japanese touch.
After his Bourbon 'old fashioned', Father,
bronzed, breezy, a shade too ruddy,
swayed as if on deck duty
under his six pointed star-lantern –
last July's birthday present.
He smiled his oval Lowell smile,
he wore his cream gaberdine dinner-jacket,
and indigo cummerbund,
his head was efficient and hairless,
his newly dieted figure was vitally trim.

Father and mother moved to Beverly Farms
to be a two-minute walk from the station,
half an hour by train from the Boston doctors.
They had no sea-view,
but sky-blue tracks of the commuters' railroad shone
like a double-barreled shotgun
through the scarlet late August sumac,
multiplying like cancer
at their garden's border.

Father had had two coronaries.
He still treasured underhand economies,
but his best friend was his little black Chevy,
garaged like a superficial steer
with gilded hooves,
yet sensationally sober,
and with less side than an old dancing pump.
The local dealer, a 'buccanneer',

had been bribed a 'king's ransom'
to quickly deliver a car without chrome.

Each morning at eight-thirty,
inattentive and beaming,
loaded with his 'calc' and 'trig' books,
his clipper ship statistics,
and his ivory slide rule,
father stole off with the Chevie
to loaf in the Maritime Museum at Salem.
He called the curator
'the commander of the Swiss Navy.'

Father's death was abrupt and unprotesting.
His vision was still twenty-twenty.
After a morning of anxious, repetitive smiling,
his last words to Mother were:
'I feel awful.'

As He Came Near Death
Roy Fisher (1964)

As he came near death things grew shallower for us:
we'd lost sleep and now sat muffled in the scent of tulips, the medical
        odours, and the street sounds going past, going away;
and he, too, slept little, the morphine and the pink light the curtains let
        through floating him with us,
so that he lay and was worked out on to the skin of his life and left there,
and we had to reach only a little way into the warm bed to scoop him up.

A few days, slow tumbling escalators of visitors and cheques, and something
        like popularity;
during this time somebody washed him in a soap called *Narcissus* and mounted
        him, frilled with satin, in a polished case.

Then the hole: this was a slot punched in a square of plastic grass rug, a slot
        lined with white polythene, floored with dyed green gravel.
The box lay in it; we rode in the black cars round a corner, got out into our
        coloured cars and dispersed in easy stages.

After a time the grave got up and went away.

Mid Term Break
Seamus Heaney (1966)

I sat all morning in the college sick bay
Counting bells knelling classes to a close.
At two o'clock our neighbours drove me home.

In the porch I met my father crying –
He had always taken funerals in his stride –
And Big Jim Evans saying it was a hard blow.

The baby cooed and laughed and rocked the pram
When I came in, and I was embarrassed
By old men standing up to shake my hand

And tell me they were 'sorry for my trouble';
Whispers informed strangers I was the eldest,
Away at school, as my mother held my hand

In hers and coughed out angry tearless sighs.
At ten o'clock the ambulance arrived
With the corpse, stanched and bandaged by the nurses.

Next morning I went up into the room. Snowdrops
And candles soothed the bedside; I saw him
For the first time in six weeks. Paler now,

Wearing a poppy bruise on his left temple,
He lay in the four foot box as in his cot.
No gaudy scars, the bumper knocked him clear.

A four foot box, a foot for every year.

A Flat One
W. D. Snodgrass (1967)

Old Fritz, on this rotating bed
For seven wasted months you lay
Unfit to move, shrunken, gray,
No good to yourself or anyone
But to be babied – changed and bathed and fed.
    At long last, that's all done.

Before each meal, twice every night,
We set pads on your bedsores, shut
Your catheter tube off, then brought
The second canvas-and-black-iron
Bedframe and clamped you in between them, tight,
    Scared, so we could turn

You over. We washed you, covered you,
Cut up each bite of meat you ate;
We watched your lean jaws masticate
As ravenously your useless food
As thieves at hard labor in their chains chew
    Or insects in the wood.

Such pious sacrifice to give
You all you could demand of pain:
Receive this haddock's body slain
For you, old tyrant; take this blood
Of a tomato, shed that you might live.
        You had that costly food.

You seem to be all finished, so
We'll plug your old recalcitrant anus
And tie up your discouraged penis
In a great, snow-white bow of gauze.
We wrap you, pin you, and cart you down below,
        Below, below, because

Your credit has finally run out.
On our steel table, trussed and carved,
You'll find this world's hardworking, starved
Teeth working in your precious skin.
The earth turns, in the end, by turn about
        And opens to take you in.

Seven months gone down the drain; thank God
That's through. Throw out the four-by-fours,
Swabsticks, the thick salve for bedsores,
Throw out the diaper pads and drug
Containers, pile the bedclothes in a wad,
        And rinse the cider jug

Half-filled with the last urine. Then
Empty out the cotton cans,
Autoclave the bowls and spit pans,
Unhook the pumps and all the red
Tubes – catheter, suction, oxygen;
        Next, wash the empty bed.

– All this Dark Age machinery
On which we had tormented you
To life. Last, we collect the few
Belongings: snapshots, some odd bills,
Your mail, and half a pack of Luckies we
        Won't light you after meals.

Old man, these seven months you've lain
Determined – not that you would live –
Just to not die. No one would give
You one chance you could ever wake
From that first night, much less go well again,
        Much less go home and make

Your living; how could you hope to find
A place for yourself in all creation? –
Pain was your only occupation.
And pain what should content and will
A man to give it up, nerved you to grind
    Your clenched teeth, breathing, till

Your skin broke down, your calves went flat
And your legs lost all sensation. Still,
You took enough morphine to kill
A strong man. Finally, nitrogen
Mustard: you could last two months after that;
    It would kill you then.

Even then you wouldn't quit.
Old soldier, yet you must have known
Inside the animal had grown
Sick of the world, made up its mind
To stop. Your mind ground on its separate
    Way, merciless and blind,

Into these last weeks when the breath
Would only come in fits and starts
That puffed out your sections like the parts
Of some enormous, damaged bug.
You waited, not for life, not for your death,
    Just for the deadening drug

That made your life seem bearable.
You still whispered you would not die.
Yet the nights I heard you cry
Like a whipped child; in fierce old age
You whimpered, tears stood on your gun-metal
    Blue cheeks shaking with rage

And terror. So much pain would fill
Your room that when I left I'd pray
That if I came back the next day
I'd find you gone. You stayed for me –
Nailed to your own rapacious, stiff self-will.
    You've shook loose, finally.

They say this was a worthwhile job
Unless they tried it. It is mad
To throw our good lives after bad;
Waste time, drugs, and our minds, while strong
Men starve. How many young men did we rob
    To keep you hanging on?

I can't think we did you much good.
Well, when you died, none of us wept.
You killed for us, and so we kept
You, because we need to earn our pay.
No. We'd still have to help you try. We would
　　　Have killed for you today.

In Praise of Darkness
Jorge Luis Borges (1967)[9]

Old age (this is the name that others give it)
may prove a time of happiness.
The animal is dead or nearly dead;
man and soul go on.
I live among vague whitish shapes
that are not darkness yet.
Buenos Aires,
which once broke up in a tatter of slums and open lots
out toward the endless plain,
is not again the graveyard of the Recolets, the Retiro square,
the shabby streets of the old Westside,
and the few vanishing decrepit houses
that we still call the South.
All through my life things were too many.
To think, Democritus tore out his eyes;
time has been my Democritus.[10]
This growing dark is slow and brings no pain;
it flows along an easy slope
and is akin to eternity.
My friends are faceless,
women are as they were years back,
one street corner is taken for another,
on the pages of books there are no letters.
All this should make me uneasy,
but there's a restfulness about it, a going back.
Of the many generations of books on earth
I have read only a few,
the few that in my mind I go on reading still –
reading and changing.
From south and east and west and north,

---

[9]Trans. Norman Thomas di Giovanni.
[10]Democritus (c. 460–c. 370 BC), meaning 'chosen of the people', was a Greek pre-Socratic philosopher, and is considered by many as the father of modern science. He allegedly blinded himself, because he believed sight hindered thought.

roads coming together have led me
to my secret centre.
These roads were footsteps and echoes,
women, men, agonies, rebirths,
days and nights,
falling asleep and dreams,
each single moment of my yesterdays
and of the world's yesterdays,
the firm sword of the Dane and the moon of the Persians,
the deeds of the dead,
shared love, words,
Emerson,[11] and snow, and so many things.
Now I can forget them. I reach my centre,
my algebra and my key,
my mirror.
Soon I shall know who I am.

After the Funeral: Cleaning out the Medicine Cabinet
Ted Kooser (1980)

Behind this mirror no new world
opens to Alice. Instead, we find
the old world, rearranged in rows,
a dusty little chronicle
of small complaints and private sorrows,
each cough caught dry and airless
in amber, the sore feet powdered
and cool in their yellow can.
To this world turned the burning eyes
after their search, the weary back
after its lifting, the heavy heart
like an old dog, sniffing the lids
for an answer. Now one of us
unscrews the caps and tries the air
of each disease. Another puts
the booty in a shoe box: tins
of laxatives and aspirin,
the corn pads and the razor blades,
while still another takes the vials
of secret sorrows – the little pills
with faded, lonely codes – holding
them out the way one holds a spider

---

[11]Ralph Waldo Emerson (1803–1882) was an American poet, social critic, and a leader in the Transcendentalist movement.

pinched in a tissue, and pours them down
the churning toilet and away.

from C
Peter Reading (1984)

The list goes on and on interminably...
rectal Bleeding, Chemotherapy
('Oh, how I dread the fortnightly injection –
the pain of it *itself*, and after that
ill for a week from the after-effects.
Anger is what I feel at dying, *anger* –
why can't the dropouts and the drunks get This?
I've always led such a clean, simple life...'),
Mastectomy, Metastases, Dyspnoea...
the list goes on and on and on and on...
(Some die in agony of mind and body
described by Hospice staff 'Dehumanized'.)
'Grief Work', 'Death Work', smug 'Terminal Caregivers'...
    I close my eyes but weep under the lids.

The Autopsy Room
Raymond Carver (1986)

Then I was young and had the strength of ten.
For anything, I thought. Though part of my job
at night was to clean the autopsy room
once the coroner's work was done. But now
and then they knocked off early, or too late.
For, so help me, they left things out
on their specially built table. A little baby,
still as a stone and snow cold. Another time,
a huge black man with white hair whose chest
had been laid open. All his vital organs
lay in a pan beside his head. The hose
was running, the overhead lights blazed.
And one time there was a leg, a woman's leg,
on the table. A pale and shapely leg.
I knew it for what it was. I'd seen them before.
Still, it took my breath away.

When I went home at night my wife would say,
'Sugar, it's going to be all right. We'll trade
this life in for another.' But it wasn't
that easy. She'd take my hand between her hands
and hold it tight, while I leaned back on the sofa

and closed my eyes. Thinking of... something.
I don't know what. But I'd let her bring
my hand to her breast. At which point
I'd open my eyes and stare at the ceiling, or else
the floor. Then my fingers strayed to her leg.
Which was warm and shapely, ready to tremble
and raise slightly, at the slightest touch.
But my mind was unclear and shaky. Nothing
was happening. Everything was happening. Life
was a stone, grinding and sharpening.

In Memoriam Roland Barthes (Killed in a road traffic accident 1980)[12]
Raymond Tallis (1987)

*Combien de temps faudra-t-il à
la nature pour refaire un cerveau pareil?*[13]

Profundity's like happiness – a castle built of cards,
its paper henges stalked by hurricanes;
Venetian glass where earthquakes buck the streets.
The simplest things can cancel subtlest minds:
a crack across the head unselves a man,
a single blow split Barthes from space and time.

The impact bricked the windows lit by thought
as *maître à penser* curdled into flesh;
and if his senses lingered for a while,
they tasted senseless absolutes of pain
in darkness where the spaces of his mind
were groping strangeness stripped of native tongue.

The fender kicked the language from his brain,
a tapestry of signs was ripped to shreds.
The tarmac shattered sentences to sounds
and disconnected every sound from sense.
And signifiers, shook from signifieds,
dissolved like skyward birds in nullity.

The body and its name went separate ways:
the flesh returned to earth, the word to words.
So 'Roland Barthes' is sentenced for all time:
a word among those words he half unmasked,
he sorts with tokens, meets them noun to noun,
is tyrannised by grammar like the rest.

---

[12]The French philosopher, linguist and cultural theorist Roland Barthes (b. 1915) was hit by a laundry van, when walking in Paris, on 25 February, 1980. He later died of his injuries.
[13]'How long will it take for nature to make such a brain?'

No-one will use his name to call him near,
or meet his gaze in bedroom, class or street,
or see his eyes decode a common world.
Poor Barthes is printed words and others' talk –
else something suffers there, beneath the light,
that absolute, alone, outside of signs.

When I Grow Up
Hugo Williams (1990)

When I grow up I want to have a bad leg.
I want to limp down the street I live in
without knowing where I am. I want the disease
where you put your hand on your hip
and lean forward slightly, groaning to yourself.

If a little boy asks me the way
I'll try and touch him between the legs.
What a dirty old man I'm going to be when I grow up!
What shall we do with me?

I promise I'll be good
if you let me fall over in the street
and lie there calling like a baby bird. Please,
nobody come. I'm perfectly all right. I like it here.

I wonder would it be possible
to get me into a National Health Hospice
somewhere in Manchester?
I'll stand in the middle of my cubicle
holding onto a piece of string for safety,
shaking like a leaf at the thought of my suitcase.

I'd certainly like to have a nervous tic
so I can purse my lips up all the time
like Cecil Beaton.[14] Can I be completely bald, please?
I love the smell of old pee.
Why can't I smell like that?

When I grow up I want a thin piece of steel
inserted into my penis for some reason.
Nobody's to tell me why it's there. I want to guess!
Tell me, is that a bottle of old Burgundy
under my bed? I never can tell
if I feel randy any more, can you?

---

[14]Sir Cecil Beaton CBE (1904–80) was a photographer and designer.

I think it's only fair that I should be allowed
to cough up a bit of blood when I feel like it.
My daughter will bring me a special air cushion
to hold me upright and I'll watch
in baffled admiration as she blows it up for me.

Here's my list: nappies, story books, munchies,
something else. What was the other thing?
I can't remember exactly,
but when I grow up I'll know. When I grow up
I'll pluck at my bedclothes to collect lost thoughts.
I'll roll them into balls and swallow them.

The Glass
Sharon Olds (1990)

I think of it with wonder now,
the glass of mucus that stood on the table
in front of my father all weekend. The tumor
is growing fast in his throat these days,
and as it grows it sends out pus
like the sun sending out flares, those pouring
tongues. So my father has to gargle, cough,
spit a mouth full of thick stuff
into the glass every ten minutes or so,
scraping the rim up his lower lip
to get the last bit off his skin, then he
sets the glass down, on the table, and it
sits there, like a glass of beer foam,
shiny and faintly yellow, he gargles and
coughs and reaches for it again,
and gets the heavy sputum out,
full of bubbles and moving around like yeast –
he is like a god producing food from his own mouth.
He himself can eat nothing, anymore,
just a swallow of milk, sometimes,
cut with water, and even then
it cannot, always, get past the tumor,
and the next time the saliva comes up
it is ropey, he has to roll it in his throat
a minute to form it and get it up and dis-
gorge the oval globule into the
glass of phlegm, which stood there all day and
filled slowly with compound globes and I would
empty it, and it would fill again,

and shimmer there on the table until
the room seemed to turn around it
in an orderly way, a model of the solar system
turning around the sun,
my father the old earth that used to
lie at the center of the universe, now
turning with the rest of us
around his death, luminous glass of
spit on the table, these last mouthfuls of his life.

Lament
Thom Gunn (1992)

Your dying was a difficult enterprise.
First, petty things took up your energies,
The small but clustering duties of the sick,
Irritant as the cough's dry rhetoric.
Those hours of waiting for pills, shot, X-ray
Or test (while you read novels two a day)
Already with a kind of clumsy stealth
Distanced you from the habits of your health.
    In hope still, courteous still, but tired and thin,
You tried to stay the man that you had been,
Treating each symptom as a mere mishap
Without import. But then the spinal tap.
It bought a hard headache, and when night came
I heard you wake up from the same bad dream
Every half-hour with the same short cry
Of mild outrage, before immediately
Slipping into the nightmare once again
Empty of content but the drip of pain.
No respite followed: though the nightmare ceased,
Your cough grew thick and rich, its strength increased.
Four nights, and on the fifth we drove you down
To the Emergency Room. That frown, that frown:
I'd never seen such rage in you before
As when they wheeled you through the swinging door.
For you knew, rightly, they conveyed you from
Those normal pleasures of the sun's kingdom
The hedonistic body basks within
And takes for granted – summer on the skin,
Sleep without break, the moderate taste of tea
In a dry mouth. You had gone on from me
As if your body sought out martyrdom

In the far Canada of a hospital room.
Once there, you entered fully the distress
And long pale rigours of the wilderness.
A gust of morphine hid you. Back in sight
You breathed through a segmented tube, fat, white,
Jammed down your throat so that you could not speak.
  How thin the distance made you. In your cheek
One day, appeared the true shape of your bone
No longer padded. Still your mind, alone,
Explored this emptying intermediate
State for what holds and rests were hidden in it.
  You wrote us messages on a pad, amused
At one time that you had your nurse confused
Who, seeing you reconciled after four years
With your grey father, both of you in tears,
Asked if this was at last your 'special friend'
(The one you waited for until the end).
'She sings,' you wrote, 'a Philippine folk song
To wake me in the morning... It is long
And very pretty.' Grabbing at detail
To furnish this bare ledge toured by the gale,
On which you lay, bed restful as a knife,
You tried, tried hard, to make of it a life
Thick with the complicating circumstance
Your thoughts might fasten on. It had been chance
Always till now that had filled up the moment
With live specifics your hilarious comment
Discovered as it went along; and fed,
Laconic, quick, wherever it was led.
You improvised upon your own delight.
I think back to the scented summer night
We talked between our sleeping bags, below
A molten field of stars five years ago:
I was so tickled by your mind's light touch
I couldn't sleep, you made me laugh too much,
Though I was tired and begged you to leave off.

Now you were tired, and yet not tired enough
– Still hungry for the great world you were losing
Steadily in no season of your choosing –
And when at last the whole death was assured,
Drugs having failed, and when you had endured
Two weeks of an abominable constraint,
You faced it equably, without complaint,

Unwhimpering, but not at peace with it.
You'd lived as if your time was infinite:
You were not ready and not reconciled,
Feeling as uncompleted as a child
Till you had shown the world what you could do
In some ambitious role to be worked through,
A role your need for it had half-defined,
But never wholly, even in your mind.
You lacked the necessary ruthlessness,
The soaring meanness that pinpoints success.
We loved that lack of self-love, and your smile,
Rueful, at your own silliness.
                                        Meanwhile,
Your lungs collapsed, and the machine, unstrained,
Did all your breathing now. Nothing remained
But death by drowning on an inland sea
Of your own fluids, which it seemed could be
Kindly forestalled by drugs. Both could and would:
Nothing was said, everything understood,
At least by us. Your own concerns were not
Long-term, precisely, when they gave the shot
– You made local arrangements to the bed
And pulled a pillow round beside your head.
And so you slept, and died, your skin gone grey,
Achieving your completeness, in a way.

Outdoors next day, I was dizzy from a sense
Of being ejected with some violence
From vigil in a white and distant spot
Where I was numb, into this garden plot
Too warm, too close, not enough like pain.
I was delivered into time again
– The variations that I live among
Where your long body too used to belong
And where the still bush is minutely active.
You never thought your body was attractive,
Though others did, and yet you trusted it
And must have loved its fickleness a bit
Since it was yours and gave you what it could,
Till near the end it let you down for good,
Its blood hospitable to those guests who
Took over by betraying it into
The greatest of its inconsistencies
This difficult, tedious, painful enterprise.

Dead Kids
Dorothy Porter (1994)

Dead kids upset me.

There's no drink
to take away the taste
of a fresh face rotting.

Useless
to tremble and vomit
and howl it's not fair.

You look at the spots
on the back of your hand
you look at the lines
fraying your face.

But you're still glad
it's the kid
not you.

A Death
Thomas Lynch (1994)

In the end you want the clean dimensions of it mentioned:
to know the thing adverbially – *while asleep,*
after long illness, tragically in a blaze –

as you would the word of any local weather:
where it gathered, when it got here, how it kept
the traffic at a standstill, slowed the pace,

closed the terminals. Lineage & Issue, Names & Dates –
the facts you gain most confidence in facing –
histories and habits and whereabouts.

Speak of it, if you speak of it at all, in parts.
The C. V. A.[15] or insufficiency or growth
that grew indifferent to prayer and medication.

Better a tidy science for a heart that stops
than the round and witless horror of someone who
one dry night in perfect humour ceases measurably to be.

---

[15]CVA (Cerebrovascular Accident), or a stroke.

Deathbeds
Billy Collins (1994)

The ancients were talkative on theirs,
so many agencies needed to be addressed:
the gods of departure who controlled
the seven portals of the world,
the ferrymen leaning on their smooth oars.
the eternal pilots, immortal conductors,
and that was just the transportation.

Japanese monks would motion for a tablet,
sometimes, an inkwell and a brush
so they could leave behind the dark,
wet strokes of a short poem,
a drop of rain on a yellow leaf.
One described the nigh clouds
and the moon making its million-mile journey.

Medieval Christians who could read
could read a treatise on the subject:
De Arte Moriendi, On the Art of Dying,
pages of instruction on what to do in bed,
how to set the heart right
how to point the soul upward
and listen to the prayer of one's own breathing.

Some pale Victorians in their tubercular
throes would ask for a looking glass
so they could behold the seraphic glow
the dry fever brought to their faces.
A few even had a photographer summoned
to open his tripod in the sickroom
and disappear under the heavy black cloth
as the subject, more or less, was doing the same.

Then there were the wits,
using their last breath to exhale a line,
a devastating capper, as if the world
were simply a large gallery full of people
and now it was time to throw on a long scarf
and make an exit, leaving
it to someone else to close the door.

Some lie on their backs for months,
students of the ceiling,
others roll over once and are gone.
Some scream for a priest

and make the one confession no one doubts.
And you, and I too, may lie on ours,
the vigilant family in a semicircle,
or the night nurse holding our hand
in the dark, or alone.
There will be no ink, mirror, or Latin book,
though the wallpaper may be tasteless
and you may feel yourself entering a myth.

I would hope for a window,
the usual frame of reference,
a clear sky, or thin high clouds,
an abundance of sun, a cool pillow.
And I would expect at the end a moment
of pure awareness
when I can feel the pea under my mattress
and pick out the dot of a hawk lost in the blue.

Geriatric
R. S. Thomas (1995)

What god is proud
    of this garden
of dead flowers, this underwater
    grotto of humanity,
where limbs wave in invisible
    currents, faces drooping
on dry stalks, voices clawing
    in a last desperate effort
to retain hold? Despite withered
    petals, I recognise
the species: Charcot, Ménière,
    Alzheimer.[16] There are no gardeners
here, caretakers only
    of reason overgrown
by confusion. This body once,
    when it was in bud,
opened to love's kisses. These eyes,

---

[16] Jean-Martin Charcot (1825–93) was a French professor of anatomical pathology, known as the founder of modern neurology, and also the namesake of Charcot's disease (Motor Neurone Disease). Prosper Ménière (1799–1862), a French physician-in-chief at the institute for deaf-mutes, researched diseases of the ear. Dr Aloysius 'Alois' Alzheimer (1864–1915) was a German psychiatrist and neuropathologist, credited with identifying the first published case of 'presenile dementia', later identified as Alzheimer's disease – a chronic neurodegenerative disease, accounting for 60–70 per cent of all cases of dementia.

cloudy with rheum,
were clear pebbles that love's rivulet
    hurried over. Is this
the best Rabbi Ben Ezra[17]
    promised? I come away
comforting myself, as I can,
    that there is another
garden, all dew and fragrance,
    and that these are the brambles
about it we are caught in,
    a sacrifice prepared
by a torn god to a love fiercer
    than we can understand.

My Father's Deaths
David Kennedy (2004)

My father, dying, didn't tell us
he was going to pass the time learning a new language.
He just started talking like people in phrasebooks do,
with a skewed sense of proportion,
frightfully certain
about things of little or no consequence.
'This tea is too hot', he would say too loudly
or 'This water is far too cold'.

My father, dying, simplified his mind
until it was so thin
it was able to pass through its own bars
and escape.

My father, dying, was a room
full of deep snow pocked
with footprints that suddenly stopped
so no one knew where they went.

---

[17]'Rabbi Ben Ezra' is a poem by Robert Browning, about Abraham ibn Ezra (1092–1167), one of the great poets, mathematicians and scholars of the twelfth century, who wrote on grammar, astronomy and the astrolabe. Browning's poem explores the paradox in Ben Ezra's teaching that good might lie in the inevitability of its absence:

For thence – a paradox
Which comforts while it mocks –
Shall life succeed in that it seems to fail:
What I aspired to be,
And was not, comforts me:
brute I might have been, but would not sink i' the scale.

My father, dying, was neither an ocean liner at night
nor the paper streamers falling from it into the water
and still held in the hands of the people
waving goodbye from the dock
but just its wake
left on the water a long time.

My father, dying, was a hole
made by a railway ticket nipper
in a ticket that didn't exist
and all the members of the on-train team
gathered round but none of them knew
if they were supposed to be looking at the hole
or at the space where the ticket should have been.

My father, dying, was a piece of my unbroken skin
where a healed scar appeared
which scabbed over then opened,
stitch by stitch, to a raw, fresh wound.

My father, dying, was a commentary
on a text that no longer existed
or, some scholars argued,
had never been written.

My father, dying, was a locked glass case
that neither of us had the key for
containing my life's work to date:
the scrawled and battered bundles
of the manuscript of a book of questions.

My father, dying, was a page
where all the letters slipped
to the bottom and lay in a heap
mumbling and whispering
and then dropped off.

from _The Unfinished_
Christopher Reid (2004)

No imp or devil
but a mere tumour
squatted on her brain.
Without personality
or ill humour,
malignant but not malign,
it set about doing –
not evil,

simply the job
tumours have always done:
establishing faulty
connections, skewing
perceptions, closing down
faculties and functions
one by one.

Hobgoblin, nor foul fiend;
nor even the jobsworth slob
with a slow, sly scheme to rob
my darling of her mind
that I imagined;
just a tumour.

Between which and the neat
gadget with the timer
that eased drugs into her vein,
she contrived to maintain
her identity

unimpaired and complete,
resolved to meet
death with all gallantry
and distinction.

Instruction
Sally Read (2005)

Check: water, soap, a folded sheet, a shroud.
Close cubicle curtains; light's swallowed
in hospital green. Our man lies dense
with gravity: an arm, his head, at angles
as if dropped from a great height. There is
a fogged mermaid from shoulder to wrist,
nicotine-stained teeth, nails dug with dirt –
a labourer then, one for the women.
A smooth drain to ivory is overtaking
from the feet. Wash him, swiftly, praising
in murmurs like your mother used,
undressing you when asleep. Dry carefully.
If he complained at the damp when alive, dry
again. Remove teeth, all tags, rip off elastoplast –
careful now, each cell is snuffing its lights,
but black blood still spurts. Now,
the shroud (opaque, choirboy ruff), fasten

it on him, comb his hair to the right. Now
he could be anyone. Now wrap in the sheet,
like a parcel, start at his feet. Swaddle (not
tight nor too loose) – it's an art, sheafing
this bundle of untied, heavy sticks. Hesitate
before covering his face, bandaging warm
wet recesses of eyes, mouth. Your hands
will prick – an animal sniffing last traces
of life. Cradle the head, bind it with tape
and when it lolls, lovingly against your chest,
lower it gently as a bowl brimmed with water.
Collect tags, teeth, washbowl. Open
the window, let the soul fly. Through
green curtains the day will tear: cabs, sun-
glare, rain. Remember to check:
tidied bed, emptied cabinet, sheeted form –
observe him recede to the flux between seconds,
the slowness of sand. Don't loiter. Slide
back into the ward's slipstream: pick up
your pace immediately.

A Scattering
Christopher Reid (2009)

I expect you've seen the footage: elephants,
finding the bones of one of their own kind
dropped by the wayside, picked clean by scavengers
and the sun, then untidily left there,
    decide to do something about it.

But what, exactly? They can't, of course,
reassemble the old elephant magnificence;
they can't even make a tidier heap. But they can
hook up bones with their trunks and chuck them
    this way and that way. So they do.

And their scattering has an air
of deliberate ritual, ancient and necessary.
Their great size, too, makes them the very
embodiment of grief, while the play of their trunks
    lends sprezzatura.

Elephants puzzling out
the anagram of their own anatomy,
elephants at their abstracted lamentations –
may their spirit guide me as I place
    my own sad thoughts in new, hopeful arrangements.

Golden Mothers Driving West
Paul Durcan (2009)

The inevitable call came from the Alzheimer's nursing home.
Mummy had been sitting there in an armchair for two years
In a top-storey room with two other aged ladies,
Deborah O'Donoghue and Maureen Timoney.
The call was to say that between 3 and 5 a.m.
The three of them had gone missing from the room.
At first it was thought that all three had slipped
Out the window, ajar in the hot, humid night.
But, no, there were no torsos in the flowerbed.
It transpired that a car had also gone missing.
Was it thinkable they had commandeered a car?
At five in the afternoon the police called
To say that a Polish youth in a car wash in Kinnegad
Had washed and hot-waxed a car for three ladies,
All of whom were wearing golden dressing gowns –
Standard issue golden dressing gowns
Worn by all the inmates of the Alzheimer's nursing home.
Why he remembered them was that he was struck
By the fact that all three ladies were laughing
For the ten minutes it took him to wash the car.
'I am surprised,' he stated, 'by laughter.'
At 9 p.m. the car was sighted in Tarmonbarry
On the Roscommon side of the River Shannon,
Parked at the jetty of the Emerald Star marina.
At 9.30 p.m. a female German child was taken
To the police station at Longford by her stepfather.
The eleven-year-old had earlier told her stepfather
In the cabin of their hired six-berth river cruiser
That she had seen three ladies jump from the bridge.
Her stepfather had assumed his daughter imagined it
As she was, he told police, 'a day-dreamer born'.
The girl repeated her story to the police:
How three small, thin, aged ladies with white hair
Had, all at once, together, jumped from the bridge,
Their dressing gowns flying behind them in the breeze.
What colours were the dressing gowns? she was asked.
'They are wearing gold,' she replied.
Wreathed on the weir downstream from the bridge
Police sub-aqua divers retrieved the three bodies,
One of whom, of course, was my own emaciated mother,
Whose fingerprints were later found on the wheel of the car.
She had been driving west, west to Westport,
Westport on the west coast of Ireland

In the County of Mayo,
Where she had grown up with her mother and sisters
In the War of Independence and the Civil War,
Driving west to Streamstown three miles outside Westport,
Where on afternoons in September in 1920,
Ignoring the roadblocks and the assassinations,
They used to walk down Sunnyside by the sea's edge,
The curlews and the oystercatchers,
The upturned black currachs drying out on the stones,
And picnic on the machair grass above the seaweed,
Under the chestnut trees turning autumn gold
And the fuchsia bleeding like troupes of crimson-tutu'd ballerinas
    in the black hedgerows.
Standing over my mother's carcass in the morgue,
A sheep's skull on a slab,
A girl in her birth-gown blown across the sand,
I shut my eyes:
Thank you, O golden mother,
For giving me a life,
A spear of rain.
After a long life searching for a little boy who lives down the lane
You never found him, but you never gave up;
In your afterlife nightie
You are pirouetting expectantly for the last time.

The Deaths
Jo Shapcott (2010)

I thought I knew my death.
I thought he would announce
himself with all the little creaks
and groans you hear of,
that we'd get friendly and walk
our walk of two drunkards
with him chattering inside me
about lumps and arteries
and his gift of pain which would be
too big to wrap properly,
that some way into our courtship
he'd give me the look and
I'd implode like a ripe mango.

I thought I knew my death
so when, after a bee buzz
of an afternoon, the rain started
and the fine hairs rose on my neck

and the long hairs tugged my scalp
and my mouth stank of seaweed
and a tingle ran round my wrists,
I didn't recognise her. She lit
a green flame over my head
and even then I didn't get it. She threw
me yards back, traced her filigree
red cartoons on my palms until
I was gone and still didn't know.

MEDICAL WRITING:

An Essay of Health and Long Life
George Cheyne (1724)

There is nothing more certain, than that the greater superiority the concoctive powers have, over the food, or the stronger the concoctive powers are, in regard of the things to be concocted; the finer the chyle[18] will be, the circulation the more free, and the spirits more lightsome; that is, the better will the health be. Now from these general propositions, taking in their own particular complexion and habits, valetudinary, studious, or contemplative persons may easily fix upon these particular vegetable or animal foods, that are fittest for them. And if any error should be committed, 'tis best to err on the safest side, and rather chuse those things that are under our concoctive powers, than those that are above them. And in the choice of animals for our food, we must not pass over the manner of fattening and fitting them up for the table.

About London we can scarce have any, but cramm'd poultry, or stall-fed butchery meat. It were sufficient to disgust the stoutest stomach, to see the foul, gross, and nasty manner, in which, and the fetid, putrid and unwholesome materials, with which they are fed. Perpetual foulness and cramming, gross food and nastiness, we know, will putrify the juices and mortify the muscular substance of human creatures; and sure they can do no less in brute animals, and thus make even our food poison. The same may be said of hot beds, and forcing plants and vegetables. The only way of having sound and healthful animal food, is to leave them to their own natural liberty, in the free air, and their own proper element, with plenty of food, and due cleanness, and a shelter from the injuries of the weather, when they have a mind to retire to it.

I add nothing about cookery: plain roasting and boiling is as high, as valetudinary, tender, studious, and contemplative persons, or those who would preserve their health, and lengthen out their days, ought to presume on. Made dishes, rich soup, high sauces, baking, smoaking, salting, and pickling, are the inventions of luxury, to force an unnatural appetite, and encrease the load, which nature, without incentives from ill habits, and a vicious palate, will of itself make more than sufficient for

---

[18]Chyle is the milky fluid containing fat droplets which drains from the lacteals of the small intestine into the lymphatic system during digestion.

health and long life. Abstinence and proper evacuations, due labour and exercise, will always recover a decayed appetite, so long as there is any strength and fund in nature to go upon. And 'tis scarce allowable to provoke an appetite, with medicinal helps, but where the digestive faculties have been spoiled and ruined by acute or tedious chronical distempers. And as soon as 'tis recovered to any tolerable degree, nature is to be left to its own work, without any spurs from cookery or physick.

The next consideration is the quantity of food that is necessary to support nature, without overloading it, in a due plight: that is indeed various, according to the age, sex, nature, strength, and country the party is of, and the exercise he uses. In these northern countries, the coldness of the air, the strength and large stature of people, demand larger supplies than in the eastern and warmer countries. Young growing persons, and those of great strength and large stature, require more than the aged, weak, and slender. But persons of all sorts will live more healthy and longer by universal temperance, than otherwise.

...

Most of all the chronical diseases, the infirmities of old age, and the short periods of the lives of Englishmen, are owing to repletion. This is evident from hence; because evacuation of one kind or another is nine parts of ten in their remedy: for not only cupping, bleeding, blistering, issues, purging, vomiting, and sweating, are manifest evacuations, or drains to draw out what has been superfluously taken down; but even abstinence, exercise, alteratives, cordials, bitters, and alexipharmicks,[19] are but several means to dispose the gross humours to be more readily evacuated by insensible perspiration.

...

I advise therefore all gentlemen of a sedentary life, and of learned professions, to use as much abstinence as possibly they can, consistent with the preservation of their strength and freedom of spirits: which ought to be done as soon as they find any heaviness, inquietudes, restless nights, or aversion to application; either by lessening one half of their usual quantity of animal food and strong liqours, 'till such time as they regain their wonted freedom and indolence; or by living a due time wholly upon vegetable diet, such as sago, rice, pudding, and the like, and drinking only a little wine and water. And if they would preserve their health and constitution, and lengthen out their days; they must either inviolably live low (or maigre, as the french call it) a day or two in the week; or once a week, fortnight, or month at farthest, take some domestick purge, which shall require neither diet, nor keeping at home; but may at once strengthen the bowels, and discharge superfluous humours.

...

Those who have written about health have given many rules, whereby to know when any person has exceeded at a meal: I think, there needs but this short one, which is; if any man has eat or drank so much, as renders him unfit for the duties and studies of his profession (after an hour's sitting quiet to carry on the digestion;) he has overdone. I mean only of those of learned professions and studious lives; for those of mechanical employments must take the body, the other part of the

---

[19]Alexipharmicks: antidotes against poisons or miasmic (bad) air.

compound, into consideration. If tender people, and those of learned professions would go by this rule, there would be little use for physick or physicians in chronical cases. Or if they would but eat only one part of animal food, at the great meal, and make the other two of vegetable food; and drink only water with a spoonful of wine, or clear small beer; their appetites would be a sufficient rule to determine the quantity of their meat and drink. But variety of dishes, the luxurious artfulness of cookery, and swallowing rich wine after every bit of meat, so lengthen out the appetite; the fondness of mothers, and the cramming of nurses have so stretched the capacities of receiving, that there is no security from the appetite among the better sort. 'Tis amazing to think how men of voluptuousness, laziness, and poor constitutions, should imagine themselves able to carry off loads of high-seasoned foods, and inflammatory liquors, without injury or pain; when men of mechanic employments, and rubust constitutions, are scarcely able to live healthy and in vigour to any great age, on a simple, low, and almost vegetable diet.

The Old Man's Guide to Health and Longer Life
John Hill (1771)

Of a regulation of temper; and of the passions

Without entering into the province of the moralist or preacher, we may affirm here, that the passions demand great regard in preserving the health of old men. The motion of the blood in circulation is greatly affected and altered by them: and the nerves may suffer yet more. The whole frame is disordered by violent passions: and I have often seen diseases; and sometimes immediate death has been the consequence of giving full scope to them.

Nothing in this world is worth the trouble and distress men bring upon themselves by giving way to immoderate passions. Life is the greatest blessing; and health the next; and these both suffer by that fond indulgence.

That the circulation is disordered by passions, we know from the true and certain indication of the pulse. In anger, it is violent and hard; in grief, faint, and slow; terrors make it irregular; and shame impedes its motions.

These are sure notices of a disordered circulation: and old men cannot bear this, even for a time, without damage. The strength of youth restores all to its former state, when the sudden gust is over: but age is weak, and cannot. Philosophy teaches the governing our passions; and that is true wisdom. The old man should love himself too well to indulge them: it is not worth his while. Quiet and regularity of Life in every respect are his business: and as he is past the fluttering pleasures of youth, let him place himself above its troubles.

Good humour, and a happy satisfaction of mind, will give the aged many years; and much happiness in them. Discontent and disturbance wear out nature: but the quiet we advise, preserves her in good condition.

Of all passions let the old man avoid a foolish fondness for women. This never will solicit him: for nature knows her own time; and the appetite decays with the power: but if he will solicit that which he cannot enjoy, he will disturb his constitution more

than by any other means whatever: and while he is shortening his life; and robbing
the poor remainder he allows, of peace; he will be only making himself the ridicule
of those who seem to favour his vain, and ineffectual desires.

In passionate people, what we blame as their fault is often their misfortune. Some
indeed, from a tyrannical disposition, have fixed this humour upon themselves by
custom with no other cause; but for one of these, there are a hundred whose fury of
temper is owing to a disorder in their body.

We know madness is a disease: and violent passion is a temporary madness. This
also arises often from a redundance of humours; and medicines will cure it.

Let the passionate old man consider, that he hurts himself more than anybody
else, by his anger; and he will then wish to be cured of its tyranny. Let him examine
himself, whether it be a disorder of his mind; and then his physician, whether it lie in
the body. In the first case the remedy is philosophy: but in the latter, a few medicines
will restore him to temper; to that temper on which his life and happiness depend.

Let the hasty old man cool himself by physic and a low diet: and let him who
is melancholy and gloomy, banish the everlasting fear of death by warmer foods,
cordial medicines, and that best of cordials, wine.

These will drive away much more than the apprehension of death; they will put
off the reality: for melancholy would have sunk the feeble, long before his time.

Of all states of the mind, a disturbed hurry of the spirits is most to be avoided.
The blood and the nerves are disordered by this much more than by labour, or
bodily motion; and they are much longer in coming to themselves again. Labour
ceases absolutely when 'tis over: but the storms of the mind leave a swelling sea,
which strength of body alone can calm; and in age this strength is faint.

No disease is more mischievous to weak old persons than a purging: and I have
seen this brought on instantly by a fit of passion; or by a fright. Medicines have
attempted to relieve the patient in vain. That flux which would have been stopped,
if natural, by a spoonful of chalk julep, or a dose of diascordium,[20] has in this case
reduced the person to a skeleton, and sunk him into the grave in spite of all help.

Why should the old man disturb his mind with anger? or what should he dread?
death is his great terror; and he is very absurd who brings that on by lesser fears.

Joy, though it be only a greater share of satisfaction, is, in a violent or outrageous
degree, as hurtful as the other passions: it hurries the circulation vehemently and
irregularly; it exhausts the spirits; and when excessive it has often occasioned sudden
death. It is a violence of youth; it belongs to that period of life more properly: that
can bear it; and to that let us leave it. Let the old man be as the Quakers in this point;
always cheerful but never merry.

Last let us caution also the aged man who would be happy, and would live longer,
to combat with all his power that dangerous enemy covetousness. 'Tis known
universally, and we have sacred attestation of it, that too great carefulness brings age
before its time; and in age it brings death prematurely. The old are in no danger of

---

[20]In premodern medicine, diascordium was a preparation of scordium, a strong-smelling plant, to treat
malignant fevers, the plague, worms, colic and sleeplessness. At the time of Hill's article, diascordium was
offered with or without opium.

extravagance, and the care of heaping up for others, when it shortens their own life, is more than any heir deserves.

Ease and good humour are the great ingredients of a happy life: and the principal means of a long one. Our whole lesson extends but thus much farther; that the old man love his life so well; and value so little all the accidents which belong to it, that he do not give a vain attention to a part, which may rob him of the whole.

The Art of Beauty
Anonymous (1825)

'Wrinkles'

One of the chief causes of wrinkles arises from the obliteration of the blood vessels in old age, or in the premature advances of senility from dissipation or disease; for wrinkles are not so much an indication of years, as of the march of the constitution. It is palpably wrong, indeed, in ninety-nine cases out of a hundred, to reckon a person's age by the number of years, rather than by the marks of decay, which cannot be mistaken. Have you ever remarked the countenance of any of your friends on recovering from a course of mercury, which some bilious disorder may have rendered indispensable? If you have not, our strongest language cannot picture to you the haggard look, the hollow eye, the wasted cheek, the bloodless and wrinkled skin, and aged-like features of those, who, in the bloom of youth, or the prime of life, have been subjected to this infallible destroyer of beauty.

Though one of the first marks of old age is a failure in the power of the stomach and liver to prepare good blood from the food and drink taken for that purpose; yet, you must remark, that blood may be manufactured by the stomach and liver, and of the freshest and healthiest kind too, and yet may be, in a great measure, useless, from the obstruction, or obliteration, of the blood vessels. Now, this is precisely what happens in advanced years, or premature old age; for the fine hair-like blood vessels, which branch-off in every direction through the texture of the skin, become obstructed and imperforate, and, consequently, the skin, not being supplied with its nourishment of fresh blood, shrinks, withers, and becomes, first, sallow, and then wrinkled. In such cases, when the smaller blood vessels are obstructed, the larger ones swell with the blood which cannot get vent, and this is the reason why you see old people's veins swell, as on the back part of the hand.

Another cause of wrinkles, of precisely the same kind, is, the obstruction of the small pipes which we have described above, as conveying moisture to the skin, to keep it smooth and soft. The little glands, also, or fountains, which supply the moisture, are diminished, or dried up, in consequence of being stinted in their supply of fresh blood, from which they manufacture, or filter, the moisture destined to soften the skin.

It requires but small observation to remark, that the thin and meagre are more liable to wrinkles than the plump and corpulent. *Embonpoint*,[21] indeed, is one of the

---

[21]*Embonpoint* refers to fleshy plumpness.

best preservatives against wrinkles, properly so called, for, though a certain kind of wrinkles are formed in this state of the system, they are very different from the dry, withered, wrinkles of old age.

A Lecture Delivered over the Remains of Jeremy Bentham
Thomas Southwood Smith (1832)

No one now disputes that the dissection of the human body, to such an extent as is necessary to afford an intimate acquaintance with its structure, and with the mutual relations of all its parts, is indispensable to the surgeon and physician. To undertake the duties of either department of the healing art without having acquired such knowledge is now considered not a folly, but a crime. The diseases of blood-vessels, the wounds of arteries, the mode of stopping haemorrhage, the displacement of the viscera by external violence or internal disease, the return of these viscera to their natural situations, the retention of them there by appropriate means, the morbid changes which take place in the progress of disease in the alimentary canal, especially of children, and which lead to the effusion of water into the brain, the various modifications of fever, the diversities of treatment required by each modification of this prevalent and fatal malady, would afford, were there time to enter into the requisite details, striking illustrations of the absolute necessity of dissection, to guide the surgeon and physician: but as these details have been entered into elsewhere,[22] it is now only necessary that I should advert to the sources of that unreasonable disgust at dissection, which has so greatly obstructed, and which does still to so large an extent obstruct, the acquisition of the knowledge of anatomy and physiology.

At the bottom of this prejudice is the vulgar notion that, after death, the features undergo some repulsive change, and that the body becomes an object of disgust. On the contrary, after the last struggles of expiring life are over, whatever be the nature of the change which the fluids and solids immediately undergo, the first effect is to increase and soften the delicacy of the skin to such a degree, as to render it in a manner transparent; while the calm and placid aspect which the features assume, gives to the countenance an expression of beauty not before possessed by it – a beauty increasing in proportion to the exquisiteness of the form, and the mildness and dignity of the expression natural to the individual. This has not escaped the eye of the poet, and can have escaped the notice of no observing person who has ever contemplated the form and features of the dead.

> He who hath bent him o'er the dead,
> Ere the first day of death is fled –
> Before Decay's effacing fingers
> Have swept the lines where beauty lingers,
> And mark'd the mild angelic air –

---

[22]Southwood Smith refers to his polemic in support of the Anatomy Act (1832), 'Use of the Dead to the Living' (1827).

The rapture of repose that's there –
The fix'd yet tender traits that streak
The languor of the placid cheek;
And, but for that sad shrouded eye,
That fires not – wins not – weeps not – now;
And but for that chill, changeless brow, ...
He still might doubt the tyrant's power,
So fair – so calm – so softly seal'd
The first – last look – by death reveal'd![23]

Where the dread of being in the presence of the dead has amounted to an exceedingly painful feeling, I have more than once succeeded in removing it by prevailing on the person labouring under the wrong impression, to contemplate steadily, for a few minutes, the countenance of the friend he has lost. I have always observed the effect on the afflicted mind to be soothing in a high degree, and never in a single instance have I witnessed the production of any thing approaching to the feeling of disgust. If there be any one present who has never looked on death before, let him now behold it as it appears in that revered and beloved countenance... Pallid as it now is in death, can you look on the sweetness, the dignity of its expression, and ever forget it? Can you dread the aspect of death assuming such a shape? Can you conceive that any thing bearing the remotest resemblance to degradation can attach to that body, devoted, by the mind that animated it, to the illustration, for the sake of human happiness, of the still more beautiful structure that lies concealed beneath that beautiful exterior?

But you will tell me, that it is not the aspect of death which renders the thought of the dissection of the body painful, so much as the associations which are connected with the person of whomsoever we regard with respect and affection. It is with the corporeal frame that our senses have been familiar; it is on this that our eye has so often rested with pleasure; it is this which has so often been the medium of conveying to our hearts delicious emotions. By no effort can we separate our idea of the peculiarities and actions of our friend from the idea of his person: the two impressions have been so constantly excited together, that they have mixed and mingled until they are one. For this very reason it is, that every thing which has been associated with my friend acquires a value from *that* consideration – his ring, his watch, his books, and his habitation. The value of these, as having been his, is not merely fictitious; they have an empire over my mind.

Euthanasia
William Munk (1887)

The common belief that the act of dying is one of severe bodily suffering is due probably in part to theoretical views of the nature of the event itself; but, principally, to the occurrence of conditions, physiological or pathological, which precede or accompany that act, and the nature and import of which are misinterpreted. Doubtless

---

[23]Lord Byron's poem 'The Giaour' (1813).

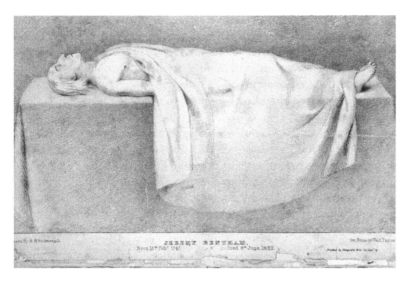

FIGURE 6: Weld Taylor, after H. H. Pickersgill, *The Mortal Remains of Jeremy Bentham*, *laid out for public dissection*, 1832. Courtesy Wellcome Library, London.

also, it is due in no small degree to confounding the actual stage of dying, with those urgent symptoms of disease that precede and lead up to it, and which are often as severe or more so in those who are to recover, as in those who are to die. As a rule, to which there are doubtless exceptions, the urgent symptoms of disease subside, when the act of dying really begins. 'A pause in nature, as it were, seems to take place, the disease has done its worst, all strong action has ceased, the frame is fatigued by its efforts to sustain itself, and a general tranquillity pervades the whole system.'[24]

Again, convulsions, which so often attend the process of dying, are accepted in evidence of suffering, when in fact they are the reverse, for they imply a loss of consciousness and sensibility, and therefore, of the capacity to feel pain. They are automatic, and in all essential respects like the convulsions of epilepsy, of which the subject is wholly unconscious. The convulsive movements that sometimes attend the last moments, and with which the person expires, constituting the so-called 'death struggle,' are doubtless of the same painless character.

Some few, however, do really suffer grievously in dying, and expire in great bodily torture. This occurs in some diseases of the heart and great vessels of the chest, in angina pectoris, and in ileus.[25] But especially in that most fearful of diseases, hydrophobia, in tetanus, and in spasmodic cholera[26] – in maladies characterized by

---

[24]Munk quotes the eighteenth-century royal physician Sir Henry Halford.

[25]Angina pectoris is a condition marked by severe pain in the chest, often also spreading to the shoulders, arms and neck, owing to an inadequate blood supply to the heart. Ileus refers to an obstruction of the ileum, or any part of the intestine.

[26]Hydrophobia is now called rabies. Tetanus is a bacterial disease marked by rigidity and spasms of the voluntary muscles. Asiatic cholera is a disease that became pandemic three times in the nineteenth century.

spasm of the external muscles, as distinguished from their convulsion, for spasm implies no such unconsciousness as does convulsion, but the reverse. Such cases are rare, but they are so terrible that they fix themselves in the memory, exert an undue influence on the judgment, and, although really exceptional in occurrence, and in the sufferings they entail, come to be regarded as but extreme instances of what is assumed to be the universal and inevitable lot of the dying. Happily for mankind it is not so.

So long as consciousness and intelligence continue, and they often do so to the last, the influence of mind and of the emotions on the bodily process of dying must be kept steadily in view. They are well-nigh as potential in the dying man as they are in the healthy. Hope is as soothing and fear as depressing in the one condition as in the other. To the dying there is no greater solace and cordial than hope – it is the most soothing and cheering of our feelings, and if, when all hope of life and in the present has fled, the dying man can dwell with hope and confidence upon his future, it will be well for him. The retrospect of a well-spent life, *memoria bene actae vitae, multorumque benefactorum recordatio*, is a cordial of infinitely more efficacy than all the resources of the medical art; but a firm belief in the mercy of God, and in the promises of salvation will do more than anything in aid of an easy, calm, and collected death. To those who are sceptical on this point, and such there are, I would remark, that unless a man has himself felt the influence of religion on his own mind, he is unable fully and accurately to understand its influence on others. If I may trust my own experience I should say, that in the aggressive *dis*believer, as in the mere passive agnostic, doubt and anxiety as to his future is all but sure to obtrude itself on his last conscious moments, disturb them, and render such an euthanasia as we contemplate, impossible.

...

The nature of the disease and the mode of death exert a marked influence on the expression of face of the dying, and this is often retained by the features after death. 'In some we observe the impress of the previous suffering, as in peritonitis and in cases of poisoning by irritants; in others the character is derived from a peculiar affection of some part of the respiratory apparatus; or from an affection of the facial muscles themselves, as in tetanus and paralysis. But the condition of the mind is perhaps more often concerned in the expression than even the physical circumstances of the body. For, as some kind of intelligence is frequently retained, and strong emotions are experienced till within a few moments of dissolution, the features may be sealed by the hand of death in the last look of rapture or of misery, of benignity or of anger. Every poetical reader knows the picture of the traits of death (no less true than beautiful) drawn by the author of "The Giaour."[27] But such observations are not confined to poets. Haller could trace in the dying countenance the smile which had been lighted by the hope of a happier existence.'[28]

---

[27]The Romantic poet George Gordon, Lord Byron; the passage Munk refers to is in the previous selection (Southwood Smith).
[28]This paragraph quotes J. A. Symonds' *The Cyclopædia of Anatomy and Physiology*, vol. 1 (1836) at length. Albrecht von Haller (1708–77) was a Swiss anatomist, physiologist, naturalist and poet, who is often referred to as the father of modern physiology.

The Needs and Rights of Old Age
I. N. Love (1897)

At the present rate of advancement the time will soon come when no one need die before his allotted time, save by accident. When we realize that the bulk of those who die in the world today, in spite of the progress of the sciences, die before they are five years old, we can see how much is left undone, and we are safe in saying that if the laws of health were properly observed and there was a proper application of the definite knowledge that we now have, all of these deaths prior to the age of five years old need not occur at all.

'Careless Living invites Early Death'

More and more we are having impressed upon us the fact that various microscopic forms of life, known as microbes, are present in the world here, there, and everywhere, seeking whom they may devour, and as time advances and investigation is more complete, we find more and more that many diseases, particularly in the early periods of life, are dependent upon these micro-organisms. It is pretty clearly established that not only are the infectious diseases to which children are particularly susceptible dependent on special germs, but many others are now found to come under that head, notable tuberculosis, the great 'white plague,' the disease from which one-seventh of all humankind die, the plague which would make the 'black plague' of the ancient regime turn pale with envy. And yet we must remember that every individual, of no matter what age, would be able to resist this invading army, and the diseases resulting therefrom would be unknown, were it not for the fact that the victims have invited the enemy by their own indiscretions. In other words, all would be safe, even against infectious germs, did they observe the rules of health and not develop in themselves susceptibility to attack. Commencing then at an early period of life we are safe in saying that the individual is rendered susceptible to disease in general, and incompetent to cope with the dangers that surround him, only on account of not having husbanded his resources. By errors of diet, improper clothing, and the failure to correctly regulate the heat of the body, conditions are developed which invite disease and death, so we are safe in saying emphatically that from the beginning did we all eat proper food at the proper times in the proper way, and properly clothe ourselves and guard against inequalities of the temperature, 'Othello's occupation' as related to the doctor would be gone.[29]

The ideal condition can not be secured, but it may be approximated just in so far as hygienic laws are respected, while the individual progresses favourably along the lines of development, maintenance and repair. Let us recognize ourselves, then, as animated mechanisms, needing constant regulation; and to the extent of this regulation will we live healthy happy lives and progress to a delightful old age.

No person properly equipped in a proper state of health should want to die, or should we have any other thought than that life is worth living, and that this is a beautiful world filled with very pleasant people.

---

[29]William Shakespeare, *Othello*: 'Farewell the pluméd troops and the big wars ... Othello's occupation's gone' (III: 3: 49).

The Art and Science of Embalming
Carl Lewis Barnes (1898)

'The Reasons for Embalming the Dead'
    A great many reasons have been advanced for embalming the dead. Some of these are plausible, while some are, perhaps, fanciful, but in the majority of cases the principle reason is to prevent the appearance of putrefaction until such time that the body may be viewed by the friends of the deceased, or until it can be conveyed to a suitable resting place. This is the first and prime reason why embalming is practiced so extensively in this country. Since the discovery of the cause of putrefaction in animal tissues, and also since the discovery of the germ theory of disease, we have added the second, but by no means the least important cause, viz.: that of disinfecting the body. The importance of this subject can hardly be overestimated, since, by the introduction of the disinfecting fluids into the body by means of the arterial system, the fluid penetrates every tissue, and by the aid of osmotic action, percolation and imbition,[30] enters even those tissues not supplied by the blood current, killing the germs of contagion and putrefaction, and thus preventing the spread of contagious or infectious diseases and the development of poisonous gases which might have serious effect on the living.

    ...
'The Funeral Director Himself'
    A large part of your success will come from your work on the face of the dead. I must assume that this has been done carefully from the first; false teeth put in before the jaws become rigid, and eyes closed by eye-caps, or otherwise, in proper time. It is simply wonderful what an amount of modelling can be done on the face of the dead by the use of cotton batting, face powder, cochineal red and the manipulation of the lips with the fingers. You can take a face which is showing age and make it look younger. You can take away the traces of pain or suffering from the corners of the mouth, and put in place a smile. You can actually do what face powders and lotions claim to do (but cannot), restore youth to the face and bloom to the cheek; and the principal aid to success in this is, work, trial, experiment; you do not know what or how much you can do until you try. A little cotton placed under the lips restores the full-teethed jaw of young life, or a little cotton placed at the corner or end of the mouth raises it and takes out the wrinkle which denotes despondency or pain. A little red put on the lips, under the eye, in the ear, and then rubbed in underneath the powder, shows the colour but does not show what put it there. In using paint or powder, use plentifully, put on more than you intend to use, then rub it off. But the most important thing of all is, always rub it in with your fingers.

---

[30]Imbition (or imbibition): absorption.

BIBLIOGRAPHY

POETRY: BIBLIOGRAPHY

Anonymous. (1770), 'On the Dissection of a Body', *The Scots Magazine*, vol. 32, 441, Edinburgh: A. Murray.

Anonymous. (c.1819), 'Spurzheim and Lavater', Archives & Manuscripts, WMS 5465/1 Wellcome Library, London.

Anonymous. (1849), 'The Water That John Drinks', London: *Punch*, July to December.

Abse, Dannie. (2003), 'Carnal Knowledge' and 'In the Theatre', *New and Collected Poems*, London: Hutchinson.

Adcock, Fleur. (1997), 'Against Coupling', *Selected Poems*, Oxford: Oxford University Press/Oxford Poets.

Allen, Grant. (1881), 'A Ballade of Evolution', *The Evolutionist at Large,* London: Chatto & Windus.

Amis, Kingsley. (1980), 'To A Baby Born Without Limbs', *Collected Poems 1944–1979*, London: Viking.

Andrews, Nin. (2000), 'Monogamous Orgasms', *The Book of Orgasms*, Cleveland, OH: Cleveland State University Poetry Centre.

Appleman, Philip. (1996), 'Alive' and 'Vasectomy', *New and Selected Poems 1956–1996*, Fayetteville, AR: University of Arkansas Press.

Armitage, Simon. (2002), 'Salvador' and 'The Straight and Narrow', *The Universal Home Doctor*, London: Faber & Faber.

Armitage, Simon. (2006), 'Ankylosing Spondylitis' and 'Hand-Washing Technique – Government Guidelines', *Tyrannosaurus Rex Versus the Corduroy Kid,* London: Faber & Faber.

Armstrong, John. (1745), *The Oeconomy of Love: A Poetical Essay,* new ed., London: M. Cooper.

Armstrong, John. (1761), 'Diet', *The Art of Preserving Health*, London: A. Millar.

Arnold, Matthew. (1867), 'Growing Old', *New Poems*, London: Macmillan & Co.

Atkinson, Tiffany. (2006), 'The Anatomy Lesson of Dr Nicolaes Tulp, 1632', *Kink and Particle*, Bridgend: Seren.

Atwood, Margaret. (1998), 'Heart Test With an Echo Chamber', 'I Was reading A Scientific Article' and 'The Woman Who Could Not Live With Her Faulty Heart', *Eating Fire: Selected Poetry 1965-1995*, London: Virago.

Auden, W. H. (1976), 'A New Year Greeting', 'The Art of Healing', and 'Surgical Ward', *Collected Poems*, London: Faber & Faber.

Auden, W. H. (1977), 'Death like his is right and splendid', *The English Auden*, London: Faber & Faber.

Bamforth, Iain. (1996), 'Unsystematic Anatomy', *Open Workings*, Manchester: Carcanet.

Barker, Jane. (1688), 'A Farewell to Poetry, with a Long Digression about Anatomy', *Poetical Recreations Consisting of Original Poems, Songs, Odes &c.* London: Printed for Benjamin Crayle.

Barlow, George. (1884), 'The Sons of Science', *Poems Real and Ideal*, London: Remington & Co.

Beadle, Samuel Alfred. (1899), 'Yellow Jack of '97', *Sketches from Life in Dixie,* Chicago: Scroll Pub. & Literary Syndicate.

Bell, Martin. (1998), 'Ode to Psychoanalysis', *Collected Poems: 1937-1966*, London: Macmillan.

Bell, Marvin. (1990), 'Frankenstein's Monster', *Iris of Creation*, Port Townsend, WA: Copper Canyon.

Benn, Gottfried. (1987), 'Appendectomy' and 'Man and Woman Go through the Cancer Ward', *Prose, Essays, Poems, The German Library,* Vol. 73., ed. Volkmar Sander, New York: Continuum.

Best, Clare. (2011), 'Intersession' and 'Account', *Excisions,* Hove: Waterloo Press.

Betjeman, John. (2006), 'The Cottage Hospital' and 'Death in Leamington', *Collected Poems*, London: John Murray.

Bierds, Linda. (2008), 'The Anatomy Lesson of Dr. Nicolaas Tulp: Amsterdam, 1632', *Flight: New and Selected Poems*, New York: G.P. Putnam's Sons/Penguin.

Bishop, Elizabeth. (2011), 'In the Waiting Room', *Poems: The Centenary Edition*, London: Chatto & Windus.

Bogan, Louise. (1995), 'Evening in the Sanitarium', *The Blue Estuaries: Poems 1923-1968*, London: Josef Weinberger Plays.

Boland, Eavan. (2008), 'Anorexic' and 'Fever', *New Collected Poems*, New York: W. W. Norton.

Borges, Jorge Luis. (1975), 'In Praise of Darkness', *In Praise of Darkness,* London: Allen Lane/Penguin.

Brooks, Gwendolyn. (1963), 'The Mother', *Selected Poems,* New York: Harper & Row.

Brown, Andy. (2014), 'Ecorché', *Poor Yorick!*, Western Connecticut State University, http://www.pooryorickjournal.com.

Brown, Andy. (2014), 'Public Speaking', *The Warwick Review*, vol. 7, 4, Coventry: University of Warwick.

Brown, Sterling A. (1980), 'Parish Doctor', *The Collected Poems of Sterling A. Brown*, ed. Michael S. Harper, Evanston, IL: Northwestern University Press.

Brown, Thomas. (1700), 'To a Gentleman that cut off his hair … in his old age', *A Collection of Miscellany Poems*, London: J. Nutt.

Browne, Isaac Hawkins. (1768), 'On a Fit of Gout: An Ode', *Poems Upon Various Subjects*, London: Printed for J. Nourse.

Browning, Robert. (1855), 'An Epistle Containing the Strange Medical Experience of Karshish, the Arab Physician', *Men and Women*, 1 of 2 vols., rev. 1863, Boston: Ticknor and Fields.

Buck, Stephen. (1734), 'Geneva', *Geneva: A Poem in Blank Verse*, London: T. Cooper.

Buckley, Alan. (2009), 'Anusol®', *Shiver*, London: Tall-lighthouse.

Burnside, John. (2005), *'De Humani Corporis Fabrica'*, *The Good Neighbour*, London: Jonathan Cape.

Bush, Duncan. (1993), 'Pneumoconiosis', *The New Poetry*, eds. Michael Hulse, David Kennedy and David Morley, Hexham, Northumberland: Bloodaxe Books.

Butler, Samuel. (1706), *Dildoides, A Burlesque Poem*. London: J. Nutt.

Campo, Rafael. (2000), 'What the Body Told', *The World In Us: Lesbian and Gay Poetry of The Next Wave*, New York: St. Martin's Press/Macmillan.

Campo, Rafael. (2002), 'What I Would Give', *Landscape with Human Figure*, Durham, NC: Duke University Press.

Carkesse, James. (1679), 'The Poetical History of Finnesbury Mad-House', *Lucida Intervalla, Containing Divers Miscellaneous Poems, Written at Finsbury and Bethlem by the Doctors Patient Extraordinary*, London: n.p.

Carey, Mary. (1720), 'Upon the Sight of my Abortive Birth the 31st December 1657', *Lady Carey's Meditations, & Poetry*, Bodleian Library: MS Rawlinson D. 1308.

Carpenter, Peter. (2002), 'Double Helix', *Just Like That*, Sheffield: Smith/Doorstop.

Carver, Raymond. (1997), 'The Autopsy Room', 'Circulation', 'Medicine' and 'What the Doctor Said', *All Of Us: The Collected Poems*, London: Harvill.

Chandler, Mary. (1733), *A Description of Bath*, 3rd ed., London: James Leake.

Clifton, Lucille. (2012), 'Poem to My Uterus', 'To My Last Period' and 'Dialysis', *The Collected Poems*, Rochester, NY: BOA Editions.

Coleridge, S. T. (1834), 'Cholera Cured Before-Hand', *The Complete Works*, vol. 2 of 2, London: W. Pickering.

Collins, Billy. (1994), 'Deathbeds', *Poetry*, 165:1, October, 29–30.

Cook-Lynn, Elizabeth. (1994), 'Grandfather at the Indian Health Clinic', *Unsettling America: An Anthology of Contemporary Multicultural Poetry*, eds. Maria Mazziotti Gillan and Jennifer Gillan, New York: Penguin.

Corcoran, Kelvin. (2004), 'The Ingliss Touriste Patient', *New and Selected Poems*, Exeter: Shearsman Books.

Corcoran, Kelvin. (2010), 'The Vaccination Queue', *Hotel Shadow*, Exeter: Shearsman Books.

Cowper, William. (1836), 'Lines Written During a Period of Insanity', *The Works of William Cowper, With a Life of the Author*, vol. 1, London: Baldwin and Cradock.

Crabbe, George. (1810), 'Professions: Physic', *The Borough: A Poem in Twenty-four Letters*, London: J. Hatchard.

Dacre, Charlotte. (1805), 'Mildew', *Hours of Solitude*, vol. 2 of 2, London: Hughes et al.

Darling, Julia. (2003), 'Too Heavy', *Sudden Collapses in Public Places*, Todmorden: Arc Publications.

Darwin, Erasmus. (1803), *Temple of Nature*, London: Joseph Johnson.

Davidson, Lucretia Maria. (1841), 'The Fear of Madness', *Poetical Remains of the Late Lucretia Maria Davidson, Collected and Arranged by Her Mother*, Philadelphia: Lea and Blanchard.

Dawes, Kwame. (2003), 'Fat Man', *New & Selected Poems: 1994-2002*, Leeds: Peepal Tree Press.

Dibdin, Charles. (1825), 'The Maniac's Funeral', *Comic Tales and Lyrical Fancies*, London: G. B. Whittaker.

Dickey, James. (1969), 'Diabetes', *The Eye-beaters, Blood, Victory, Madness, Buckhead and Mercy*, Garden City, NY: Doubleday.

Dickinson, Emily. (1924), 'I had been Hungry', 'Much Madness is Divinest Sense' and 'Surgeons must be Very Careful', *The Complete Poems of Emily Dickinson*, ed. Martha Dickinson Bianchi, Boston: Little, Brown & Co.

Doak, SuAnne. (1994), 'Hands', *The Viet Nam Generation Big Book* Vol.5: 1-4, March 1994, http://www2.iath.virginia.edu/sixties/HTML_docs/Index_entry_title.html.

Dobell, Sydney. (1855), 'The Wounded', *Sonnets on the War*, London: David Bogue.

Doty, Mark. (1995), 'Fog', *My Alexandria*, London: Jonathan Cape.

Doty, Mark. (2004), 'Theory of the Soul', *Theories and Apparitions*, London: Jonathan Cape.

Douglas, Evelyn (John Barlas). (1887), 'Behold the Plague-wind, from some Orient Fen', *Holy of Holies: Confessions of an Anarchist*, Chelmsford: J. H. Clarke.

Downman, Hugh. (1790), *Infancy, or the Management of Children*, Edinburgh: Printed for J. Bell and J. Bradfute et al.

Downman, Hugh. (1799), 'To Dr. William Hunter', on flyleaf of Hunter's copy of printed book, *Hugh Downman, Poems to Thespia* (Exeter, 1781), Hunterian Eh.2.2, University of Glasgow Special Collections.

Dugdale, Sasha. (2003), 'Anatomy Class', *Notebook*, Manchester: Carcanet.

Dunbar-Nelson, Alice Moore. (1988), 'To Madam Curie', *The Works of Alice Dunbar-Nelson, Vol. 2, The Schomburg Library of Nineteenth-Century Black Women Writers*, Oxford: Oxford University Press.

Durcan, Paul. (2009), 'Golden Mothers Driving West', *Life Is A Dream: 40 Years Reading Poems 1967-2007*, London: Harvill Secker.

Eliot, T. S. (1963), 'East Coker' and 'Hysteria', *Collected Poems 1909–1962*, London: Faber & Faber.

Enright, D. J. (1987), 'Confessions of an English Opium Smoker', *Collected Poems*, Oxford: Oxford University Press.

Farley, Paul. (2006), 'A Great Stink', *Tramp In Flames,* London: Picador.

Fawkes, Francis. (1761), 'The Smoking Doctor's Soliloquy over his Pipe', *Original Poems and Translations*, London: Printed for the author and sold by R. and J. Dodsley et al.

Finch, Anne (Kingsmill), Countess of Winchilsea. (1713), 'The Spleen', *Miscellany Poems, on Several Occasions*, London: John Barber.

Fisher, Roy. (2005), 'As He came Near Death' and 'The Hospital in Winter', *The Long and The Short Of It: Poems 1955-2005*, Hexham, Northumberland: Bloodaxe Books.

Flint, Sally. (2015), 'The Hospital Punch', *The Hospital Punch*, Exeter: Maquette Press.

Gilbert, Sandra M. (1984), 'Metastasis', *Emily's Bread*, New York: W. W. Norton.

Ginsberg, Allen. (2009), 'Hospital Window', *Collected Poems 1947-1997*, London: Penguin.

Gould, Hannah F. (1829), 'To the Automaton Chess Player', *Specimens of American Poetry*, vol. 3 of 3, ed. Samuel Kettell, Boston: S. G. Goodrich.

Gould, Hannah F. (1832), 'To the Siamese Twins', *Poems,* Boston: Hilliard, Gray, Little & Wilkins.

Graves, Robert. (2003), 'The Halls of Bedlam' and 'Twins', *The Complete Poems*, London: Penguin.

Green, Matthew (1737), *The Spleen, An Epistle*, London: A. Dodd.

Greenlaw, Lavinia. (1993), 'The Man Whose Smile Made Medical History', *Night Photograph*. London: Faber & Faber.

Gross, Philip. (1998), 'The Wasting Game', *The Wasting Game*, Hexham, Northumberland: Bloodaxe Books.

Gross, Philip. (2013), 'Nimzo-Indian', *Later*, Hexham, Northumberland: Bloodaxe Books.

Gunn, Thom. (1993), 'Lament' and 'The Man With Night Sweats', *Collected Poems*, London: Faber & Faber.

Haas, Robert. (1989), 'A Story About the Body', *Human Wishes*, New York/London: Harper Collins.

Halliday, James. L. (c.1920), 'The Sanitary Three', *Scot's Poesie* (unbound notebook), Wellcome Library, London, MS Gen 1669/120.

Hardy, Thomas. (2001), 'Heredity', *The Complete Poems*, London: Palgrave Macmillan.

Harper, Michael. (1973), 'Maalox Bland Diet Prescribed', *Debridgement*, New York: Doubleday.

Harrison, Tony. (1984), 'Pain-Killers', *Selected Poems*, London: Penguin Books.

Hay, William. (1794) 'The Immortality of the Soul', *The Works of William Hay, Esq.,* vol. 2 of 2, London: J. Dodsley.

Heaney, Seamus. (1966), 'Mid Term Break', *Death of a Naturalist*, London: Faber & Faber.

Heaney, Seamus. (2001), 'Out of the Bag', *Electric Light*, London: Faber & Faber.

Henley, William Ernest. (1889), 'Enter Patient' and 'Waiting', *Poems*, 2nd ed., London: David Nutt.

Hicok, Bob. (1995), 'Duke', *The Legend of Light*, Madison, WI: University of Wisconsin Press.

Hicok, Bob. (1998), 'Alzheimers', *Plus Shipping*, New York: BOA Editions.

Hill, Selima. (2008), 'In a Hedge', *Gloria: Selected Poems*, Hexham, Northumberland: Bloodaxe Books.

Holmes, Oliver Wendell. (1895), 'The Stethoscope Song: A Professional Ballad', *The Complete Poetical Works of Oliver Wendell Holmes,* Boston: Houghton, Mifflin & Co.

Holub, Miroslav. (1990), 'What the Heart is Like', 'Brief Reflection on the Word Pain', and 'Suffering', *Poems Before & After*, Hexham, Northumberland: Bloodaxe Books.

Hood, Thomas. (1827), 'Craniology', *Whims and Oddities*, 2nd series, London: Charles Tilt.

Hood, Thomas. (1870), *Miss Kilmansegg and her Precious Leg*, London: F. Moxon Son & Co.

Hood, Thomas. (1905), 'Fragment, Probably Written During Illness', *The Complete Poetical Works*, London: Henry Frowde.

Hopkins, Lemuel. (1793), 'Epitaph on a Patient Killed by a Cancer Quack', *American Poems, Selected and Original,* Litchfield: Collier & Buel.

Hopkinson, Francis. (1789), *An Oration which Might have been Delivered to the Students in Anatomy, on the Late Rupture Between the Two Schools in this City,* Philadelphia: T. Dobson & T. Lang.

Huard. (1786), 'On the Education of the Blind', *An Essay on the Education of the Blind*, ed. René Just Haily, London: Sampson Low, Marston & Co.

Hughes, Langston. (1995), 'Interne at Provident', *The Collected Poems of Langston Hughes*, London/New York: Vintage.

Hughes, Ted. (1995), 'The Tender Place', *New Selected Poems*, London: Faber & Faber.

Jennings, Elizabeth. (2002), 'Genes, Likenesses', *New Collected Poems*, Manchester: Carcanet.

Johnson, Alexander. (1789), *Relief from Accidental Death*, London: Logographic Press.

Jones, Mary. (1750), 'After the Small Pox', *Miscellanies in Prose and Verse*, Oxford: Dodsley.

Justice, Donald. (2006), 'Counting the Mad', *Collected Poems*, New York: Knopf.

Kasdorf, Julia. (1998), 'Lymphoma', *Eve's Striptease*, Pittsburgh, PA: University of Pittsburgh Press.

Keats, John. (1820), 'Ode on Melancholy', *Lamia, Isabella, The Eve of St Agnes and Other Poems,* London: Taylor and Hessey.

Kennedy, David. (2004), 'My Father's Deaths', *The Roads*, Cambridge: Salt Publishing.

Kenyon, Jane. (2005), 'Having it out with Melancholy', *Constance*, Minneapolis, MN: Graywolf Press.

Kinnell, Galway. (2001), 'Parkinson's Disease', *A New Selected Poems*, Boston: Mariner/Houghton Mifflin.

Kipling, Rudyard. (1910), 'Our Fathers of Old', *Rewards and Fairies*, Garden City, NY: Doubleday, Page & Co.

Kipling, Rudyard. (1919), 'A Death Bed', *The Years Between*, Garden City, NY: Doubleday, Page & Co.

Kipling, Rudyard. (1937–9), 'Doctors', *The Works of Rudyard Kipling*, vol. xxv, London: Macmillan.

Kooser, Ted. (1980), 'After the Funeral: Cleaning out the Medicine Cabinet', *Sure Signs: New And Selected Poems*, Pittsburgh, PA: University of Pittsburgh Press.

Kooser, Ted. (1985), 'The Urine Sample', *One World at a Time*, Pittsburgh, PA: University of Pittsburgh Press.

Lamb, Charles. (1818). 'A Farewell to Tobacco', *The Works of Charles Lamb*, 1 of 2 vols., London: Ollier.

Lamb, Charles. (1903), 'Cleanliness' (vol. 3) and 'On an Infant Dying as Soon as Born' (vol. 5), *The Works of Charles and Mary Lamb*, ed. E. V. Lucas, London: Methuen.

Lane, Joel, (2002). 'Insulin', *The Gift: New Writing for the NHS,* ed. David Morley, Exeter: Stride Publications.

Larkin, Philip. (1988), 'Ambulances', 'The Building', and 'Faith Healing', *Collected Poems*, London: Faber & Faber.

Lasdun, James. (1997), 'Plague Years', *Woman Police Officer in Elevator*, New York: W. W. Norton.

Lawrence, D. H. (1916), 'Malade', *Amores*, New York: B. W. Huebsch.

Lawrence, D. H. (1932), 'Healing', *Last Poems*, Florence: G. Orioli.

Lee-Hamilton, Eugene. (1894), 'Siamese Twins', *Sonnets of Wingless Hours*, London: Elliot Stock.

Lifshin, Lyn. (1997), 'The Man Who is Married to Siamese Twins Joined at the Skull', *Cold Comfort: Selected Poems 1970–1996*, Boston, MA: Black Sparrow Press.

Lowell, Robert. (2003), 'Fetus', 'Terminal Days at Beverly Farms', 'Waking in the Blue' and 'Watchmaker God', *Collected Poems*, London: Faber & Faber.

Linton, W. J. (1865), 'The Hunchback', *Claribel and Other Poems*, London: Simpkin, Marshall, & Co.

Loy, Mina. (1997), 'An Aged Woman' and 'Auto-Facial-Construction', *The Lost Lunar Baedecker: Poems of Mina Loy*, New York: Farrar, Strauss, Giroux.

Lux, Thomas. (2001), 'The Blister Test' and 'The Nerve Doctors', *The Street of Clocks*, Todmorden: Arc Publications.

Lykiard, Alexis. (2007), 'The Dirty Thirties', *Judging By Disappearances*, Bristol: Bluechrome Publishing.

Lynch, Thomas. (1994), 'A Death', 'The Old Operating Theatre, All Souls Night' and 'These Things Happen in the Lives of Women', *Grimalkin and Other Poems*, London: Jonathan Cape.

Mackay, Charles. (1848), 'The Mowers: An Anticipation of Cholera', *Town Lyrics, and other Poems*, London: D. Bogue.

Macphee, Kona. (2004), 'IVF', *Tails*, Hexham: Northumberland: Bloodaxe Books.

Madhubuti, Haki R. (1996), 'Abortion', *Groundwork: New and Selected Poems, Don L. Lee/Haki R. Madhubuti from 1966 – 1996*, Chicago, IL: Third World Press.

Maguire, Sarah. (1997), 'Psoriasis', *The Invisible Mender*, London: Jonathan Cape.

Matthews, Aidan, (1998), 'At the Nurses' Station', *According to the Small Hours*, London: Jonathan Cape.

McAuliffe, John. (2007), 'Tinnitus', *Next Door,* Dublin: Gallery Press.

McCabe, Brian. (1999), 'Small Intestine' and 'Donor', *Body Parts,* Edinburgh: Canongate.

McClatchey, J. D. (1998), 'My Mammogram', *Ten Commandments*, New York: Knopf.

Meinke, Peter. (1977), 'The Patient', *The Night Train and the Golden Bird*, Pittsburgh, PA: University of Pittsburgh Press.

Merriam, Eve. (1995), 'The Plague of Painlessness', *Embracing the Dark*, Halifax: Garden Street Press.

Mew, Charlotte. (1916), 'On the Asylum Road', *The Farmer's Bride*, London: The Poetry Bookshop.

Mitchell, Adrian. (2008), 'A Puppy Called Puberty' and 'A Dog Called Elderly', *Come On Everybody: Poems 1953–2008*, Hexham, Northumberland: Bloodaxe Books.

Mitchell, Silas Weir. (1896), *The Birth and Death of Pain*, Boston: Merrymount Press.

Molloy, Dorothy. (2006), 'Gethsemane Day', *Gethsemane Day*, London: Faber & Faber.

Montagu, Lady Mary Wortley. (1747), 'Saturday: The Small-pox', *Six Town Eclogues*, London: n.p.

Montagu, Lady Mary Wortley. (1748, 1768), 'A Receipt to Cure the Vapors', *The Poetical Works of the Right Honorable Lady Mary Wortley Montagu*, Dublin: J. Williams.

Morgan, Edwin. (1996), 'De Quincey in Glasgow', *Collected Poems*, Manchester: Carcanet.

Muldoon, Paul. (1973), 'The Cure for Warts', *New Selected Poems 1968–1994*, London: Faber & Faber.

Murray, Les. (2003), 'Travels With John Hunter', *New Collected Poems*, Manchester: Carcanet.

Naden, Constance Woodhill. (1887), 'Evoltionary Erotics', *A Modern Apostle*, London: Kegan, Paul, Trench & Co.

Nash, Ogden. (1961), 'The Germ', *Collected Verse*, London: J. M. Dent.

Neaves, Lord Charles. (1875), 'Dust and Disease', *Songs and Verses Social and Scientific*, Edinburgh: Blackwood.

Neruda, Pablo. (1956), 'Ode to the Liver', *Nuevas Odas Elementales (New Elemental Odes)*, Buenos Aires: Losada Publishers.

O'Donoghue, Bernard. (1991), 'The Weakness', *The Weakness*, London: Chatto & Windus.

O'Hara, Frank. (1995), 'Anxiety', The *Collected Poems of Frank O'Hara,* ed. Donald Allen, Oakland, CA: University of California Press.

Olds, Sharon. (1996), 'History of Medicine', *The Wellspring*, London: Jonathan Cape.

Olds, Sharon. (2005), 'The Glass' and 'The Moment the Two World's Meet', *Selected Poems*, London: Jonathan Cape.

O'Reilly, Caitriona. (2001), 'Thin', *The Nowhere Birds*, Hexham, Northumberland: Bloodaxe Books.

Ostriker, Alicia. (1998), 'Mastectomy', *The Little Space: Poems Selected and New, 1968–1998*, Pittsburgh, PA: University of Pittsburgh Press.

Outram, George. (1916), 'The Barley Fever', *Legal and Other Lyrics*, London: T. N. Foulis.

Owen, Wilfred. (2013), 'Disabled' and 'Mental Cases', *The Complete Poems and Fragments*, London: Chatto & Windus.

Peirce, Kathleen. (1991), 'Obesity', *Mercy*, Pittsburgh, PA: University of Pittsburgh Press.

Pinsky, Robert. (1975), 'Essay on Psychiatrists', *Sadness and Happiness*, Princeton: Princeton University Press.

Plath, Sylvia. (1981), 'Face Lift', 'Fever 103', 'Paralytic', 'Thalidomide', 'Two Views of a Cadaver Room' and 'The Surgeon at 2 a.m.', *Collected Poems*, London: Faber & Faber.

Plutzik, Hyam. (1987), 'Cancer and Nova', *The Collected Poems*, New York: BOA Editions.

Porter, Dorothy. (1997), 'Dead Kids', *The Monkey's Mask*, New edition, London: Serpent's Tail.

Porter, Peter. (1984), 'Anatomy Lesson', *Collected Poems,* Oxford/New York: Oxford University Press.

Queneau, Raymond. (1948), 'The Human Species', *L'instant fatal*, Paris: Editions Gallimard.

Quillet, Claude. (1710), *Callipædia: Or, the Art of Getting Beautiful Children. A Poem, in Four Books*, trans. W. Oldisworth, London: Bernard Lintott.

Randall, Dudley. (2009), 'Old Witherington', *Roses and Revolutions: The Selected Writings of Dudley Randall*, ed. Melba Joyce Boyd, Detroit, MI: Wayne State University Press.

Read, Sally. (2005), 'Instruction', *The Point of Splitting*, Hexham, Northumberland: Bloodaxe Books.

Reading, Peter. (1981), 'The Euphemisms', *Tom O'Bedlam's Beauties*, London: Martin Secker & Warburg.

Reading, Peter. (1984), 'Talking Shop' and selections, *C*, London: Martin Secker & Warburg.

Rees-Jones, Deryn. (1998), 'Calcium' and 'My Father's Hair', *Signs Round A Dead Body*, Bridgend: Seren.

Reid, Christopher. (2009), 'A Scattering' and 'The Unfinished', *A Scattering*, Oxford: Areté Books.

Reznikoff, Charles. (1995), 'On the Kitchen Shelf', 'The Dusty Medicine Bottles', and 'Pestilence [Epidemic]', *The Complete Poems of Charles Reznikoff*, Boston, MA: Black Sparrow Press.

Rich, Adrienne. (1987), 'A Woman Dead in Her Forties', *The Fact of a Doorframe: Poems 1950–2001*, New York: W. W. Norton.

Rilke, Rainer Maria. (1989), 'Going Blind', *The Selected Poetry of Rainer Maria Rilke*, ed. Stephen Mitchell, New York: Vintage.

Rilke, Rainer Maria. (1994), 'The Song of the Dwarf', *The Book of Images*, ed. Edward Snow, New York: North Point/Farrar, Straus and Giroux.

Rilke, Rainer Maria. (2001), 'Corpse-Washing', *New Poems: a Revised Bilingual Edition*, ed. Edward Snow, New York: North Point Press/Farrar, Straus and Giroux.

Riordan, Maurice. (1995), 'The Doctor's Stone', *A Word from the Loki*, London: Faber & Faber.

Robertson, Robin. (1997), 'Lithium', *A Painted Field*, London: Picador.

Robertson, Robin. (2013), 'The Halving' and 'A & E', *Hill of Doors*, London: Picador.

Robinson, Anna. (2010), 'Operation at St Thomas' Hospital for Poor Women', *The Finders of London*, London: Enitharmon.

Robinson, A. Mary. (1888, 1902), 'Neurasthenia', *The Collected Poems, Lyrical and Narrative*, London: T. F. Unwin.

Roethke, Theodore. (2011), 'Dolor', 'Epidermal Macabre', and 'My Papa's Waltz', *The Collected Poems of Theodore Roethke*, New York: Knopf.

Ross, Sir Ronald. (1911), 'Indian Fevers' and 'Malaria', *Philosophies*, London: John Murray.

Rukeyser, Muriel (2006), 'Two Years', *The Collected Poems of Muriel Rukeyser*, Pittsburgh, PA: University of Pittsburgh Press.

Rossetti, Christina. (1906), 'The Plague', *The Poetrical Works of Christina Georgina Rossetti*, ed. William Michael Rossetti, London: Macmillan and Co., Ltd.

Satyamurti, Carole. (1998), 'Knowing Our Place' and 'Prognoses', *Selected Poems*, Oxford: Oxford University Press.

Scott, David. (1998), 'Heart', *Selected Poems*, Hexham, Northumberland: Bloodaxe Books.

Scott, John. (1782), 'To Disease', *The Poetical Works of John Scott*, London: J. Buckland.

Sexton, Anne. (1999), 'The Addict', 'Noon Walk on the Asylum Lawn', 'The Operation' and 'You, Doctor Martin', *The Complete Poems,* Boston: Mariner/Houghton Mifflin.

Shapcott, Jo. (2002), 'Twin Found in Man's Chest', *The Gift: New Writing for the NHS.* ed. David Morley, Exeter: Stride Publications.

Shapcott, Jo. (2010), 'The Deaths', *Of Mutability*, London: Faber & Faber.

Shelley, Percy Bysshe. (1833), 'The Magnetic Lady to her Patient', *The Shelley Papers*, ed. T. Medwin, London: Whittaker, Treacher & Co.

Simpson, Louis Aston Marantz. (1988), 'Typhus', *Collected Poems,* St Paul, MN: Paragon House.

Snodgrass, W. D. (1967), 'A Flat One', *After Experience*, New York: Harper & Row.

Southey, Robert. (1799), 'The Surgeon's Warning', *Poems*, vol. 2 of 2., Bristol: Biggs and Cottle.

Southgate, Christopher. (2006), 'Crick, Watson and the Double Helix', *Easing the Gravity Field*, Nottingham: Shoestring Press.

Sprackland, Jean. (2013), 'Supra-Ventricular Tachycardia', *Sleeping Keys*, London: Jonathan Cape.

Standfast, Richard. (c.1750, c. 1780, c. 1790), *A Dialogue Between a Blind-man and Death*, London: n.p.

Stevenson, Anne. (2005), 'A Ballad for Apothecaries' and 'Fragments: Mrs Reuben Chandler writes to her husband during a cholera epidemic', *Poems: 1955–2005*, Hexham, Northumberland: Bloodaxe Books.

Stone, John. (1972), 'Cadaver' and 'To a Fourteen-Year-Old Girl in Labor and Delivery', *The Smell of Matches*, Baton Rouge: Rutgers University Press.

Stringer, Arthur. (1914), 'Anaesthesia', *Open Water*, London: John Lane.

Sweeney, Matthew. (1992), 'Artificial Blood', *Cacti*, London: Secker & Warburg.

Symmons Roberts, Michael. (1999), 'The Lung Wash', *Raising Sparks*, London: Jonathan Cape.

Symmons Roberts, Michael. (2004), 'Post-Mortem' and 'Mapping the Genome', *Corpus*, London: Jonathan Cape.

Symonds, John Addington. (1880), 'The Camera Obscura', *New and Old*, London: Smith, Elder & Co.

Symons, Arthur. (1889), 'The Opium Smoker', *Days and Nights*, London: Macmillan.

Symons, Arthur. (1896), 'The Absinthe Drinker', *Silhouettes,* 2nd ed., London: Leonard Smithers.

Tabb, John Bannister. (1895), 'With Cholera Morbus', *Quips and Quiddits, Ques for the Qurious*, Washington, DC: Library of Congress.

Tallis, Raymond. (1987), 'In Memoriam Roland Barthes', *Glints of Darkness*, Liverpool: Windows Project.

Tate, Nahum. (1686), *Syphilis: Or, a Poetical History of the French Disease*, London: Jacob Tonson.

Tate, Nahum. (1696), 'Upon the Sight of an Anatomy', *Miscellanea Sacra, or, Poems on Divine & Moral Subjects*, London: Henry Playford.

Taylor, John. (1635), *The Old, Old, Very Old Man*, London: Henry Gosson.

Thomas, Edward. (1915), 'Melancholy', *Poems,* New York: H. Holt & Co.

Thomas, R. S. (1995), 'Geriatric', *No Truce with the Furies*, Hexham, Northumberland: Bloodaxe Books.

Tucker, Mary Eliza Perine. (1867), 'The Opium Eater', *Poems,* New York: M. Doolady.

Tupper, Martin. (1838), 'The Stammerer's Complaint', *Geraldine, a Sequel to Coleridge's 'Christabel', with other Poems,* London: Joseph Rickerby.

Turnbull, Gael. (1965), 'Twenty Days: Twenty Cases: A Sketchbook and a Morula,' *Poetry*, vol. 106, 1/2, Apr–May, 136–59.

Turner, Charles. (1873), 'Gout and Wings', *Sonnets, Lyrics and Translations*, Brighton: Henry S. King & Co.

Wagoner, David. (1983), 'Their Bodies', *First Light*, Boston: Little Brown.

Wallace, Ronald. (1987), 'The Anatomy of the Hand' and 'Metaphor as Illness', *People and Dog in the Sun,* Pittsburgh, PA: University of Pittsburgh Press.

Ward, Frederick William Orde, (F. Harald Williams). (1894), 'The Scourge of God', *Confessions of a Poet,* London: Hutchinson & Co.

Warsh, Lewis. (1971), 'Gout', *Dreaming As One*, New York: Corinth Books.

Whitman, Walt. (1860), 'To Think of Time', *Leaves of Grass*, Boston: Thayer and Eldridge.

Whitman, Walt. (1867), 'I Sing the Body Electric', *Leaves of Grass*, Boston: Thayer and Eldridge.

Whitman, Walt. (1881–2), 'A March in the Ranks Hard-Prest, and the Road Unknown' and 'The Wound-Dresser', *Leaves of Grass*, Boston: James R. Osgood & Co.

Whittier, John Greenleaf. (1930), 'Fat Man', *A Study of Whittier's Apprenticeship as a Poet: Dealing with Poems Written Between 1825 and 1835 not Available in the Poet's Collected Works,* ed. Frances Mary Pray, Bristol, NH: Musgrove Printing House.

Williams, C. K. (2006), 'The Coma', 'Dissections' and 'Saint Sex', *Collected Poems*, Hexham, Northumberland: Bloodaxe Books.

Williams, Hugo. (2002), 'Bath Night', 'Sex' and 'When I grow Up', *Collected Poems*, London: Faber & Faber.

Williams, Miller. (1999), 'Thinking about Bill, Dead of AIDS', *Some Jazz a While: Collected Poems*, Champaign, IL: University of Illinois Press.

Williams, William Carlos (1991), 'Io Baccho!' and 'Complaint', *Collected Poems*, vol. 2 of 2, ed. Christopher MacGowan, London: Paladin/Grafton.

Wilmott, John, Earl of Rochester. (1705), 'A Song of a Young Lady to her Ancient Lover', *Poems on Several Occasions*, London: J. Tonson.

Wilson, Anthony. (2012), 'Blood', *Riddance*, Tonbridge: Worple Press.

Wright, Kit. (2000), 'The Day Room', *Hoping It Might Be So*, Oxford: Leviathan.

Young, Francis Brett. (1919), 'On a Subaltern Killed in Action', *Poems, 1916–18*, London: W. Collins & Sons.

MEDICAL WRITINGS: BIBLIOGRAPHY

Anonymous. (1747–57), Petitions to the London Foundling Hospital, *London Metropolitan Archives*, A/FH/A/9/1/4; A/FH/A/9/1/6; A/FH/A9/1/55x.

Anonymous. (1825), *The Art of Beauty,* London: Knight & Lacey.

Anonymous. (1884), 'Dr Koch on the Cholera', *The Lancet,* 124 (3180), 9 August 1884, 249–50.

Anonymous. (1918), 'Spanish Influenza – Three-Day Fever – The Flu', *United States Public Health Service*, Washington: Government Printing Office.

Acton, William. (1867), *The Functions and Disorders of the Reproductive Organs*, 2nd American ed., Philadelphia: Lindsay and Blakiston.

Alcott, Louisa May. (1863), *Hospital Sketches,* Boston: James Redpath.

Alderson, John. (1788), 'An Essay on the Nature and Origin of the Contagion of Fevers', Hull: G. Prince.

Barnes, Carl Lewis. (1898), *The Art and Science of Embalming*, Chicago: Trade Periodical Company.

Beard, George Miller. (1881), *American Nervousness: Its Causes and Consequences*, New York: Putnam.

Beddoes, Thomas. (1802), *Hygeia*, 1 of 2 vols., Bristol: R. Phillips.

Boyston, Zabdiel. (1726), *An Historical Account of the Small-Pox Inoculated in New England*, London: S. Chandler.

Brown, John. (1795), *The Elements of Medicine*, 1 of 2 vols., trans. and revised Thomas Beddoes, Portsmouth, NH: William & Daniel Treadwell.

Burney, Fanny. (March to June 1812), *Frances Burney D'Arblay Collection of Papers*, Berg Collection, New York Public Library, MSS Arblay.

Cadogan, William. (1771), *A Dissertation on the Gout*, 2nd ed., London: J. Dodsley.

Cadogan, William. (1749), *An Essay upon Nursing and the Management of Children*, 3rd ed., London: J. Roberts.

Carlyle, Thomas. (1858), 'Signs of the Times', *The Collected Works of Thomas Carlyle*, vol. 3 of 16, London: Chapman & Hall.

Carpenter, William B. (1875), *Principles of Mental Physiology*, London: Henry S. King.

Chambers, Thomas King. (1850), *Corpulence: Or, Excess of Fat in the Human Body*, London: Longman.

Charcot, Jean-Martin. (1877), *Lectures on the Diseases of the Nervous System*, 2nd series, trans. George Sigerson, London: The New Sydenham Society.

Cheyne, George. (1724), *An Essay of Health and Long Life,* London: George Strahan.

Cheyne, George. (1733), *The English Malady*, London: G. Strahan.

Cheyne, George. (1742), *The Natural Method of Curing the Diseases of the Body, and the Disorders of the Mind, Depending on the Body*, London: George Strahan.

Cobbe, Francis Power. (1866), 'The Fallacies of Memory', *The Galaxy*, 1(2), 15 May, 85–180.

Darwin, Charles. (1859), *On The Origin of Species,* London: John Murray.

de Bienville, M. D. T. (1775), *Nymphomania, or a Dissertation Concerning the Furor Uterinus,* trans. Edward Sloane Wilmot, London: J. Bew.

Defoe, Daniel. (1722), *A Journal of the Plague Year,* London: E. Nutt et al.

Diderot, Denis. (1905), 'Letter on the Blind', *Diderot's Early Philosophical Works,* trans. Margaret Jourdain, Chicago: Open Court Publishing Co.

Ellis, Havelock. (1905), *Sexual Selection in Man,* Philadelphia: F. A. Davis & Co.

Freud, Sigmund. (1910), *Three Contributions to the Sexual Theory,* trans. A. A. Brill, New York: The Journal of Nervous and Mental Disease Publishing Company.

Hammond, William A. (1879), *Fasting Girls: Their Physiology and Pathology,* New York: Putnam & Sons.

Hill, John. (1771), *The Old Man's Guide to Health and Longer Life,* 6th enlarged and corrected ed., London: E. & C. Dilly.

Holmes, Oliver Wendell. (1891), 'Currents and Cross-Currents in Medical Science', and 'Border Lines of Knowledge in Some Provinces of Medical Science', *The Writings of Oliver Wendell Holmes: Medical Essays, 1842-1882,* Cambridge, MA: Riverside Press.

Hume, David. (1748, 1777), *An Enquiry Concerning Human Understanding,* London: A. Millar.

Hunter, John. (1839), *Lectures on the Principles of Surgery,* Philadelphia: Haswell, Barrington and Haswell.

Huxley, T. H. (1869), *On the Physical Basis of Life,* New Haven: Yale College Courant.

James, William. (1902), 'Religion and Neurology', *The Varieties of Religious Experience,* London and New York: Longmans, Green & Co.

James, William. (1914), *Habit,* New York: Henry Holt & Co.

Jenner, Edward. (1798), *An Inquiry into the Causes and Effects of the Variolae Vaccinae, or Cow-pox,* London: for the author.

Laycock, Thomas. (1860), *Mind and Brain,* 2 of 2 vols., Edinburgh: Sutherland & Knox.

Lister, Joseph. (1867), 'Illustrations of the Antiseptic System of Treatment in Surgery', *The Lancet,* 90 (2309), 30 November 1867, 668–69.

Love, I. N. (1897), 'The Needs and Rights of Old Age', *Journal of the American Medical Association,* 20 November, 1033–39.

Mandeville, Bernard. (1730), *Treatise of the Hypochondriack and Hysterick Diseases,* London: J. Tonson.

Marten, John. (1709), *Gonosologium Novum,* London: N. Crouch et al.

Marten, John. (1723), *Onania,* 9th edition, London: Elizabeth Rumball.

Mettrie, Julian Offray de la. (1749), *Man a Machine,* London: W. Owen.

Montagu, Lady Mary Wortley. (1796), 'Letter on Smallpox in Turkey' (letter 36, to Mrs S.C. from Adrianople, 1717), *Letters of the Right Honourable Lady Mary Wortley Montagu,* Aix: Anthony Henricy, 167–9.

Munk, William. (1887), *Euthanasia,* London and New York: Longmans, Green & Co.

Nightingale, Florence. (1860), *Notes on Nursing,* New York: D. Appleton and Company.

Osler, William. (1920), *The Old Humanities and the New Science, Presidential Address to the Classical Association,* Boston and New York: Houghton Mifflin Co.

Pseudo-Aristotle. (1784), 'Aristotle's Masterpiece', *The Works of Aristotle in Four Parts*, London: Printed for all booksellers.

Quincey, Thomas De. (1821), 'Confessions of an English Opium-Eater', *London Magazine*, vol. iv, July to December, London: Taylor & Hessey.

Rivers, W. H. (1918), 'On the Repression of War Experience', *Lancet*, 191 (927), orig. 1 (4927), 2 February, 169–204.

Röntgen, W. C. (1896), 'On a New Kind of Rays, December 28, 1895', *Nature*, 53, 23 January, 274–6.

Rush, Benjamin. (1892), *Old Family Letters, Copied from the Originals for Alexander Biddle*, Philadelphia: J. B. Lippincott.

Shaftesbury, Anthony Ashley Cooper, Earl of. (1732), *Characteristicks*, vol. 1 of 3, London: John Darby.

Sharp, Jane. (1725), *The Compleat Midwife's* Companion, 4th ed., London: John Marshall.

Smellie, William. (1765), *A Collection of Preternatural Cases and Observations in Midwifery*, 3 of 3 vols., 3rd ed., Dublin: T. and J. Whitehouse.

Snow, John. (1855), *On the Mode of Communication of Cholera*, London: John Churchill, New Burlington Street, England.

Southwood Smith, Thomas. (1832), *A Lecture Delivered over the Remains of Jeremy Bentham*, London: Effingham Wilson.

Stretzer, Thomas. (1741), *A New Description of Merryland*, 4th ed., Bath: W. Jones.

Stopes, Marie. (1919), *Wise Parenthood*, 4th ed., London: A. C. Fifield.

Trotter, Thomas. (1804), *An Essay Medical, Philosophical and Chemical on Drunkenness*, London: T. N. Longman & O. Rees.

Virchow, Rudolf. (1863), *Cellular Pathology*, 2nd ed., trans. Frank Chance, Philadelphia: J. B. Lippincott.

Whytt [Whyte], Robert. (1765), *Observations on the Nature, Causes, and Cure of those Disorders ... Nervous, Hypochondriac or Hysteric*, London: T. Becket and P. A. de Hondt.

Williams, Carlos William. (1948), 'Of Medicine and Poetry', *The Autobiography of William Carlos Williams*, New York: New Directions.

Willich, A. F. M. (1800), *Lectures on Diet and Regimen*, Boston: Manning & Loring.

INDEX